PAEDIATRIC OPERATIVE DENTISTRY

A DENTAL PRACTITIONER HANDBOOK
SERIES EDITED BY DONALD D. DERRICK, D.D.S., L.D.S., R.C.S.

PAEDIATRIC OPERATIVE DENTISTRY

D. B. KENNEDY

B.D.S., L.D.S., R.C.S. (Eng.), M.S.D., F.R.C.D. (Can.)

Private practitioner in paediatric dentistry, Vancouver, British Columbia, Canada;

Part-time instructor, Department of Restorative Dentistry, Faculty of Dentistry, University of British Columbia, Vancouver;

Formerly Lecturer in Dental Department for Children, Guy's Hospital, London

Second Edition

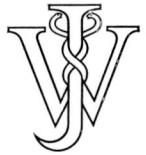

BRISTOL: JOHN WRIGHT & SONS LTD.
1979

First edition, 1976
Second edition, 1979
Spanish edition, 1977

CIP Data
Kennedy, David Bernard
  Paediatric operative dentistry. – 2nd ed.
  – (A dental practitioner handbook; no. 21).
  1. Pedodontics   2. Dentistry, Operative
  I. Title   II. Series
  617.6'45   RK55.C5

ISBN 0 7236 0525 4

PRINTED IN GREAT BRITAIN BY HENRY LING LTD., A SUBSIDIARY OF
JOHN WRIGHT & SONS LTD., AT THE DORSET PRESS, DORCHESTER

PREFACE TO THE SECOND EDITION

A SECOND edition gives an author the chance to respond to the many and varied critiques of the first edition. This is coupled with the opportunity to update material and to correct errors in the first edition. For this, the author is very grateful. While some criticism has been ignored, it was so that the original goals of the text, namely to discuss operative dentistry for the child patient, are maintained.

Pat Parsons drew the additional line diagrams in Chapters 2 and 17 while Bob Paton again assisted greatly in the other illustrations. The typing was done by Reva Lander. Throughout the preparation for the second edition, my partner, Dr. Richard Kramer, undertook many of the daily tasks involved with running a busy practice to allow me the time to update the text.

April 1979

PREFACE TO THE FIRST EDITION

MANY parents do not recognize the importance of restoring the primary dentition. Yet malocclusions can sometimes be attributed to the premature loss of primary teeth, or aggravated by that loss. Paediatric dentistry can play a vital role in the dental development of the young patient by providing natural space maintainers for the permanent teeth and by instilling in the child positive attitudes towards oral health.

Operative dentistry is just one aspect of overall dental health care for the child. However, it requires the utmost in technical skill and attention to detail. It cannot be divorced from epidemiology, diagnosis, treatment planning, behaviour management, and preventive care. This book in no way attempts to cover all aspects of paediatric dentistry—rather it is limited to all facets of operative dentistry concerning the primary and young permanent dentition. Cavity preparations are described in detail and variations from previously accepted norms justified. An attempt has been made to justify each particular procedure by identifying the indications, contra-indications, and reasons for success or failure.

The book is subdivided into chapters dealing with specific topics so that the practitioner can quickly refer to a particular area to find assistance with his problem. The glossary may help remind or update him regarding terminology which may be hazy in his memory. This subdivision may also be of value to the dental student, either during his review or as supplementary reading for a technique course on paediatric operative dentistry. Because of the organization of material by topic, there will be repetition in areas which overlap; perhaps the reader will consider this as reinforcement of important information.

The philosophy of providing the highest standard of care is presented, together with practical hints which help attain this goal. Whilst references to scientific studies support the text, every effort has been made to make the book of practical value by providing solutions to everyday problems. These practical hints can be readily incorporated into a busy practice.

ACKNOWLEDGEMENTS

THE author wishes to thank Dr. Donald Derrick for inviting him to undertake the project and for his help throughout; also John Wright & Sons Ltd. have been most understanding and patient. I was fortunate enough to consult frequently with Peter Stevenson Moore throughout the preparation of the manuscript; his insight and constructive criticism were much appreciated. Dr. Paul Starkey and Professor Paul Barton of Indiana University read and edited the manuscript, respectively; their assistance was greatly valued. Malcolm Williamson from the Faculty of Dentistry at the University of British Columbia kindly lent me his D.D.P.H. thesis which was most useful for the section on fissure sealants. It was pleasant to have Pat Parsons undertake the task of producing the line diagrams; her enthusiasm, her attention to detail, and her expertise were much appreciated. The line diagrams in Chapter 17 were prepared by the Medical Illustrations Department at Guy's Hospital under my direction in 1972. Bob Paton, from the Faculty of Dentistry at the University of British Columbia, was of great assistance with many of the clinical photographs. Individual acknowledgement of borrowed illustrations is given in the appropriate legends. The unpleasant job of typing the various drafts of the manuscript was graciously undertaken by Anne Smith, Jean Currie, Lesley Cook, from the practice, Sue Southern, from the University of British Columbia, Pauline McClafferty and Linda Smallshaw. Thanks are due to Dr. Trevor Harrop, Chairman of the Restorative Department at the University of British Columbia, for allowing me the use of secretarial and technical assistance.

This work was possible only because of the nature of my professional environment. I am indebted to Dr. Gordon Jinks and our staff for providing pleasant working conditions in our paediatric dentistry practice which left me the energy after a day's clinical work to embark on the manuscript. Specifically my dental assistants Judy Pearson, Lesley Cook and Blythe Footit provided humour and encouragement throughout. The motivation for this work is more deeply rooted; the desire to perpetuate high standards of paediatric dentistry was instilled during my graduate training at Indiana University by Dr. James Roche. His expertise and enthusiasm for paediatric dentistry have been a model for this author.

CONTENTS

CHAPTER 1

THE BASIS FOR
PAEDIATRIC OPERATIVE DENTISTRY

THE preservation of the primary dentition until their normal anti-cipated exfoliation can be justified on the following grounds:
Maintenance of arch length.
Maintenance of a healthy oral environment.
Prevention and relief of pain.
Maintenance and improvement of appearance.

MAINTENANCE OF ARCH LENGTH

Premature loss of primary molars is a local aetiological factor in the development of a malocclusion. Usually orthodontists recommend the preservation of primary teeth since the best space maintainer is the retained healthy primary tooth. While the preservation of the primary dentition will not always prevent a malocclusion it usually will make it less severe; also the permanent molar relation-ship will be symmetrically maintained, an important consideration when assessing the difficulty of active orthodontic treatment. On the other hand, the premature loss of primary molars often aggra-vates a developing malocclusion. The effect of the premature loss is to reveal and localize any crowding that is present (Tulley and Campbell, 1970). This can be used to the patient's advantage in the planned extraction of primary teeth, as in a serial extraction programme, so that permanent teeth are later removed. Hopefully, much space closure and concurrent correction of crowding will occur spontaneously to reduce the need for subsequent appliance therapy.

Early loss of primary molars causes more severe effects than the early loss of primary incisors. As a rule, the earlier the tooth is lost the more severe the effects; conversely, the older the child, the less serious the effects. It is more harmful to lose a second primary molar at age 3 than at age 8. The location of the lost primary tooth is also significant. In the mixed dentition, the loss of those primary teeth adjacent to permanent teeth produces a more serious problem. At the distal aspect of the primary dentition the first permanent molar is prevented from mesial migration by the presence of the primary molars. Therefore the premature loss of the second primary molar can have drastic consequences if it occurs before or during the eruption of the first permanent molar. The mesial migration of the

1

first permanent molar, if unchecked, will result in the second premolar (which erupts later) being blocked out from the arch, usually to the lingual.

Adjacent to the permanent incisors in the mixed dentition is the primary canine. Its premature loss can, under conditions of crowding and adverse musculature, encourage deviation of the centre line and deepening of the overbite by tipping of the permanent incisors distally and lingually. Although this discussion has been mainly directed towards the effects of extraction, it should be recognized that mesial migration of posterior teeth can occur as a result of interproximal caries.

The effects of premature loss of primary incisors on the developing occlusion are usually negligible. Once the primary canines are fully erupted (at about age 3 years), no space loss is likely to occur following removal of primary incisors. This does not apply to the infancy period (under 3 years) when the retention of primary incisors prior to the eruption of primary canines is justified since their early removal would encourage the primary canines to assume a more mesial position and thus impinge upon space for the permanent incisors. Their maintenance is also justified on the basis of appearance.

MAINTENANCE OF A HEALTHY ORAL ENVIRONMENT

Two micro-organisms, *Lactobacillus acidophilus* and *Streptococcus mutans*, have been closely linked with the carious process as based on Miller's acidogenic theory. Although at present no one organism has been positively incriminated, their presence in the oral cavity in excessive numbers is not considered beneficial. It has been proven that restoration of carious lesions reduces the micro-organism count in the oral flora (Elliot, 1964). The same study showed that children with a low prevalence of decay also have low micro-organism counts. Thus, reducing oral micro-organisms by restorative dentistry to the primary dentition may indirectly reduce the incidence of decay in the permanent dentition. Nikiforuk and Pulver (1969), in a review article, reported that there was an infective transmissible factor in dental caries; it may be that the organisms present in untreated primary tooth lesions are partially responsible for the caries in adjacent permanent teeth. Irrespective of this, there is a proportional relationship between caries in the primary dentition and the caries which occur later in the same child's permanent dentition (Hargreaves, 1964; Hill and Blayney, 1967).

Restoring carious primary teeth will certainly improve the health of the oral environment, and a sound, healthy dentition may be far reaching in its good effects. For example, parents frequently complain that their child has a poor appetite. The physician's response may well be to prescribe a tonic while the real problem lies in the child's carious teeth. A child does not want to eat if his teeth hurt every time he chews; he cannot be blamed for wanting mashed foods. While many children manage to eat without a full complement of teeth, few can function properly when their teeth are ravaged by caries. The restoration to correct occlusion and contour can allow the child to enjoy proper function during mastication. Once function is restored, pain is removed, and the infection is eliminated, these children will be able to enjoy more detergent food. With their full nutritional needs satisfied, their whole outlook on life is improved.

PREVENTION AND RELIEF OF PAIN

From the viewpoint of both the child and the dentist, the prevention of pain is more desirable and easier to handle than its relief. One of the most difficult problems that the dentist faces daily is the need to provide emergency treatment for patients in pain. Management of the child presents a great problem since the child's awareness of dental problem is significantly correlated with a negative behavioural response (Wright and Alpern, 1971); lack of sleep, restlessness and distress from toothache unfavourably influence the child's behaviour. The dentist must then attempt to relieve the pain of a child who is not at his best. Furthermore, the emergency patient often has to be accommodated into an already busy daily schedule for the dentist, often at the expense of other patients presenting for routine care. Depending on the ability of the child, the dentist, and the parent to cope with the situation, a traumatic early dental experience may occur which can unfavourably condition the child against dentistry for a lifetime.

Prevention of pain is the key to success. Treatment can then be performed on a more cooperative child; furthermore, when lesions are diagnosed early, the operative dentistry is less extensive, easier to perform and less time-consuming.

MAINTENANCE AND IMPROVEMENT OF APPEARANCE

No one can be sure of the real value of the dentition to an individual since different people have different attitudes towards their own teeth, both in terms of appearance and function. Parents are certainly aware of the cosmetic value of orthodontic treatment and of the aesthetic restoration of anterior teeth. Children, too, are becoming more aware of their appearance, perhaps because they live

3

very much in an era of peer evaluation. Children want to be like everyone else; they want to avoid ridicule and criticism from their peers. Such criticism may be directed towards unsightly teeth and may be psychologically traumatic. The older child can certainly express his desires for an aesthetic smile to be like his peers; however, the younger pre-school child seldom has that ability because of his limited vocabulary and the strong parental influence exerted over him at this age. The author's personal experience in the aesthetic restoration of primary incisors has been most favourable.

PRIMARY TEETH AND SPEECH

Parents often associate the premature loss of primary incisors with the development of speech problems such as lisping. They should be reassured that usually no permanent habits result from premature loss of primary incisors; any lisping that might occur following primary incisor removal will be often reversible when the permanent incisors erupt. All children go through a transition period from primary to mixed dentition when they are without incisors; and during this period most of them do not develop permanent speech anomalies, which demonstrates the adaptability of the tongue. It should be remembered that the child's speech is developed between 18 and 36 months.

Paediatric operative dentistry cannot be divorced from the following topics: epidemiology, diagnosis, behaviour guidance, treatment planning and preventive care. It is impossible for the dentist to diagnose carious lesions if he doesn't know where to look for them; therefore a working knowledge of the epidemiology of dental caries in children is essential.

EPIDEMIOLOGY

Prevalence of a disease refers to the percentage showing evidence of that disease, i.e. the percentage of decayed teeth or the percentage of children affected by decay.

Incidence of dental caries is the rate of occurrence of new lesions.

Decay experience in a community is measured by evaluating the total effects of the carious process (past and present) up to the time of the examination. It is measured in terms of Decayed, Missing, or Filled Teeth or Surfaces, i.e. DMFT or DMFS. For permanent teeth capital letters are used while small letters (dmft or dmfs) are used for the primary dentition.

The above definitions (modified from Holloway, Swallow and Slack, 1969) serve as references for the following material. Epidemiological surveys indicate that the dental needs of young children are high. The results are presented by age groups.

4

Primary Dentition (age 0–5 years)

About 10 per cent of 2-year-olds exhibit dental caries (Hennon et al., 1969). The results of two studies of pre-school children are shown in the following table.

Age Group (in months)	Caries Free (percentage)	Average def	Reference
12–23	98·0	0·04	1
18–23	91·7	4·65	2
24–35	82·0	0·76	1
36–47	64·0	1·41	1
36–39	42·0	6·16	2
48–60	42·0	3·07	1

1. Winter et al., 1971a, b.
2. Hennon et al., 1969.

Hennon and co-workers (1969) found a greater prevalence of caries in each age group than Winter and co-workers (1971a, b). The reason for this was that their diagnostic techniques were more refined since they used sharp explorers and bite-wing radiographs while Winter et al. relied solely upon visual examination. The radiographic findings of Hennon et al. indicate that 75 per cent of all posterior interproximal lesions would have remained undiagnosed without the use of bite-wing radiographs (*Fig. 1*). These studies show that caries in pre-school children can be effectively diagnosed only with an explorer and with radiographs when posterior contacts are closed. Failure to use them in clinical practice is really turning one's back on a potential problem.

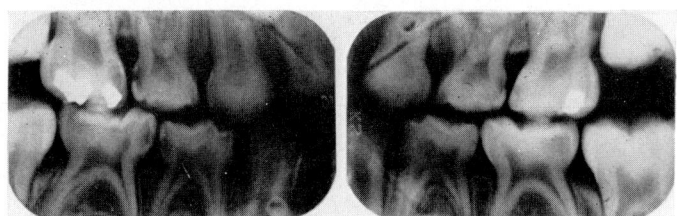

Fig. 1.—Bite-wings of 5-year-old demonstrating interproximal lesions in all four quadrants.

Two other interesting facts arise from the study of Winter et al. (1971a, b). First, a greater caries prevalence was noted in the lower social groups. Second, the aetiological role of certain feeding habits was identified. These feeding habits may produce a condition in infants and young children known as *nursing bottle mouth syndrome*. The aetiology is traced to prolonged ingestion of sucrose-containing fluids that are often syrupy in texture from a nursing bottle, a reservoir feeder, pacifier, or dinky cup (Winter et al., 1971a, b).

5

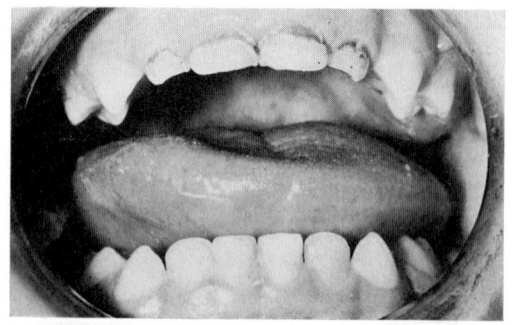

a

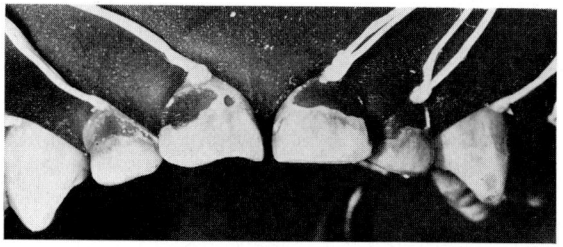

b

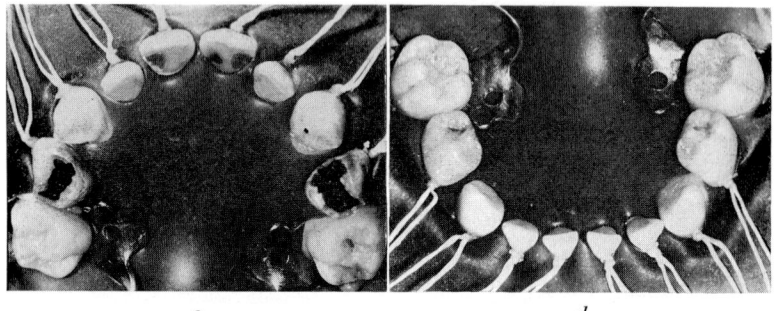

c   *d*

Fig. 2.—Nursing bottle caries. *a*, Anterior view: caries affects
maxillary but not mandibular incisors. Age 20 months. Apple
juice in bottle to bed.
b,c,d. More extensive case. Age 26 months. Apple juice in bottle
to bed. *b*, Anterior view: class 5 lesions. *c*, Maxillary view: caries
affects first primary molar more than primary canine or second
primary molar. *d*, Mandibular view. Incisors are not affected.
Occlusals of D's carious.
e,f,g, Severe case. Age 18 months. Juice in bottle to bed and honey
on soother. *e*, Anterior view. Crowns destroyed to gingival margin.
f, Maxillary view. Note destruction of D's also. *g*, Mandibular view.
h,i, Nursing caries. At-will breast feeding. Age 19 months. *h*,
Anterior view. *i*, Maxillary view.

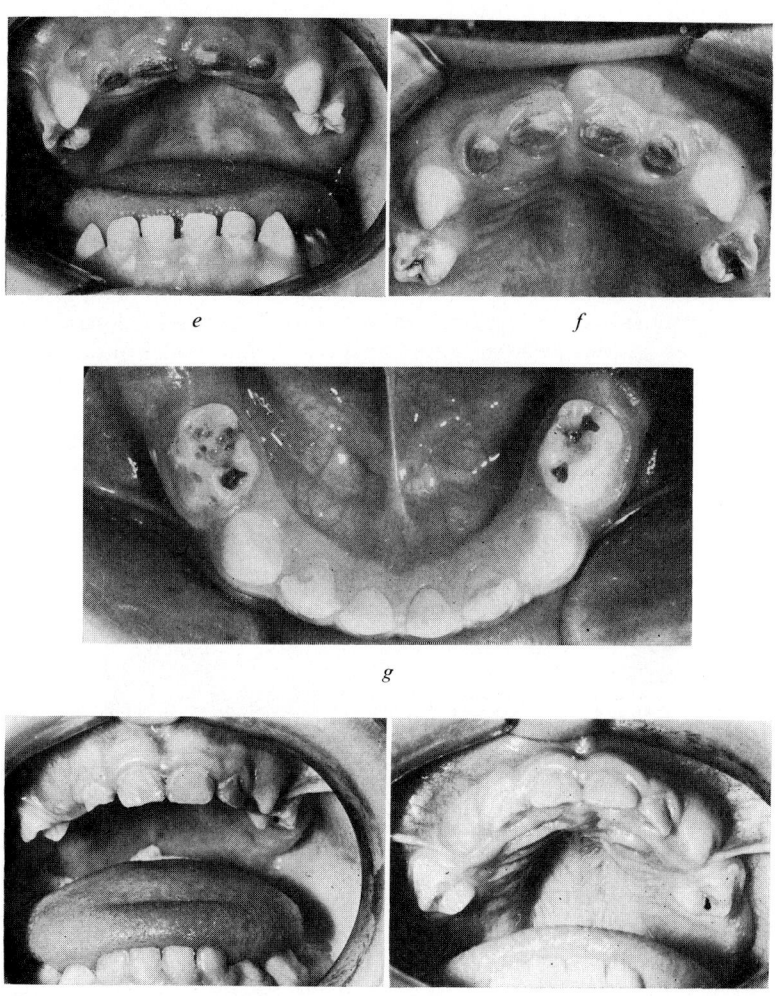

e

f

g

h

i

Although sweetened syrups and juices are the most common culprits, unsweetened milk has the potential to produce dental caries if left stagnant over the tooth surface for a sufficient time (Vianna, 1971). Indeed, prolonged nursing with human milk from 'at-will' breast feeding can also produce decay in infants (Gardner et al., 1977). The pattern of carious attack is identical to nursing bottle caries (*Fig. 2*). Indeed, parents may require exhaustive questioning to reveal the true aetiology of the condition. The carious lesion affects primarily the labial surfaces of the maxillary primary incisors and

7

the occlusal surfaces of the first primary molars (Picton and Wiltshear, 1970) (*Fig. 2*). The anterior lesion, if untreated, will encompass the lingual and interproximal areas of the maxillary incisors in a circumferential manner. By nature of the suckling habit, the lower lip protects the mandibular incisors; the primary canines and second primary molars are rarely affected due to the eruption sequence combined with the cessation of the feeding habit. Decreased salivary flow during sleep aggravates the condition by reducing the diluting and buffering effects of the saliva. The previous description refers to the initial clinical appearance of nursing bottle mouth. If the lesions are left untreated, tooth destruction continues so that eventually the maxillary primary incisors may be flush with the gingivae (*Fig. 2e,f,g*). The parents may present their child for treatment at this stage reporting that 'the teeth came in soft and brown and just broke off.' Such a history may lead to the inaccurate diagnosis of a developmental anomaly of the primary dentition.

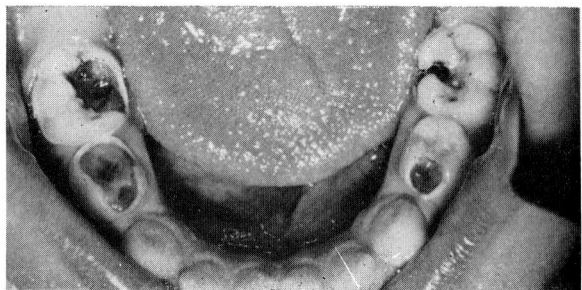

Fig. 3.—Gross destruction of mandibular primary molars in a 3-year-old child.

This condition differs in aetiology from the extensive carious lesions often seen in the primary molars of pre-school children and school-age children (*Figs. 3, 4*). In this latter instance, the extensive tooth destruction may not necessarily be traced to infant feeding habits if the second primary molars are decayed. Rather, a detailed account of the child's dietary habits may reveal a craving for sucrose-containing foods, often as snacks; this has been shown to be responsible for a higher incidence of decay (Gustafson et al., 1954).

When the parents are apathetic about seeking dental care at an early age, the tooth destruction will continue unimpeded. This condition may be inaccurately labelled as rampant caries while it is actually a result of neglect in seeking care. By contrast, rampant caries is defined by Massler (1945) as 'a suddenly appearing, widespread, rapidly burrowing type of caries resulting in early involvement of the pulp and affecting those teeth usually regarded as

8

immune to ordinary decay'. This often affects the teenager and young adolescent (McDonald, 1974).

After infancy, caries prevalence increases until only 42 per cent of 3-year-olds are caries-free while the average def is 6·16 (Hennon et al., 1969). It should be emphasized that these caries prevalences refer to children who have had no systemic exposure to fluoride.

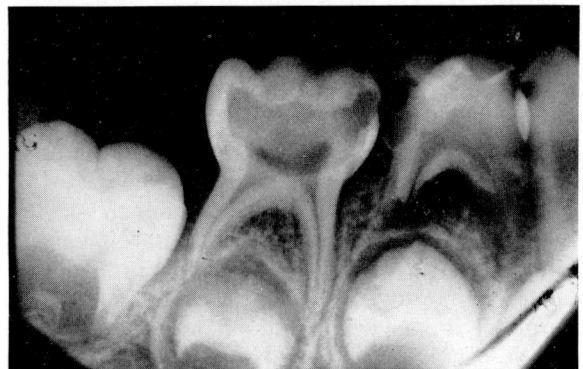

Fig. 4.—Mandibular primary molar periapical radiograph demonstrating large lesions in primary molars of a 3-year-old.

Among 5-year-old British children, 21·6 per cent are caries-free and the mean def per child is 4·5 (Health of the School Child, 1969). These findings are consistent with those of Timmis (1971), who reported that 24 per cent of 5-year-olds living in non-fluoride areas were caries-free. However, bite-wings were not used in his study and the supposition is made that some interproximal lesions were undiagnosed.

Location of Caries—Primary Dentition

Since the location and diagnosis of individual lesions are discussed in subsequent chapters, an outline only will be given here. Occlusal lesions in primary molars are more common than interproximal lesions in pre-school children (Parfitt, 1956). In these young children posterior contacts may not close until age 3 years, which may explain this observation; however, once posterior contacts close, the prevalence of interproximal lesions will increase. Second primary molars have more occlusal lesions than first primary molars, likewise the mandibular molars have more than the maxillary because of the depth and anatomy of the occlusal fissures. The labial and lingual surfaces of primary teeth seldom decay, except in the nursing bottle mouth syndrome. Mandibular primary incisors seldom decay, probably because of the spacing that occurs in the area and their

9

close proximity to the ducts of the submandibular salivary gland, which means that they benefit from the diluting and buffering properties of saliva.

Hennon et al. (1969) found the following areas of primary teeth to be most commonly affected by caries (from McDonald, 1974):

	Maxillary	*Mandibular*
Second molar	occlusal-lingual	occlusal-buccal
First molar	occlusal	occlusal-buccal
Canine	buccal	buccal
Lateral	mesial	mesial
Central	mesial	mesial

The Mixed Dentition (*age 6–12 years*)

The eruption of first permanent molars and permanent incisors introduces additional areas which are susceptible to decay. Furthermore, primary molar contacts will be closed throughout the mixed dentition; if the primate space* also closes with the eruption of the first permanent molar, two other surfaces (between first primary molar and primary canine in the mandibular arch) are in close contact and are thus susceptible to interproximal caries. No attempt will be made to quote dmf and DMF values in the mixed dentition age groups for British children, although these figures are available from the Health of the School Child Reports, published by H.M.S.O. annually. Critical analysis of these reports reveals that a disappointingly small number of bite-wing radiographs are taken compared to the total number of examinations; this author believes that many interproximal lesions therefore remain undiagnosed and that the real dmf and DMF would be higher than those reported in these publications. However, it can be said with certainty that 75 per cent of school-age children will exhibit dental caries, although this figure may indeed be closer to 100 per cent in unfluoridated communities.

Location of Caries—Mixed Dentition

The newly erupted first permanent molars and permanent incisors have morphologic areas which are susceptible to plaque retention and subsequent development of caries. These are the occlusal surfaces in permanent molars, the lingual development pit and groove in maxillary permanent molars, the buccal development pit and groove in mandibular permanent molars, and lingual pits in maxillary permanent incisors, notably the lateral incisor. Probably because of the depth and inclination of the occlusal fissures, the mandibular permanent molars decay more frequently than maxillary

---

* *See* Glossary.

molars. In a non-fluoridated community the following prevalence of occlusal caries in first permanent molars can be expected (Walsh and Smart, 1948):

Age	Maxillary	Mandibular
7 years	12 per cent	25 per cent
9 years	35 per cent	50 per cent
12 years	52 per cent	70 per cent

It is alarming to note that half of the mandibular first permanent molars are carious within three years of eruption.

In addition to these susceptible areas, the closing of posterior contacts will result in the development of Class 2 lesions. At age 7 years, there will be more molar interproximal lesions than occlusal lesions; this prevalence is reversed at age 9 years (Parfitt, 1956). There are probably two reasons for this: more permanent molars will exhibit occlusal decay at age 9, and secondly, some primary molars will be exfoliated to reduce the prevalence of posterior interproximal lesions. In the mixed dentition the mesial surface of the first permanent molar is placed at risk if dental caries affects the second primary molar. Also, the interproximal surfaces of maxillary incisors may be at risk in those children with closed anterior contacts and a high dental caries incidence.

The Early Permanent Dentition (age 12–15 years)

There is an alarmingly high incidence of caries in the young permanent dentition (age 12–15 years) among British schoolchildren (Berman and Slack, 1972). The average DMF at age 11–12 years varies between 5·6 (Sutcliffe, 1966; Health of the School Child, 1963) and 6·0–7·5 (Hargreaves, 1964; Berman and Slack, 1972). This rises to 10·7–11·7 at ages 14–15 years (Berman and Slack, 1972). Almost none of the children in these age groups are caries-free. The young permanent dentition is thus a time of high caries activity (*Fig. 5*).

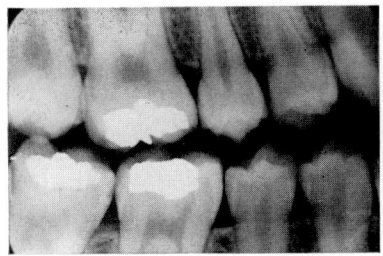 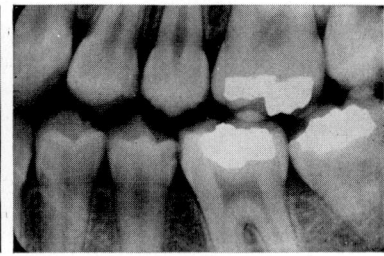

a	*b*

Fig. 5.—Bite-wings of a 13-year-old demonstrating developing interproximal lesions between several posterior teeth.

Location of Caries—Early Permanent Dentition

In this age group the order of susceptibility of teeth to caries attack (Berman and Slack, 1972) is:

1. First permanent molar (most susceptible).
2. Second permanent molar.
3. Premolars.
4. Maxillary anterior teeth.
5. Canine and mandibular incisors (least susceptible).

These researchers also noted a bilateral symmetry of caries attack in these children.

The occlusal surfaces of recently erupted second molars and premolars are susceptible to caries by virtue of their morphology. By comparison, buccal and lingual surfaces of these teeth, together with permanent canines and mandibular incisors, are seldom attacked by caries. The exception to this is the lingual pit of maxillary lateral incisors, which has been reported to be carious in 11 per cent of the 12–15-year-old age group (Berman and Slack, 1973).

There are more occlusal than interproximal lesions in the 12- and 13-year-olds due to the recent eruption and early occlusal attack of second molars and premolars. Certainly the occlusal surface of second permanent molars appears to become carious very quickly after eruption; it is also a clinical impression that the spread of occlusal decay in mandibular second permanent molars is very fast. However, after age 13 years, there is an increased percentage of interproximal compared to occlusal lesions (Berman and Slack, 1972) (*Fig. 5*).

DIAGNOSIS

Before any treatment is performed, a thorough examination including appropriate radiographs is necessary to obtain diagnostic records. Also included should be a medical, familial and dental history, an assessment of the child's cooperative ability, the occlusion, and the oral home care. From the epidemiological surveys the clincian should direct particular attention to those areas which are commonly decayed in the respective age groups. The need for bite-wing radiographs to diagnose interproximal lesions cannot be overemphasized: Hennon et al. (1969) observed that 75 per cent of these Class 2 lesions would be undiagnosed without bite-wing radiographs. When considering interproximal lesions in primary molars, the clinician must remember that the distance between external enamel surface and pulp is smaller in primary than permanent teeth (*see* Chapter 3). A Class 2 lesion into dentine on one primary molar surface is often accompanied by enamel decalcification on the adjacent primary tooth; such decalcifications, or radiographic etches of enamel, frequently exhibit histological

12

carious penetration to the dentine (Dwyer et al., 1973). On this basis, and for other reasons described in Chapter 7, the restoration of radiographic interproximal enamel etches in primary molars is both justifiable and recommended.

Symmetry of carious attack is to be expected (*Figs. 1, 5*); therefore the presence of interproximal molar lesions in one quadrant should encourage the clinician to look critically for similar lesions in other quadrants (McDonald, 1974). Even if they are not present, it is not uncommon for such lesions to become apparent clinically within a year if a truly effective preventive programme is not implemented. When deciding on the need to restore incipient lesions, the clinician should assess the child's caries incidence (from previous dental care), the anticipated response to preventive care, and the regularity of dental visits.

BEHAVIOUR GUIDANCE

Correct guidance of the child's behaviour through the dental experience favourably influences both child and parent in their attitudes towards dentistry. The dentist's objective should be to lead a child through a pleasant dental experience so that he becomes a good dental patient, accepts treatment gracefully and therefore seeks and enjoys good dental health throughout life (Starkey, 1974). The operator who is constantly evaluating his techniques of behaviour management will be able to provide the highest standard of care for the child because the success of his treatment procedures depends in part upon his ability to manage the child. When conventional measures fail, the use of premedication, nitrous oxide analgesia, intravenous sedation, and in rare instances general anaesthesia must be considered so that the necessary dentistry can be performed. No longer is it excusable to provide substandard or compromise care on the pretext that the child was 'impossible'. The dentist must aim to provide the best care, the type of care he would want for his own child, and ensure that the child's behaviour is controlled so that this goal is achieved. Also, a compromise on standards of care for primary teeth, on the basis that they will exfoliate, ignores the duration required of the restorations and the value of the teeth in maintaining arch integrity.

The parameters of this book do not include an in-depth account of child behaviour guidance. Indeed, no rigid rules can be given since both the child and the practitioner are individuals and their personal communication and interaction will be unique. The following generalizations, however, may be of practical value.

The dentist should direct his efforts to preventing behaviour problems. We should talk to the child in terms that he can understand,

13

and once communication is established the dentist should use a 'Tell–Show–Do' approach. Anticipating the child's emotions will allow the dentist to explain the procedure to be performed and the sensations that the child should expect. The timing of explanations is very important and can serve as a foundation for building trust and confidence. The child is reinforced positively and negatively for good and bad behaviour, respectively. A set of working rules should be established early and rigidly enforced so that the child knows the limits of acceptable behaviour. The calm, confident manner of the dentist conveys a sense of security to the child, who can quickly sense any nervousness, indecision or annoyance on the part of the operator. A sense of purpose that an important health service is to be provided should be transmitted to child and parent, who may respond by improved oral home care and punctual appointment keeping.

Some children may require a go-ahead approach even if their behaviour is not amenable to reason. The astute operator reserves this approach for those children who must be made to realize that their fears are unfounded and that a certain procedure is neither unpleasant nor painful. The fearful child may require the use of premedication to reduce his anxiety to a level where treatment no longer presents a major trauma in his life. In contrast, the truly resistant or defiant child needs to realize early who is 'captain of the ship'; he may use his temper tantrums to great advantage at home and not surprisingly will test out the dentist in an effort to get his own way. Once disciplined, such children are often cooperative patients and faithful admirers of the dentist, who may have been the first person ever to discipline them. The reader is referred to comprehensive articles on Child Management which also discuss the value of parental and sibling support.

PAIN CONTROL

Hand in hand with behaviour guidance goes pain control; this invariably means that local anaesthesia is required unless other forms of analgesia are used. Mink and Spedding (1966) describe the technique for an atraumatic injection procedure for the child. Infiltrations provide adequate anaesthesia for maxillary teeth but not for mandibular teeth where an inferior alveolar block is required.

A hurt child can no longer trust a dentist—the child's cooperation is founded on trust and honesty. It is inconceivable to think that anyone would consider restoring a deep lesion without a local anaesthetic, when caries removal could result in a possible pulp exposure. There is no evidence that primary teeth are any less sensitive than their permanent successors, although this has been a clinical impression.

Further, the dentist who works on primary teeth without a local anaesthetic is placed in an impossible situation if the child becomes restless, for he has no means of knowing whether the child is in pain or becoming fatigued—the treatment differing markedly for each case.

TREATMENT PLANNING

Reference has already been made to diagnostic records and treatment planning. Apart from orthodontic extractions, it is assumed that the dentist will strive to restore the primary dentition to normal contour and function, thus allowing them to be the natural space maintainer. Restorable teeth should be saved unless they do not meet the criteria outlined in Chapters 15, 16 and 17.

Dental appointments constitute inconvenience to the parents because of transport, baby-sitting responsibilities for other children, lost time from school for the child and from work for some parents. Therefore treatment should be planned effectively to minimize visits for the child. Contrary to common opinion in Great Britain, Lenchner's study (1966) does not support the hypothesis that the length of the appointment affects the child's behaviour and his attitude towards dentistry. He found that children can tolerate appointments of 48–175 minutes without significant deterioration in behaviour patterns. His experiences have been routinely duplicated in my practice. The operator should therefore be encouraged to make full use of his local anaesthetic by performing quadrant dentistry.

Full arch dentistry can be accomplished for many children, particularly recall patients who may require two Class 1 restorations in first permanent molars. Adatia and Gehring (1972) indicate no adverse effects of giving bilateral mandibular block injections. A major advantage of performing arch dentistry is that postoperative lip chewing is minimized since both sides of the mouth feel the same to the child.

The prevalence of dental caries will often determine that more than one restoration must be placed in a quadrant since interproximal caries commonly affects adjacent primary molars simultaneously. When planning treatment, dentists must also take into account the child's past decay experience and the prognosis for co-operation in the preventive recommendations. Incipient lesions should be restored in those caries-active children who require other operative work in that quadrant.

Sequencing of appointments can help in favourably conditioning the child's response to treatment. Unless emergency care is required, the following treatment sequencing is recommended since it gradually introduces the child to dentistry. The initial examination visit includes history taking and radiographs. Next comes a preventive visit which can include discussion of treatment, plaque scoring, review of oral hygiene, diet counselling, prophylaxis and topical fluoride application. The prophylaxis and fluoride treatment give both child and dentist the opportunity to establish further rapport in an essentially atraumatic setting; it also emphasizes the preventive philosophy of the practice to the parent and child. Not until the third visit is any operative dentistry performed; by this time rapport should have been established (if it has not been, the need to use other means for behaviour guidance, such as premedication, should have been determined at the second visit).

When possible, maxillary teeth should be treated first since the maxillary infiltration is easier to administer than the mandibular block. Also, infiltrations should be less painful for the child, although the experienced dentist should have no problem in administering a painless block providing topical anaesthesia is used. In so far as possible, the first and also the last appointment of the sequence should be short to give the child confidence initially, and finally to leave him with a favourable memory of dental treatment.

Unfortunately, such treatment sequencing cannot always be performed when there are extensive lesions or when emergency treatment is required. Emergency treatment should be limited to relief of pain because of the limited tolerance of the child who is distressed by pain and lack of sleep. When possible, extraction should be delayed until pain has been relieved by placement of a direct or indirect pulp treatment or opening for drainage (*see* Chapter 17). Conservative treatment at the emergency visit has substantial advantages. First, pain is relieved and yet the child and parents do not form an association between extraction and pain relief; second, the busy practitioner can schedule a further appointment for complete examination and diagnostic records. Children who present for emergency treatment frequently have many large lesions, although only one of these may cause the pain. Overzealous practitioners may be tempted to perform pulp therapy on all these; others will be horrified by the accumulation of dental neglect and recommend wholesale extractions at the emergency visit. Neither approach takes into account other potential dental problems, such as space loss and crowding. Also, many of the large open lesions have probably been present for several months; one extra week without care, until diagnostic records are made, is probably of no consequence, provided pain from the offending tooth is relieved.

PREVENTIVE CARE

However high the standard of operative dentistry may be, its success lies partially in the ability of the patient and parents to maintain a favourable oral environment for these restorations. Thus preventive dentistry must go hand in hand with any operative work. (The preventive aspects of operative dentistry are discussed in greater detail in Chapter 14.) By making projections of the future in his treatment planning, the dentist can prevent unnecessary repetition of work. For example, the astute diagnostician who sees a 4-year-old with interproximal caries in the primary molars and decalcification along the gingival margin may be wise to consider placing steel crowns on these teeth, partially as a preventive measure. This is especially true if the prognosis for home care is poor and the restorations are larger than the 'textbook ideal' since they have a long life ahead of them. Stainless-steel crowns, once placed, seldom require further treatment, and that cannot always be said of Class 2 alloys in primary molars in 4-year-olds. Thus the crown may be a more economical restoration, despite the sense of false economy given by the alloy, which may require replacement.

REFERENCES

ADATIA A. K. and GEHRING E. N. (1972) Bilateral inguinal alveolar and lingual nerve block. *Br. Dent. J.* **133**, 377.

Adult Dental Health in England and Wales in 1968 (1970) London, H.M.S.O.

BERMAN D. S. and SLACK G. L. (1972) Dental caries in English school children. *Br. Dent. J.* **133**, 529.

BERMAN D. S. and SLACK G. L. (1973) Susceptibility of tooth surfaces to carious attack. *Br. Dent. J.* **134**, 135.

DWYER D. M., BERMAN D. S. and SILVERSTONE L. M. (1973) A study of approximal carious lesions in primary molars. *J. Int. Assoc. Dent. Child.* **4**, 41.

ELLIOT R. P. (1964) Full-mouth rehabilitation retards oral lactobacilli. *J. Tenn. Dent. Assoc.* **44**, 13.

GARDNER D. E., NORWOOD J. R. and EISENSON J. E. (1977) At-will breast-feeding and dental caries: four case reports. *J. Dent. Child.* **44**, 186.

GUSTAFSSON B. E., QUESNEL C. E., LANKE L. S., LUNDQUIST C., GRAHNEN H., BANOW B. E. and KRASSE B. O. (1954) Vipeholm dental caries study. *Acta Odontol. Scand.* **11**, 232.

HARGREAVES J. A. (1964) The problem of caries in child dental health. *Br. Dent. J.* **116**, 386.

Health of the School Child, 1962 and 1963 (1963) London, H.M.S.O.

Health of the School Child, 1966/1968 (1969) London, H.M.S.O., p. 38.

HENNON D. K., STOOKEY G. K. and MUHLER J. C. (1969) Prevalence and distribution of dental caries in pre-school children. *J. Am. Dent. Assoc.* **79**, 1405.

HILL I. N. and BLAYNEY J. R. (1967) Fluorine and dental caries. *J. Am. Dent. Assoc.* **74**, 234.

HOLLOWAY P. J., SWALLOW J. N. and SLACK G. L. (1969) Deciduous teeth and future caries experience. *Child Dental Health.* Bristol, John Wright, p. 182. (2nd ed. (1975) by Holloway P. J. and Swallow J. N., p. 198.)

LENCHNER V. (1966) The effect of appointment length on behaviour of the pedodontic patient and his attitude towards dentistry. *J. Dent. Child.* **33**, 61.

McDONALD R. E. (1974) *Dentistry for the Child and Adolescent.* 2nd ed. St. Louis, C. V. Mosby, Chapters 1 & 2.

MASSLER M. (1945) Teenage caries. *J. Dent. Child.* **12**, 57.

MINK J. R. and SPEDDING R. H. (1966) An injection procedure for the child dental patient. *Dent. Clin. North Am.* Philadelphia, W. B. Saunders, p. 309.

NIKIFORUK G. and PULVER F. (1969) Practical aspects of current caries research and epidemiological data. *J. Dent. Child.* **36**, 249.

PARFITT G. J. (1956) Conditions influencing the incidence of occlusal and interstitial caries in children. *J. Dent. Child.* **23**, 31.

PICTON D. C. A. and WILTSHEAR P. J. (1970) A comparison of the effects of early feeding habits on the caries prevalence of deciduous teeth. *Dent. Pract. Dent. Rec.* **20**, 170.

STARKEY P. E. (1974) Personal communication.

SUTCLIFFE P. (1966) Caries experience and dental treatment in children. *Br. Dent. J.* **121**, 508.

TIMMIS J. C. (1971) Caries experience of 5-year-old children living in fluoride and non-fluoride areas of Essex. *Br. Dent. J.* **130**, 278.

TULLEY W. J. and CAMPBELL A. C. (1970) *A Manual of Practical Orthodontics.* 3rd ed. Bristol, John Wright, p. 66.

VIANNA R. B. C. (1971) *The Cariogenic Potential of Milk.* Typed Thesis, Indiana University.

WALSH J. P. and SMART R. S. (1948) Relative susceptibility of tooth surfaces to dental caries and other comparative studies. *N.Z. Dent. J.* **44**, 17.

WINTER G. B., RULE D. C., MAILER G. P., JAMES P. M. C. and GORDON P. H. (1971a) The prevalence of dental caries in pre-school children aged 1 to 4 years. *Br. Dent. J.* **130**, 271.

WINTER G. B., RULE D. C., MAILER G. P., JAMES P. M. C. and GORDON P. H. (1971b) The prevalence of dental caries in pre-school children aged 1 to 4 years. *Br. Dent. J.* **130**, 434.

WRIGHT G. Z. and ALPERN G. D. (1971) Variables influencing children's cooperative behaviour at the first dental visit. *J. Dent. Child.* **38**, 126.

RECOMMENDED READING

BERMAN D. S. and SLACK G. L. (1972) Dental caries in English school children. *Br. Dent. J.* **133**, 529.

HOFFDING J. and KISLING E. (1978) Premature loss of primary teeth. Parts 1 and 2. *J. Dent. Child.* **45**, 279.

McDONALD R. E. (1974) *Dentistry for the Child and Adolescent*, 2nd Ed. St. Louis, C. V. Mosby, pp. 26–37.

MINK J. R. and SPEDDING R. H. (1966) An injection procedure for the child dental patient. *Dent. Clin. North Am.* Philadelphia, W. B. Saunders, p. 309.

WINTER G. B., RULE D. C., MAILER G. P., JAMES P. M. C. and GORDON P. M. (1971) The prevalence of dental caries in pre-school children aged 1 to 4 years. 1. Etiological factors. *Br. Dent. J.* **130**, 271 and 434.

CHAPTER 2

RADIOGRAPHIC TECHNIQUES

RADIOGRAPHS are essential for the accurate diagnosis of both caries and possible pulp pathology. The value of radiographs in paediatric operative dentistry is described in other parts of the book (Chapters 1, 7, 16 and 17 in particular). Therefore, this chapter will emphasize the techniques for taking radiographs on young children. Specifically, intra-oral and simple extra-oral procedures will be described since these are commonly used by practitioners. Extra-oral radiographs, using elaborate equipment (e.g. Panorex), will not be described.

GENERAL CONSIDERATIONS

Radiographic procedures may well be one of the first 'treatment services' a child will receive. The experience should be as pleasant as possible so that it can be used as a stepping stone in properly guiding the child's behaviour through the dental experience. A brief explanation of the anticipated procedure is necessary. The 'tooth camera' and 'tooth film' are shown to the child. He is reassured that the camera will not touch his face; he is encouraged to remain very still so that the 'tooth picture doesn't come out fuzzy'. The easiest film should be taken first, leaving the most difficult until last. This usually means that the maxillary anterior occlusal film is taken first, leaving mandibular molar periapical films until last.

The radiographic techniques described in this chapter use a bisecting angle concept rather than a parallel method. They are applicable to both long and short cone machines. One of the main problems in taking radiographs of children is that of film stabilization; whenever possible the film is stabilized by occlusal pressure using a film holder. A shoulder-high lead apron should be used during all exposures.

There will never be uniform agreement of the number and type of radiographs that should be taken on children. Certainly bite-wings are essential to the early diagnosis of Class 2 primary molar lesions when the contacts are closed. Recent periapical radiographs are also essential to detect pulp pathology (e.g. internal resorption) whenever the lesion is close to the pulp; in the case of Class 2 lesions, this occurs whenever the marginal ridge is broken down. They also identify the presence of and the eruption sequence of succedaneous teeth. Anterior occlusal radiographs may assist in the diagnosis of Class 3 and 4 lesions, their proximity to the pulp and the presence

19

of physiological and pathological root resorption in primary incisors. In the pre-school child they also identify the permanent successors, including occasional supernumerary teeth, root fractures, and dilacerations. Intra-oral radiographs invariably provide greater detail than extra-oral films.

The practitioner must decide which radiographs are indicated for each individual child after his examination. It must be emphasized that radiographs are supplementary to and not a substitute for a thorough clinical examination. The techniques described are appropriate for the primary dentition and mixed dentition; modifications are described for radiographic procedures on infants.

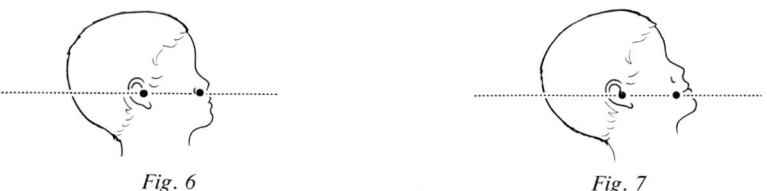

Fig. 6	*Fig. 7*

Fig. 6.—Correct head position for all maxillary films and bite-wings: ala–tragus line parallel to the floor.

Fig. 7.—Correct head position for mandibular molar films: tragus–angle of the mouth parallel to floor.

Head Position: The ala–tragus line (ala of the nose to the tragus of the ear) is parallel to the floor for all maxillary films and the bite-wings (*Fig. 6*). The tragus–angle of the mouth line is parallel to the floor for all mandibular periapical films (*Fig. 7*). Head position for the mandibular anterior occlusal film and lateral jaw are considered later.

Individual Films: All intra-oral films are placed with the edge of the film 2 mm from the incisal or occlusal surfaces of the teeth. All occlusal films are stabilized during exposure by having the child gently close his mouth to hold the film. Bite-wings for children are identical to those for adults and use bite-tabs or bite-sponges. Maxillary posterior periapical films can be held by thumb pressure; alternatively a holder can be used as with mandibular periapical films. Identification dots are placed towards the incisal edge or occlusal plane. The dots are placed in the anterior-superior corner for bite-wings. This standardization prevents misinterpretation of radiographs.

PRE-SCHOOL SURVEY—PRIMARY DENTITION

Eight intra-oral films are taken—maxillary and mandibular anterior occlusals (using Type 2 film, adult size), 4 molar periapical films and

2 posterior bite-wings (using Type 0 film, child size) (*Fig. 8*). Film placement, central ray entry point and angulations will be described. *Anterior Maxillary Occlusal:* Type 2 film is placed with its long axis running right to left and not anteroposteriorly. The anterior edge of the film is 2 mm in front of the incisal edge of the primary central

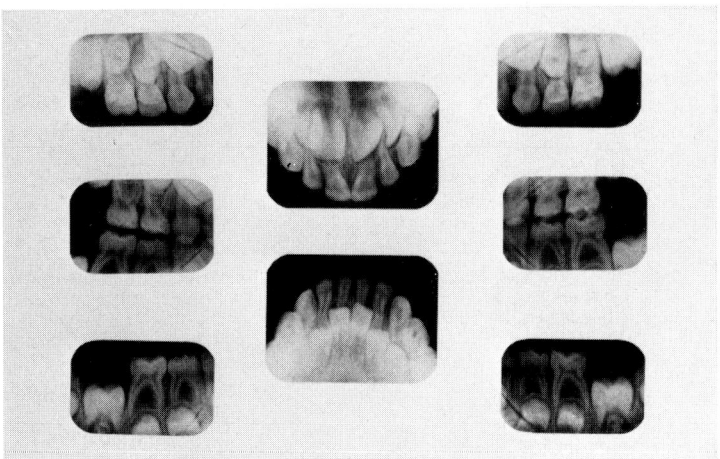

Fig. 8.—Eight film pre-school survey.

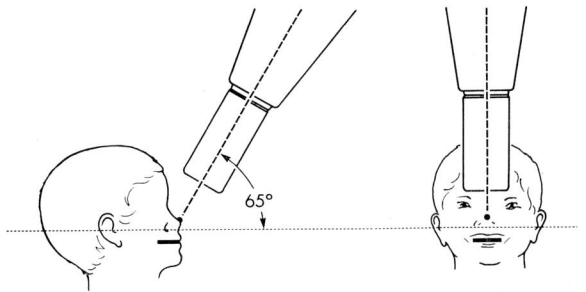

Fig. 9.—Anterior maxillary occlusal film. Cone angled at +65°.
Central ray enters at tip of nose in the midline.

incisors. It is placed symmetrically to the midline, the edges of the film extending to the primary canines. With the ala–tragus line parallel to the floor the cone is placed at a +65 degrees angulation so that the central ray enters at the midline half an inch above the tip of the nose (*Fig. 9*). The exposed developed film should demonstrate the crowns and roots of all maxillary primary incisors as well as the developing permanent incisors.

21

Anterior Mandibular Occlusal: The head is tilted backwards and upwards so that the occlusal plane is at 45 degrees to the horizontal. This correct head position is obtained by placing the X-ray cone at 45 degrees on the child's chest and moving the head until the occlusal plane is parallel to the end of the cone. Film placement is identical to the maxillary occlusal radiograph except that the film is upside down. Cone position is at 25 degrees below the horizontal (*Fig. 10*),

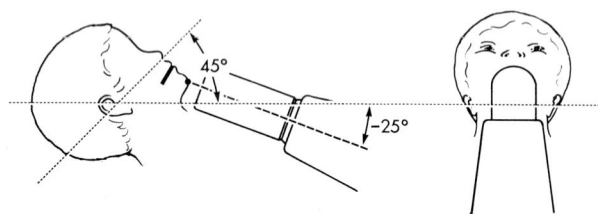

Fig. 10.—Anterior mandibular occlusal film. Occlusal plane at 45°, Cone angled at −25°. Central ray enters ½ in (23 mm) above lower border in the midline.

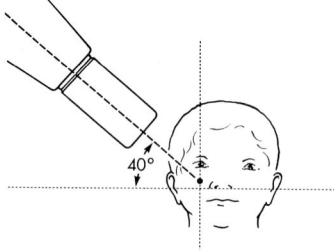

Fig. 11.—Maxillary molar periapical film, stabilized by the thumb. Cone angled at +40°. Central ray enters on line with pupil of eye.

the central ray being directed at the apices of the mandibular incisors. The completed radiograph should demonstrate the crowns and roots of the mandibular primary incisors as well as the developing permanent mandibular incisors

Maxillary Molar Periapicals: Type 0 film is bent sharply at the anterior corner that will adapt to the anterior hard palate. The long axis of the film runs anteroposteriorly with the anterior edge of the film located at the mesial of the primary canine. The film should extend an even 2 mm beyond the cusps of the primary molars. The film is stabilized during exposure by light thumb pressure from the hand opposite to the side which is being radiographed (i.e. right thumb for left side film). The thumb is placed in the middle of the film, the fingers of the hand extending out of the X-ray source. A holder can also be used; the child then bites on the plastic. With the ala–tragus line parallel to the floor, the cone is angled at

+40 degrees so that the central ray enters below the pupil of the eye on the ala–tragus line (*Fig. 11*). The crowns and apices of primary canine and primary molars as well as their permanent successors should be seen on the exposed film.

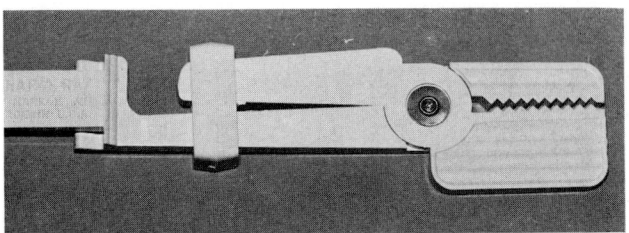

Fig. 12.—Snap-a-Ray* film holder.

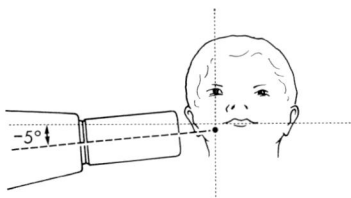

Fig. 13.—Mandibular molar periapical film. Cone angled at −5°. Central ray enters ½ in (23 mm) above lower border in line with pupil of eye.

Mandibular Molar Periapicals: Type 0 film is sharply bent at the anterior inferior corner to minimize impingement on the sublingual tissues. The film is symmetrically placed in a wooden, metal or plastic holder* (*Fig. 12*). The tongue is retracted and the film and bite-block are placed with the anterior edge extending to the mesial of the primary canine. The bite-block is usually stabilized by the first and second primary molars. The superior edge of the film should extend occlusally 2 mm from the cusps of the primary molars. As the child closes to stabilize the film there is the danger of tilting of the film. With the tragus–angle of the mouth line parallel to the floor, the cone is angled at −5 degrees so that the central ray passes half an inch above the inferior border of the mandible in line with the pupil of the eye (*Fig. 13*). The crowns and apices of the primary canine and primary molars as well as developing permanent crowns should be seen on the developed radiograph. *Posterior Bite-wings:* The anterosuperior and antero-inferior corners of a Type 0 film are bent sharply to minimize impingement on the anterior hard palate and anterior lingual tissues respectively. A

---

* Snap-a-Ray—Silverman's, Plymouth Meeting, Pennsylvania.

23

bite-tab is added to the film prior to insertion into the mouth. When the film is placed slightly across the mouth so that the anterior part is close to the midline it will be more comfortable than if it is placed closely adjacent to the lingual tissues. The child is required to close on the bite-tab in centric occlusion. The anterior part of the film should extend to the primary canine. With the ala–tragus line parallel to the floor, the cone is angled at $+8$ degrees with the central ray passing between primary molar contact areas (*Fig. 14*). The

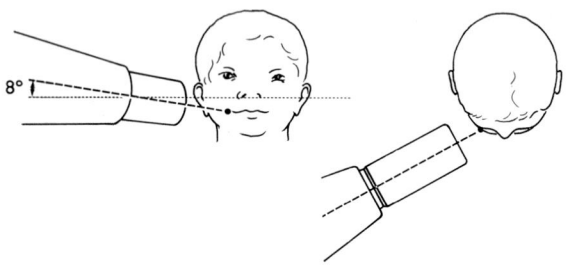

Fig. 14.—Bite-wings. *Left*, Cone angled at $+8°$. *Right*, Central ray enters between primary molar contact areas.

processed radiograph should demonstrate the maxillary and man-dibular cheek teeth from primary canine to second primary molar in occlusion. The occlusal plane should be in the middle of the film so that equal amounts of mandibular and maxillary teeth are shown. The main reason for this being tilted is movement of the film by the child's tongue. All posterior contacts must be opened by the exposure to make the radiograph of diagnostic value.

Modifications for Infants

The child under 3 years of age will usually experience difficulty with any of the pre-school survey radiographs. For these infants it may be necessary to obtain parental help in taking a film of diagnostic value. The mother should hold both the child and the film. Both child and parent face the same way with the child's head being cradled against the parent's shoulder. The parent's left hand re-strains the child's body and arms while the right hand positions and holds the film. Alternatively, the parent's right hand stabilizes the head from upward movement (to look at the X-ray head). The left hand closes the lower jaw on the film (*Fig. 15*). When the attending parent is the mother, she should be asked if she is pregnant. If she is, someone else should hold the child.

Type 0 film should be used for all intra-oral exposures in preference to the larger Type 2 film. It will often be impossible for the young child to manage the molar periapical films and the posterior bite-wings. He will be unable to adequately stabilize the maxillary molar film during exposure by digital pressure. Also, the mandibular molar film and bite-wing impinge intolerably on the sublingual tissues in these young children. The following modifications are recommended: the posterior maxillary occlusal film replaces the maxillary molar periapical, the lateral jaw replaces the mandibular molar film and the bite-wings are modified as described below.

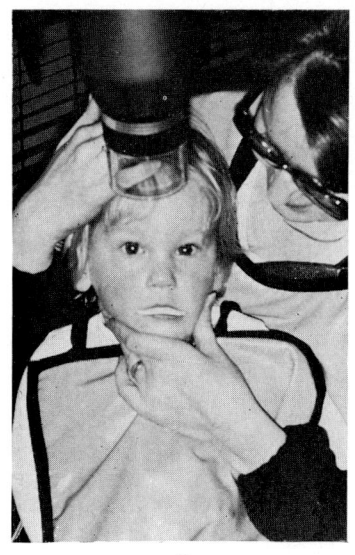 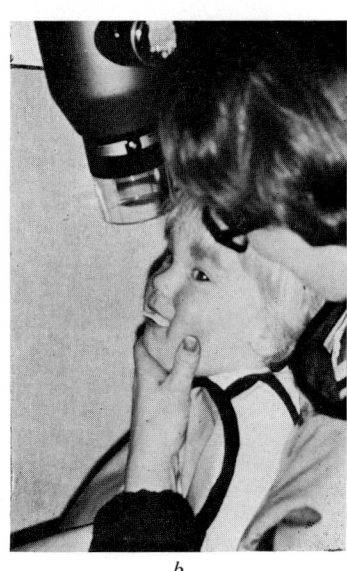

a   *b*

Fig. 15.—Parent and infant positioned for maxillary anterior film. *a*, Anterior view. *b*, lateral view.

Posterior Maxillary Occlusal: Type 0 or Type 2 film can be used depending on the age of the child and what size they can tolerate. The long axis of the film runs anteroposteriorly with the anterior part of the film located between the maxillary primary lateral incisor and the primary canine. The film should extend 2 mm beyond the primary molar crowns. It is stabilized by having the child bite or by the parent's digital pressure. With the ala–tragus line parallel to the floor, the cone is angled at +60 degrees so that the central ray passes through the apices of the primary molars (*Fig. 16*).

Lateral Jaw: The occlusal plane is parallel to the floor. The 5 × 7 lateral jaw film is held by the child's hand on the side that is being radiographed. The film is placed perpendicular to the floor along the face adjacent to the primary molars. The head is rotated so that

25

the nose and the chin touch the film. The vertical angulation of the cone is −17 degrees with the central ray perpendicular to the film passing half an inch below and behind the angle of the mandible on the side opposite to the film. Since the film is large enough to accommodate both right and left sides, metal markers should be used to identify the appropriate sides.

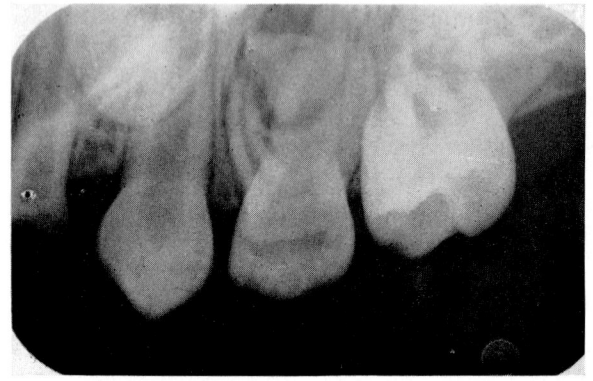

Fig. 16.—Posterior maxillary occlusal film of an infant. Note deep lesion in the first primary molar.

Posterior Bite-wing Modification: The bite-wing (Type 0 film) is placed in the buccal rather than the lingual sulcus with the bite-tab facing the occlusal surfaces of the teeth. The film is bent along its long axis so that it is easily tolerated. Head position, cone angulation and central ray entry point are identical to the lateral jaw. Essentially this is a reverse bite-wing taken like a lateral jaw film.

THE MIXED DENTITION SURVEY

Twelve intra-oral films are taken (*Fig. 17*): mandibular and maxillary permanent incisor periapicals, 4 primary canine periapicals, 4 molar periapicals and 2 posterior bite-wings. Type 2 film should be used for all exposures; Type 0 film can be used for the mandibular incisor and canine periapicals in children who cannot tolerate the larger film. The molar periapical and bite-wing radiographs are identical in film placement, cone angulation and central ray entry point to the respective pre-school survey films, except that a Type 2 film is used. Therefore they will not be described further here.

Maxillary Permanent Incisor Periapical (*Fig. 18*): Type 2 film is used with its long axis running anteroposteriorly; 2 mm of film shows anterior to the incisal edges of the permanent central incisors. The film is symmetrically placed with respect to the midline. The film is stabilized by thumb pressure as in the maxillary primary molar

26

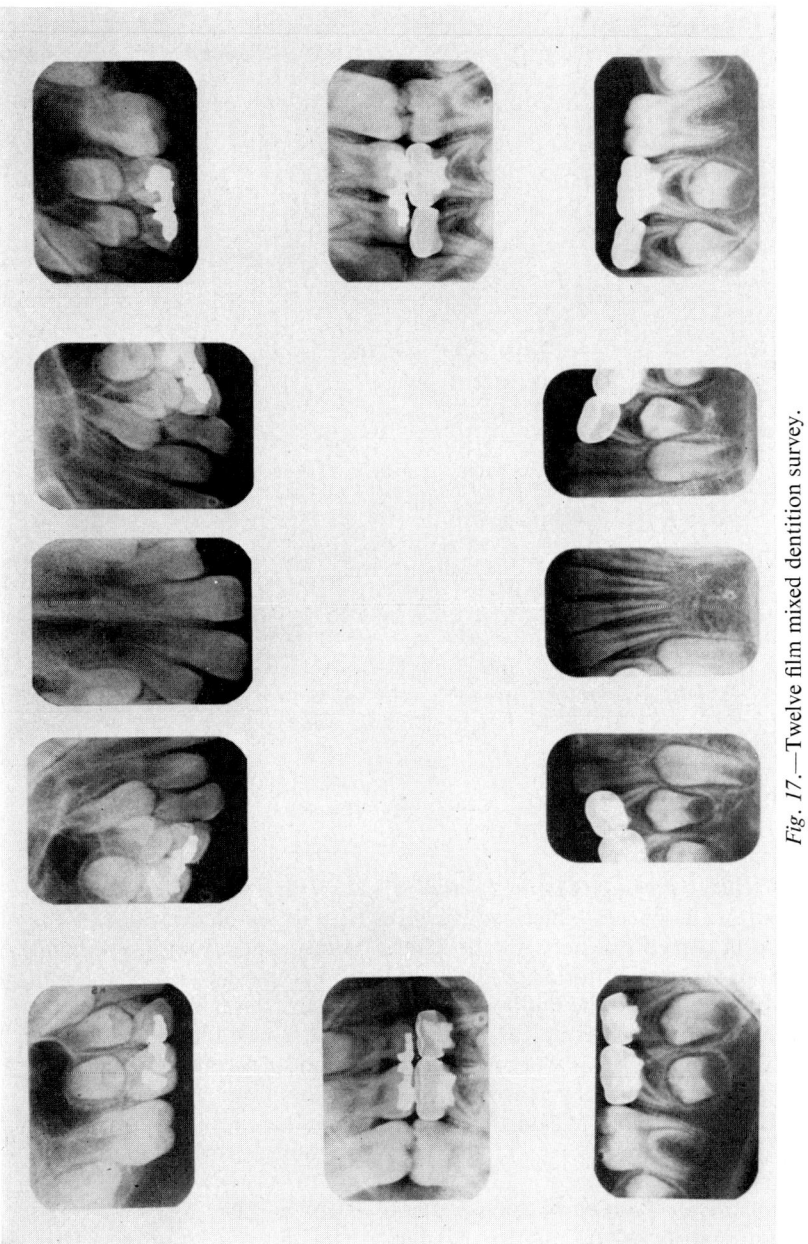

Fig. 17.—Twelve film mixed dentition survey.

periapical. If the arch is narrow the film can be bent along its length at its lateral border. With the ala–tragus line parallel to the floor, the cone angled at +55 degrees, the central ray passes through the tip of the nose. The radiograph should demonstrate the undistorted crowns and apices of the maxillary permanent central incisors.

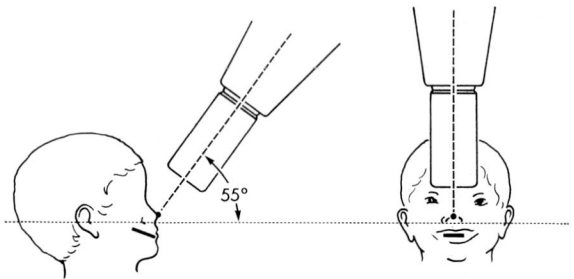

Fig. 18.—Maxillary permanent incisor periapical. Cone at 55°. Central ray enters at tip of nose in the midline.

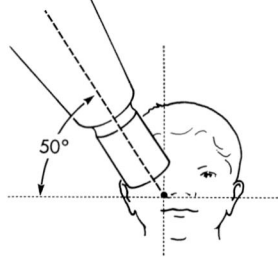

Fig. 19.—Maxillary canine periapical. Cone at +50°. Central ray enters at ala of the nose.

Maxillary Primary Canine Periapical (Fig. 19): Type 2 film is sharply bent at the corner which will fit into the midline of the palate. The film is placed in line with the lateral incisor and canine roots with 2 mm showing anterior to their crowns. The mesial part of the film should extend to the midline. Thumb pressure holds the film, as with maxillary molar periapicals; alternatively a film holder is used. The ala–tragus line is parallel to the floor, the cone angled at +50 degrees, the central ray passing through the ala of the nose. The undistorted crowns and roots of lateral incisor and canine should be shown on the radiograph; there will, however, be some overlap of the first primary molar.

Mandibular Permanent Incisor Periapical (Fig. 20): Type 2 film is bent sharply at the inferior corners to facilitate positioning of the film and to minimize impingement on the soft tissues. These bends

28

are unnecessary if the smaller Type 0 film is used. With the film symmetrically placed in the bite-holder, the inferior part of the film is placed under the tongue as far back as possible. As the superior part of the film is placed, the sublingual tissues are depressed; the further back the inferior part of the film the more comfortable it is for the child. The film is stabilized by biting pressure from the permanent central incisors on the bite-block. The tragus–angle of the mouth line is parallel to the floor, the cone angled at − 10 degrees with the central ray entering $\frac{1}{2}$ in (23 mm) above the lower border of the mandible at the midline. The processed radiograph should show the undistorted crown and roots of the permanent central incisors. This film, together with the mandibular primary canine film, is one of the most difficult for the child to tolerate. For this reason many clinicians prefer to use a mandibular anterior occlusal film until the child reaches the permanent dentition.

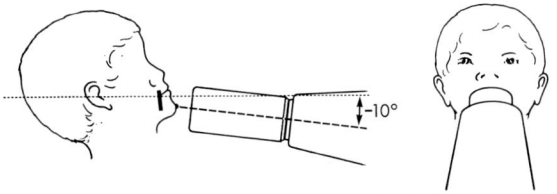

Fig. 20.—Mandibular permanent incisor periapical. Cone at − 10°. Central ray enters $\frac{1}{2}$ in (23 mm) above lower border in midline.

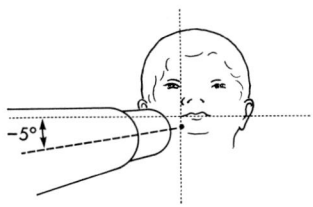

Fig. 21.—Mandibular canine periapical. Cone at − 5°. Central ray enters $\frac{1}{2}$ in (23 mm) above lower border in line with ala of the nose.

Mandibular Primary Canine Periapical (Fig. 21): Type 2 film is sharply bent at the inferior corner that will be placed closest to the midline. Alternatively, unbent Type 0 film is used. The inferior part of the film is placed first as far under the tongue as possible, the film placed in line with the crowns and roots of the lateral incisor and canine. The film is stabilized by biting pressure on the crowns of these teeth. The tragus–angle of the mouth line is parallel to the floor. The cone is angled at − 5 degrees with the central ray passing $\frac{1}{2}$ in (23 mm) above the lower border of the mandible, through the roots of the primary canine; this will usually be in line with the ala of the nose.

EXPOSURE TIMES AND DEVELOPING TECHNIQUES

Successful radiographs are dependent on correct exposure times and developing techniques as well as film placement, cone positioning and central ray entering points. Because of the variety of radiographic machines and the use of both short and long cones, no set rules will be given for exposure times and developing techniques. Rather, the practitioner is encouraged to review the manufacturer's instructions for his individual machine. He is also referred to texts on radiology to help improve the quality of his X-rays. There is an ever-increasing trend to use automatic developers. These machines can be recommended from personal use since they standardize the quality of the processed radiograph. Bent films should be straightened prior to processing to minimize being caught in developer rollers.

RECOMMENDED READING

BEAN L. R. and ISAAC H. K. (1973) X-ray and the child patient. *Dent. Clin. North Am.* **17:1**, 13.

MATLOCK J. F. (1974) In: McDonald, R. E. *Dentistry for the Child and Adolescent.* 2nd ed. St. Louis, C. V. Mosby, p. 93.

SMITH N. J. D. (1973) *Radiography and Radiology for the Dental Practitioner. Br. Dent. J.* Reprint. B.M.A. House, Tavistock Square, London.

CHAPTER 3

ANATOMY OF PRIMARY AND PERMANENT TEETH

ANATOMICAL variations between primary and permanent teeth dictate different approaches to both cavity design and pulp therapy. The basic differences are depicted in *Figs. 22* and *23* and will be discussed in relation to their clinical significance.

CROWN MORPHOLOGY

The crowns of primary teeth are more bulbous than their permanent successors. The molar crowns are wider mesiodistally than they are occluso-gingivally. The mesiodistal and incisogingival dimensions of the primary incisors and canines are similar to each other.

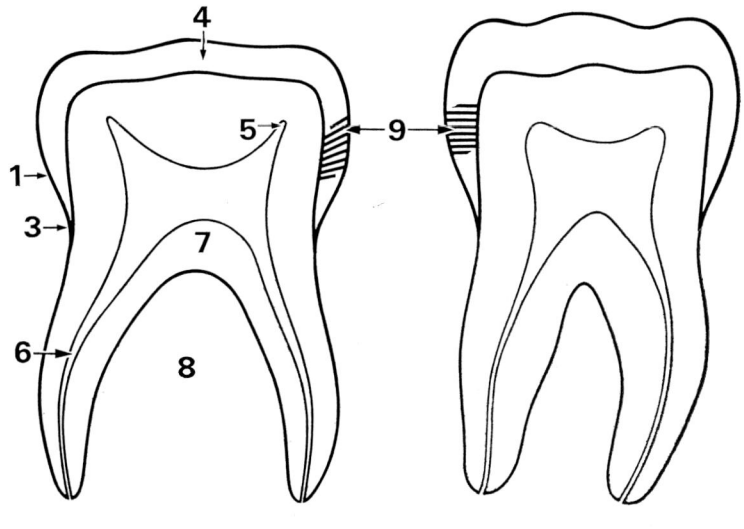

PRIMARY   **PERMANENT**

Fig. 22.—Differences between primary and permanent teeth:— Cross-sectional view in buccolingual plane. 1. Bulbous crown and cervical prominence. 2. Narrow occlusal table. 3. Cervical constriction (apical to cervical enamel prominence). 4. Thin enamel. 5. Pulp horns. 6. Fine canals. 7. Thin pulpal floor. 8. Developing permanent tooth. 9. Enamel rod inclination.

The primary molars exhibit a very narrow occlusal table in a buccolingual plane because of the occlusal convergence of the buccal and lingual walls. This narrow occlusal table is more pronounced in the first than in the second primary molar. This should automatically reduce the buccolingual dimensions of the occlusal part of any Class 1 or 2 cavity to prevent weakening of cusps. Because of the broad gingivally-located contact areas, there will be gingival divergence of buccal and lingual walls; as a result, the interproximal margins of a Class 2 cavity must extend widely at the gingival aspect of the embrasures to be self-cleansing. The isthmus area, where the interproximal box and the occlusal lock meet, is narrow—exactly at a point where strength is needed to withstand the forces of occlusion and the trauma of opposing cusps. Furthermore, the occlusal aspects of the interproximal box leave little margin for error since overextension will leave unsupported enamel or alloy.

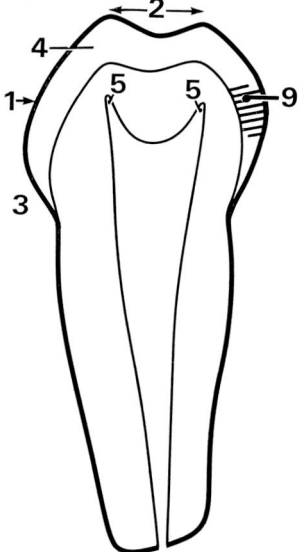

Fig. 23.—Mesiodistal view of mandibular primary molar.

These are major causes of the high failure rate of Class 2 alloys from ditched interproximal margins and fractured isthmuses. This is more noticeable in mandibular first primary molars because of their very narrow occlusal table (Castaldi, 1957).

There is a marked cervical prominence of enamel in primary molars gingival to which is an equally marked cervical constriction. The placement of the floor of the interproximal box in a Class 2 cavity is dictated by these anatomical differences. It is easy to run short of sound tooth structure when the gingival floor of the interproximal box is placed too far cervically. The operator may then be tempted to re-establish the gingival floor by moving the axial wall farther pulpally—unfortunately at the risk of closely approximating the pulp. The lingual and buccal aspects of the cervical prominence of enamel can be used to retain a stainless-steel crown, whose margins fit apical to this in the gingival sulcus. However, the marked mesiobuccal enamel bulge of the first primary molar frequently requires reduction to facilitate fitting of the stainless-steel crown; the undercut is too severe to accurately engage the margins of the crown.

The primary enamel is only half as thick as in permanent teeth. The primary teeth are usually lighter in colour; also, they give the clinical impression of being easier to cut with a bur. The thin enamel, together with the relatively large pulp horns, means that there may be only a very small distance between the outer enamel surface and the pulp. The clinical significance of this is threefold. First, it is imperative that lesions be diagnosed at an early stage since failure to do so may result in the undetected caries penetrating to the pulp between recall visits. This is especially true with Class 2 lesions, since the distance between the mesial surface of the mandibular first primary molar and the pulp may be as little as 1·6 mm (Wheeler, 1965). Bite-wing radiographs at each recall are thus mandatory when posterior contacts are closed. Second, the operator must re-evaluate the size of his burs and adapt them to the size of the primary molar; overextension either buccally or lingually at the embrasures, or pulpally, is to be avoided. The diameter of the flat fissure number 2 bur is about 1·0 mm.* Burs of this dimension are recommended. Third, care must be taken to provide restorative material in sufficient bulk for retention without exposing the pulp.

PULP AND ROOT MORPHOLOGY

The primary tooth pulp horns are larger than those in permanent teeth and are relatively closer to the surface when the thinner primary enamel is considered. Cavity design must be established around these pulp horns which are situated below the appropriate cusps. Therefore, in a Class 2 cavity with a *narrow* isthmus, tunnelling, grooving, or rounding of the axiopulpal line angle can be carried out without fear of pulp exposure. This will provide a greater bulk of alloy at the weak isthmus area. Preoperative bite-wing radiographs may give the operator an idea of the superficially placed pulp horns and allow him to plan his preparation accordingly.

The pulp horns are extensions of the bulky coronal pulp which accounts for most of the primary tooth's pulp tissue; this is particularly true of primary molars. Maxillary molars have three pulp

---

* Information provided by Amalgamated Dental Co., 26 Broadwick St., London.

horns which correspond to the three roots (mesiobuccal, distobuccal and palatal). Mandibular molars have four pulp horns located under the respective cusps: mesiobucally, mesiolingually, distobucally, and distolingually. There are two roots and usually two or three root canals; the mesial root may have one or two canals. Access to the coronal pulp chamber is best achieved through the occlusal surface by locating all the pulp horns and joining them with bur cuts. The roof of the pulp chamber can then be lifted off. The depth of the coronal pulp varies markedly; the preoperative radiograph gives the operator a good idea not only of its depth, but also of the thickness of the pulpal floor and the mesiodistal location of the entrance of the root canals. The thin pulpal floor may have accessory canals (Winter, 1962), though these are seldom visible radiographically. These accessory canals, together with the porous pulpal floor seen in non-vital primary molars (Moss et al., 1965), may account for the leakage of inflammatory products from the pulp chamber to the inter-radicular area. This may explain the high incidence of inter-radicular bone loss in non-vital primary molars compared to the periapical bone loss seen in non-vital permanent teeth.

The primary pulp ages just as the permanent pulp. Thus the root canals of a primary molar in a 3-year-old may appear radiographically very wide while they may appear very fine or obliterated in the same child at age 8. Similarly, the primary pulp is capable of physiological and pathological changes such as secondary dentine formation, internal resorption, pulp stones and calcifications. Thorough radiographic preoperative assessment is mandatory to help establish the diagnosis of pulp pathology (see Chapter 16).

The roots of primary teeth are longer and thinner mesiodistally than those of permanent successors. The roots of the primary molars are flared to allow for the development of the underlying premolars. Retention of primary molar roots following physiological resorption or extraction is due to the curved narrow roots. The radicular pulp of the primary molars follows a thin, tortuous and branching path, as shown by Hibbard and Ireland (1957). The multiple branching of the primary pulp makes conventional endodontic procedures considerably more difficult to perform than in permanent teeth. Therefore the treatment usually consists of removing part of the primary pulp and then applying some medicament either to devitalize the remaining pulp or to allow it to heal. The fact that a permanent successor is lying close to the primary molar roots means that burs, broaches, files and reamers must be handled with extreme care. At the same time, any medicament placed in the pulp chamber and/or root canals must be resorbable.

CONTACT AREAS
The contact areas between primary molars are broader, flatter and situated farther gingivally than those between permanent molars (Davies and King, 1961). The clinical significance of this is three-fold. First, interproximal lesions need to be extensive before they are clinically observable as a grey shadow undermining the marginal ridge. This, together with the larger pulp horns, thin enamel, and Stoner's observation (1967) that broken down marginal ridges are often associated with pulp exposure, makes early diagnosis of Class 2 lesions even more imperative. Because the contact areas are broad and flat, interproximal exploration may be fruitless, leaving the bite-wing radiograph as the best diagnostic aid of primary molar Class 2 lesions. Second, the buccal and lingual margins of the inter-proximal box must extend far enough towards the embrasure at the gingival to make them self-cleansing. Again, care must be taken to ensure that occlusal enamel is not left unsupported to discourage marginal failure. Third, to ensure that the gingival seat of a Class 2 lesion is self-cleansing, the gingivally located contact area must be broken. Care must be taken to prevent the gingival seat from being established apical to the cervical constriction. When the gingival seat is placed too far apically, matrix application is extremely difficult. However, when caries extends subgingivally it is impossible to establish optimal gingival floor depth.

ENAMEL RODS
The enamel rods of permanent teeth incline horizontally or apically in the gingival one-third. This requires the use of a gingival margin trimmer in permanent teeth to ensure that there will be no un-supported enamel rods. The enamel rod inclination in the gingival one-third of primary molars is towards the occlusal (*Fig. 22*). Thus, there is no need for cavo-surface bevelling since all enamel rods of the gingival wall will accordingly be supported.

REFERENCES
CASTALDI C. R. (1957) Analysis of some operative procedures currently being used in paedodontics. *J. Can. Dent. Assoc.* **23,** 377.

DAVIES G. N. and KING R. M. (1961) *Dentistry for the Pre-school Child.* London, E. & S. Livingstone, pp. 229–230.

HIBBARD E. D. and IRELAND R. L. (1957) Morphology of the root canals of the primary molar teeth. *J. Dent. Child.* **24,** 250.

Moss S. J., ADDELSTON H. and GOLDSMITH E. D. (1965) Histologic study of pulpal floor of deciduous molars. *J. Am. Dent. Assoc.* **70,** 372.

STONER J. E. (1967). Dental caries in deciduous molars. *Br. Dent. J.* **123,** 130.

WHEELER R. C. (1965) *A Textbook of Dental Anatomy and Physiology.* Philadelphia, W. B. Saunders Co.

WINTER G. B. (1962) Abscess formation in connexion with deciduous molar teeth. *Arch. Oral Biol.* **7,** 373.

RECOMMENDED READING

DAVIES G. N. and KING R. M. (1961) *Dentistry for the Pre-school child.* London, E. & S. Livingstone, Chapter 12.

MCDONALD R. E. (1974) *Dentistry for the Child and Adolescent.* St. Louis, C. V. Mosby Co., Chapter, 3.

WHEELER R. C. (1965) *A Textbook of Dental Anatomy and Physiology.* Philadelphia, W. B. Saunders Co.

CHAPTER 4

PRINCIPLES OF OPERATIVE DENTISTRY

ONE object of cavity preparation is to remove carious material. The cavity is designed with possible future sites of attack in mind, and the completed cavity is then restored to correct contour with a suitable material. Black (1924) outlined an approach to cavity preparation and identified certain principles that should be followed. His recommendations have withstood the test of time and are applicable in everyday dentistry. Both primary and permanent teeth lend themselves to these principles. It is recommended that during cavity preparation the following sequence be followed:

Gain access;
Establish outline form;
Eliminate caries;
Establish resistance and retention form;
Refine and débride the cavity.

The above steps blend together and therefore cannot really be considered as separate activities, particularly with the use of high-speed cutting instruments. However, the operator who keeps these steps in mind will be well equipped to evaluate his own cavity preparation and find ways of improving his technique.

ACCESS

Operator preference and to a certain extent patient behaviour will determine the extent of usage of high- and low-speed cutting and hand instrumentation. A bur commensurate with the tooth's size and projected cavity dimensions is recommended for use in the high-speed handpiece for cutting the majority of the preparations. Once the whistling noise and water coolant spray have been explained to the child, acceptance is seldom a problem, particularly when compared to the vibration experienced by the slow-speed handpieces. The reduced operating time and efficiency of cutting afforded by high-speed burs help shorten the appointment for the child; it is also less stressful for the practitioner who is frustrated by the comparative inefficiency of the slow-speed handpiece. The dental student, however, should be very selective in his use of the high-speed cutting instruments; his inexperience in behaviour management and sudden unexpected movements of the child may result in overextension and unnecessary pulp exposure.

For the child's comfort, as much of the cavity preparation as possible should be completed with the high-speed cutting instruments. However, the practitioner should not exceed his own self-determined boundaries with this instrument because of the danger of inadvertent pulp exposure and damage to an adjacent interproximal surface. Cutting should commence at the occlusal pits and fissures. The chance of inadvertent pulp exposure is reduced by limiting the cavity initially to 0·5 mm pulpal to the amelodental junction; this depth should be maintained on both the pulpal and axial walls. This will usually allow sufficient bulk of restorative material for both strength and retention. This depth will also ensure elimination of incipient enamel caries and possibly reveal dentinal caries undermining the enamel. Slow speed and hand instrumentation can then be used to finish the cavity.

Inadvertent pulp exposure tends to be avoided when the occlusal lock of a Class 2 cavity is prepared before the interproximal box, since visibility of the latter is improved. This also minimizes the risk of marking the adjacent tooth. If this does occur it is frequently of minimal clinical significance since it is so common to see adjacent interproximal areas on primary molars in need of simultaneous restoration. However, the situation becomes more serious when no lesion is present on the adjacent tooth, such as the mesial surface of the first permanent molar when a distal cavity is prepared in the second primary molar. Cardwell (1974) found that dental students marked the tooth adjacent to the interproximal cavity they were preparing in over 90 per cent of the cases. No statistics are available for practitioners, although it is obvious that great care needs to be taken to prevent an iatrogenic area of plaque retention and subsequent cavity formation.

The small size of the Class 3 lesion makes it desirable to use slow-speed instrumentation from the outset. Often this is the best way to keep the cavity small enough to be aesthetically acceptable. This recommendation applies to both primary and permanent teeth. Bur size must be commensurate with the tooth size, the projected cavity dimensions and the relatively superficial placement of the pulp horns in primary teeth. The diameter of the flat fissure No. 2 is 1·00 mm* (*see also* Chapter 3); this or similarly sized burs are thus recommended for Class 1 and 2 cavity preparations. The No. 2 inverted cone bur† is suitable for Class 3 and 5 cavities.

---

* Information supplied by Amalgamated Dental Co., 26 Broadwick St., London. Flat Fissure Long Head Plain Cut No. 2L (English No.) is equivalent to American No. 57L.
† Inverted Cone Bur No. 2 (English No.) = No. 35 American.

OUTLINE FORM

Black (1924) identified pits and fissures and interproximal contact surfaces as areas that were particularly susceptible to caries. He recommended that cavity preparations should include these danger areas so that the margins of the cavity and restorative material would be located in a so-called immune area; at least they would be in a self-cleansing or readily cleansed area. In effect, he was recommending extension for prevention. This means that the Class 1 cavity should not be confined to the carious defect; rather the outline form should include the pits and fissures throughout the occlusal surface. Failure to place the margins in a self-cleansing area increases the likelihood that new decay will develop later. Similarly, the interproximal box of a Class 2 cavity must allow the passage of an explorer tip between its margins and the adjacent tooth in three directions—buccally, lingually, and gingivally. Only then will the interproximal margins be self-cleansing. The results of overextension have been mentioned (Chapter 3); underextension may result in the incomplete removal of caries, predisposition to the onset of new caries, and difficulty in matrix application.

Class 3 and 5 cavities differ from Class 1 and 2 cavities because the outline form need include only the carious lesion. Maintaining the principles of Class 1 and 2 cavity preparation would result in unnecessary tooth destruction when restoring an incipient Class 3 lesion. However, enamel decalcification adjacent to a Class 5 lesion would necessitate extending the Class 5 cavity to include that area in order to prevent recurrent caries.

ELIMINATION OF DECAY

Unless indirect pulp treatment is being performed, all cavities must be rendered caries-free before any restorative material is inserted, including bases. The recommended outline form and depth may result in a caries-free cavity if the initial lesion is small. Should further caries remain, it should be removed with round burs run at slow speed and with spoon excavators. High-speed burs are less efficient than slow-speed burs for removing caries. Particular emphasis should be placed on removing all softened and stained material at the amelodentinal junction; frequently such material persists under the cusps. If it is left, it will continue to proceed pulpally, in addition to undermining the enamel until a cusp may eventually fracture. Round burs run at a very slow speed with a light touch are preferred to spoon excavators since the latter, when properly sharpened, often remove more material than is clinically necessary. This may be unfortunate if indirect pulp treatment was planned and an unwanted exposure is encountered. In asymptomatic teeth, it is acceptable to leave stained hard dentine at the base of the cavity if its removal would, in the operator's opinion, result in pulp exposure (as explained in Chapter 17).

RESISTANCE AND RETENTION FORM

The ease of manipulation, low cost, and time proven results of amalgam alloy make it the material of choice for all posterior cavity preparations in children, and in some instances for anterior restorations (particularly in primary teeth). Until adhesives have been further developed, retention of restorative materials replacing carious lesions must come from mechanical means, and further discussion of this topic is related to that concept.

The restoration will be subjected to displacing forces either occlusally or interproximally; cavity design must contend with this problem. A minimal cavity depth of 0·5 mm pulpal to amelodentinal junction will usually provide sufficient bulk of restorative material for strength. An exception is the axiopulpal line angle of Class 2 cavities which must be rounded, tunnelled, or grooved to provide additional bulk of restorative material at this point of weakness. The weakness may be aggravated by the trauma of opposing cusps and the placement of excessively deep anatomical grooves in the restoration.

Davies and King (1961) indicate that strength at the isthmus area of a Class 2 cavity is three times greater when the bulk of alloy is provided in depth rather than in width. Provided that a narrow outline form is made, the cavity can be deepened at the isthmus without fear of pulp exposure. Thus, just as with permanent teeth, there should be a tendency towards narrower and deeper preparations (Gilmore, 1964), which not only conserve maximum tooth structure but also adhere to Black's principles. This is in contrast to the recommendation that the width of the primary molar isthmus in Class 2 preparations be increased (Lampshire, 1955). Also, more effective bulk of alloy can also be provided by selective grinding of the opposing cusps; no clinically visible untoward effect on the occlusion is observed, since primary molars are normally subject to attrition.

Rounded *internal* line angles are recommended for both primary and permanent teeth. The advantages are threefold. First, they reduce the stress within the tooth that results from masticatory forces. Second, rounded line angles permit easier condensation of amalgam. Third, there is less chance of pulp horn exposure when a round bur is used compared to an inverted cone bur; however, both the bur's inclination and the outline form are variables which make this advantage a theoretical consideration. The major disadvantage of rounded line angles is that they are more difficult to see and evaluate than sharper, square line angles. For this reason the self-critical operator may elect to persist in the use of sharp internal line angles and, except for the axiopulpal line angle, he is justified in this approach since there is no clinical proof that any untoward effects occur in primary teeth. External line angles will be discussed relative to the individual cavity preparations (Chapters 7, 8 and 9).

Both round and sharp internal line angles usually result in a slight dentinal undercut which provides mechanical retention. Retention grooves are recommended for both primary and permanent Class 2 cavities (Chapter 7). Retention grooves, pits or pins can also be placed in dentine to a depth of 1–2 mm close to the amelodentinal junction so that they do not weaken the enamel. These will be discussed in the following chapters. The depth and inclination of such retentive aids (particularly pins) must relate to the size of the pulp horn, its location, and the cervical prominence of enamel in primary molars; exposure of either the pulp or periodontal membrane is to be avoided.

The 90 degree angle at the cavo-surface margin results in adequate support of alloy and enamel rods by dentine; the more acute angles are responsible for marginal deterioration (Jørgensen and Palbøl, 1965). This is because the enamel rod/prism structure runs at 90 degrees from the amelodentinal junction to enamel surface. It also facilitates carving of the alloy. The finishing of the cavity should be performed with this in mind, irrespective of the marked variation from tooth to tooth in cuspal inclines.

REFINEMENT AND DÉBRIDEMENT OF THE CAVITY

The final stage of cavity preparation is the establishment of well-supported and finished margins and a cavity that is free of debris. Hatchets and chisels can be used on the occlusal aspects of the cavity walls to test the support of the enamel and break off weakened margins. Gingival margin trimmers can be used with care on the floor of the interproximal boxes in primary molars (as described in Chapter 7) to remove weak enamel fragments; they are recommended for routine use in finishing permanent molar Class 2 cavities.

Grieve (1968) examined the smoothness of interproximal margins produced by various finishing techniques, using tracings from photomicrographs as a measuring tool. The cavity prepared by a diamond instrument in the air turbine had a very rough margin which required finishing before the restoration was inserted. The tungsten carbide plain cut fissure bur run at 20,000 rpm produced the best results at the embrasure margins. This has been confirmed by the electron microscopic evaluation of Class 2 proximal margins (Boyde and Knight, 1970); however, the direction of bur rotation and the routine use of a chisel are also responsible for the production of smooth margins. Grieve (1968) also recommended the use of chisels on the gingival floor of the interproximal box of permanent teeth Class 2 preparations. The chisels remove unsupported enamel and can also be used to refine the buccogingival and linguogingival line angles. On the basis of these results a tungsten carbide plain cut fissure bur (No. 2L)* can be recommended to finish the cavity margins and a hatchet or chisel can then be used to break away unsupported enamel.

PULP PROTECTION

Pulp-protecting bases will be discussed fully in Chapter 11. However, at this time it is important that the clinician recognize the potential insult to the pulp from cavity preparation. On the one hand, it has been documented that the most apparently atraumatic cavity preparation causes histological pulp damage; of course, the greater the use of burs during the cavity preparation, the more severe the pulp pathology. On the other hand, patients rarely complain of pain following the placement of restorations. However, this does not necessarily mean that pulp damage has not occurred, but rather that any damage is subclinical and, generally, reversible. The pulp can respond unfavourably to the following irritants:
Thermal change;
Dehydration;
Vibration/pressure.
Bacterial contamination.

Thermal Change

It is currently accepted in Great Britain that all burs run at high speed (in the air turbine) should be cooled with water or an air/water combination. The aim of this is to reduce the production of heat in the dentine, which will then be transferred to the pulp. However, high-speed burs probably remove tooth structure so fast that the heat is never allowed to penetrate close to the pulp. Furthermore, an air/water spray coolant reduces visibility when working in the maxillary arch by indirect vision. In North America, the need for an air/water spray as a coolant is not uniformly accepted. In many dental schools and practices, air coolant is used as an alternative. Thus, it seems pertinent to review the evidence in support of each method.

---

* English No. 2L = No. 170L American.

When low speeds (500 rpm) are used without any coolant, some transient disruption of the odontoblastic layer will be seen. As bur speeds increase (still without any coolant) further damage takes the form of vacuolization of odontoblasts and aspiration of their nuclei. When the uncooled bur speed exceeds 3000 rpm (still in the range of slow speed), the damage is no longer confined to that pulp immediately adjacent to the cavity preparation. Further clinical and histological evidence is provided from studies in which contralateral young permanent teeth with Class 5 cavities were cut with a bur in the air turbine, using either an air or an air/water spray coolant. These are particularly relevant since most cavity preparation is done with burs run in the air turbine. Pulpal damage in the initial post-operative period (up to 6 weeks) was more severe in the air-cooled than in the air/water cooled groups (Dachi and Stigers, 1968; Marsland and Shovelton, 1970). However, recovery from initial damage was complete in both cases.

Contrary to what might be supposed, the intrapulpal temperature is *not* raised with either method of cooling; rather it is lowered slightly (Bhaskar and Lilly, 1965). In support of air coolant, a 4-year clinical study of teeth prepared either with air or with air/water coolant revealed no clinical differences between each group; no one method caused clinically evident pulp damage (Bouschour and Matthews, 1966). Thus, there seems to be adequate evidence to support the use of air-cooled high-speed instrumentation on the basis of clinical rather than microscopic results.

The practitioner has to rely very much on the pulp's healing potential. Fortunately, in young teeth the highly cellular pulp and incompletely formed apices lend themselves freely to repair. However, the pulp may be insulted prior to operative dentistry by the size of the carious lesion. To avoid adding injury to insult, and thus to minimize pulp damage, an air/water spray coolant is recommended for all rotary instrumentation at both high and low speeds. Also, this will wash debris from the cavity preparation, help prevent dehydration, and avoid the unpleasant odour that occurs with air-cooled burs. It is assumed that all burs, particularly those run at high speed, will be used with a light touch and an intermittent gentle paintbrush motion.

Dehydration

Excessive use of air coolant during the cavity preparation or débridement can cause pulp damage (Brännström, 1960). While the cavity must be dry to obtain maximum visibility and ideal conditions for inserting restorative materials, the dentist should be alert to potential pulpal damage caused by excessive dehydration.

Vibration/Pressure

It has been suggested that the vibration of burs can produce pulp damage both immediately adjacent to the cavity floor and also on a more widespread scale through the pulp (Holden, 1962). Excessive pressure to young permanent teeth is to be avoided since their shortened roots, due to incompletely formed apices, reduce their periodontal support. Heavy instrumentation can result in unnecessary postoperative mobility, particularly in teeth with small root surface areas, such as incisors and premolars. Fortunately, the child's healing potential comes to the clinician's rescue, but this is of no consolation to the child who is subjected to unnecessary and unpleasant force during operative dentistry.

Bacterial Contamination

Recent laboratory study (Beagrie, 1979) indicates that bacteria left in cavity preparations prior to placement of the restorative material are a greater cause of pulpal inflammation than the material itself. It is, therefore, critical to ensure that cavity preparations are thoroughly washed and dried to eliminate all bacterial debris.

REFERENCES

BEAGRIE G. S. (1979) Pulp irritation and silicate cement. *J. Can. Dent. Assoc.* **45**, 67.

BHASKAR S. N. and LILLY G. E. (1965) Intrapulpal temperature during cavity preparation. *J. Dent. Res.* **44**, 644.

BLACK G. V. (1924) *A Work on Operative Dentistry*, Vol. 2, 5th ed. Chicago, Chicago Medico-Dental Publishing Co.

BOUSCHOUR C. F. and MATTHEWS J. L. (1966) A four-year clinical study of teeth restored after preparation with an air turbine handpiece with an air coolant. *J. Prosth. Dent.* **16**, 306.

BOYDE A. and KNIGHT P. J. (1970) Scanning electron microscope studies of the preparation of the embrasure walls of Class II cavities. *Br. Dent. J.* **129**, 557.

BRÄNNSTRÖM M. (1960) Dentinal and pulpal response. II. Application of an air stream to exposed dentin. Short observation period. *Acta Odontol. Scand.* **18**, 17.

CARDWELL J. A. (1974) Personal communication, results available from a study reported by Cardwell J. A. (1972). *J. Dent. Res.* **51**, 1269.

DACHI S. F. and STIGERS R. W. (1968) Pulpal effects of water and air coolants used in high-speed cavity preparations. *J. Am. Dent. Assoc.* **76**, 95.

DAVIES G. N. and KING R. M. (1961) *Dentistry for the Pre-school Child.* London, E. & S. Livingstone Ltd. p. 237.

GILMORE H. W. (1964) *Practical Dental Monographs* (Nov., 1964), 5–31, Chicago, Year Book Publishers, Inc.

GRIEVE A. R. (1968) Finishing cavity margins. *Br. Dent. J.* **125**, 12.

HOLDEN G. G. P. (1962) Some observations on the vibratory phenomena associated with high-speed air turbines and their transmission to living tissue. *Br. Dent. J.* **113,** 265.

JØRGENSEN K. D. and PALBØL O. P. (1965) Experiments on the relationship between the strength and the angle of amalgam margins. *Acta Odontol. Scand.* **23,** 513.

LAMPSHIRE E. L. (1955) Evaluation of cavity preparations in primary molars. *J. Dent. Child.* **22,** 3.

MARSLAND E. A. and SHOVELTON D. S. (1970) Repair in the human dental pulp following cavity preparation. *Arch. Oral Biol.* **15,** 411.

RECOMMENDED READING

BOYDE A. and KNIGHT P. J. (1970) Scanning electron microscope studies of the preparation of the embrasure walls of Class II cavities. *Br. Dent. J.* **129,** 557.

CHAPTER 5

ISOLATION

THE operating area has to be well isolated for two procedures—cavity preparation and placement of the restoration. Isolation improves access and visibility, and sterility should pulp treatment be performed. At its simplest, it may take the form of soft-tissue retraction by cotton rolls in the sulci and a mirror to retract the tongue when endodontics is not anticipated. For the insertion of the restoration, isolation not only improves access but, more important, keeps the operating area dry. Since about 40 per cent of failed restorations are due to faulty manipulation of the restorative material (Healey and Phillips, 1949), the practitioner must pay attention to the details of material handling. For the best results, he must obtain effective isolation.

There are two means of achieving isolation—by the rubber dam or by using cotton rolls and cotton gauze. Since the rubber dam provides the best isolation, the question arises as to why so few dentists use it. Many practitioners probably do not feel sufficiently practised in the use of the dam to place it confidently on a child. They may also feel that it takes too long to apply. The first reason for not using the rubber dam can be eliminated by practice, starting with simple cases initially. The objection that placing the dam takes too long is in fact inaccurate. Approximately 25 per cent of an operative visit is spent unproductively in conversation, watching the patient rinse, and waiting for the patient to reposition himself. The child patient may use these as delaying tactics and, in a 30-minute appointment as much as ten minutes can be wasted. Once practised, it takes less than two minutes to isolate a quadrant of two primary molars and a primary canine (Heise, 1971). If operative visits are approximately 30 minutes long, it is easy to see that the rubber dam is not time-consuming; in fact, it allows the operator to work faster because of lack of unproductive interruptions and therefore saves time. It permits quadrant dentistry to be performed efficiently at one visit.

There will never be uniform agreement about the use of the rubber dam in paedodontics; the decision to use it or not must lie with the individual practitioner. There is no clinical proof that those restorations placed under the dam endure the insults of the oral cavity better than those placed under cotton roll isolation. But there is greater expansion and corrosion of alloys contaminated with saliva, which makes them more susceptible to failure. The reader should not condemn the rubber dam without giving it a good trial of constant use over several months so that his technique is refined to the point when placing the dam is no longer a major hurdle. Only when this has been achieved can the operator properly evaluate the use of the rubber dam in paediatric dentistry. He should look seriously at those many operators in exclusive paedodontic practice who have worked both with and without it and ask himself why they are no longer using cotton roll isolation in preference to the rubber dam. The acceptance of the rubber dam by children is directly related to the acceptance of the technique by the dentist (Curzon and Barenie, 1973).

RUBBER DAM
Advantages and Indications

The advantages of the rubber dam can be listed as follows:
  1. Improvement of access.
  2. Retraction and protection of soft tissues.
  3. Provision of a dry operating field.
  4. Provision of an aseptic environment.
  5. Prevention of the ingestion and inhalation of foreign bodies.
  6. Aid to patient management.

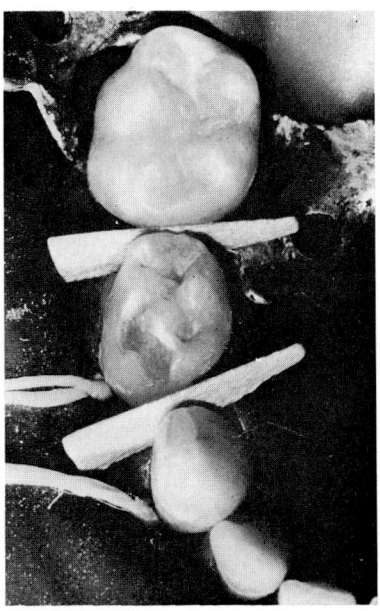

Fig. 24.—Isolated mandibular right quadrant. An 8A clamp is used.

1. *Improvement of Access*

Almost every dentist who has worked with children is familiar with the very inquisitive tongue that interferes when least wanted. The rubber dam improves access and visibility by eliminating the tongue, lips, cheeks and saliva from the operating field (*Fig. 24*). It allows the operator an unhindered view of the isolated area and permits him access so that he can proceed uninterrupted. Because of the improved access and visibility, details of cavity preparation can be refined; decalcification and minute exposures are more readily observed.

2. *Retraction and Protection of Soft Tissues*

Besides retracting the tongue and cheeks, the rubber dam both protects and retracts the gingivae. A criticism of the rubber dam is that the bur always catches in the dam. This begs the question, 'where would the bur go if there were no rubber dam?' Answer: 'into the soft tissues'.

Selective use of rubber dam clamps and ligation facilitates access to deep subgingival caries, particularly in partially erupted teeth. The mandibular second permanent molar often exhibits a Class 1 lesion with an operculum of soft tissue partially covering the distal aspect of the tooth (*Fig. 25*). The rubber dam isolates the occlusal surface of a second permanent molar by retracting soft tissues so that the restoration can be completed adequately in one visit (*Fig. 26*). When the dam is not used in such an instance, the operator cannot extend his cavity for prevention, which means that the restoration may fail and need to be replaced. Any gingival trauma from use of the dam is transient.

3. *Provision of a Dry Operating Field*

The dam can be placed immediately after local anaesthesia is administered and while it is taking effect. A dry field is impossible with the use of water-cooled high-speed cutting instruments; however, high-velocity vacuum aspirators can either be used by the dental assistant or attached to a saliva ejector fitting on the rubber dam clamp as described by Cragg (1966) to prevent flooding of the dam. The improved access is a good reason for preparing the cavities under the dam. If the rubber dam is placed following cavity preparation, the sharp cavity walls will tear it and frustrate the clinician.

The correctly placed rubber dam ensures a dry field in which the restorative material can be placed—only then can one hope to obtain the best properties of that material. Those who have endured attempts at packing an alloy in the midst of a pool of saliva will remember that increased tactile stimuli and pain increase salivation. Local anaesthesia and rubber dam placement eliminate both saliva and gingival haemorrhage contamination.

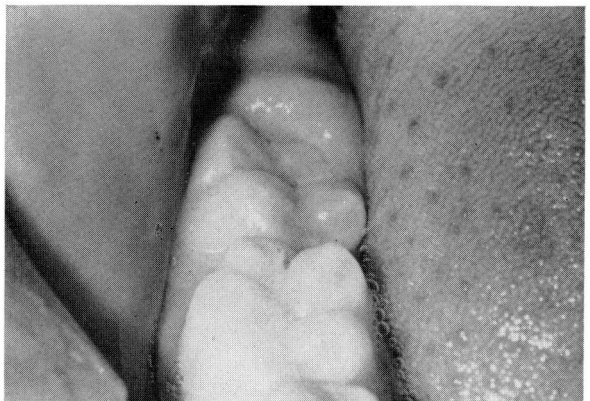

Fig. 25.—Mandibular second permanent molar with soft-tissue operculum covering distal part of the occlusal surface.

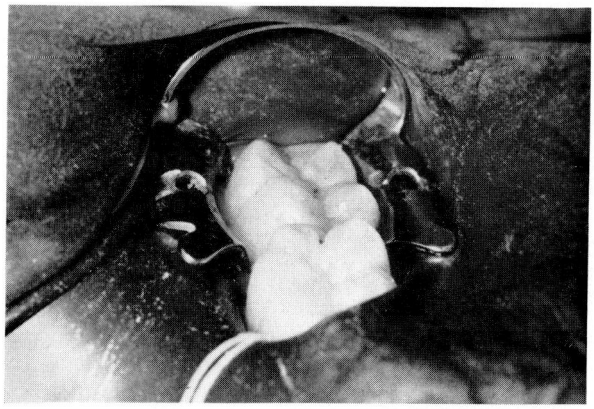

Fig. 26.—Retraction of operculum allows correct cavity extension for prevention. An Ivory 14A clamp has been used.

4. *Provision of an Aseptic Environment*

Endodontists have recommended routine use of the rubber dam for all phases of root-canal work in permanent teeth. The pulp of primary teeth is made up of the same tissues as that of the permanent tooth, and the primary tooth should have the same aseptic environment as the permanent tooth for its pulp treatment. Stoner's conclusion (1967) that a primary molar with a broken down marginal ridge will frequently exhibit a carious pulp exposure strongly

49

emphasizes the need to use a rubber dam for restoring all extensively decayed primary molars, since endodontic treatment is a distinct possibility.

5. *Prevention of the Ingestion and Inhalation of Foreign Bodies*

Malpractice insurance companies unfortunately have records of inhaled and ingested broaches, files, reamers, inlays and other foreign bodies. These serious and traumatic occurrences for both patient and dentist could have been avoided by use of the rubber dam (Grossman, 1971). Indeed, several anaesthetists in North America refuse to assist dentists performing work under general anaesthesia unless they use the rubber dam, which serves as one of the better 'throat packs' available.

Conscious children do not take kindly to particles of alloy, cement and tooth fragments resting on their tongues, palate and cheeks. In addition to the increased salivation, the added aggravation does little to relax the patient, particularly when there is a danger of ingesting or inhaling these foreign bodies.

6. *Aid to Patient Management*

Dentists who are inexperienced with the rubber dam find it difficult to believe that it aids the management of the patient, particularly the child. However, there must be a good reason why so many paediatric dentists use it routinely. Personal experience indicates that the upset child often settles down once the rubber dam is in place. It may be that the child mentally disassociates the tooth from the rest of the body, which could explain the improvement in behaviour (Jinks, 1966). More likely, the child realizes that he is in no danger of choking from the water of the high-speed air turbine; also, he is not embarrassed by the taste of particles and the like and thus responds favourably to the increased comfort afforded by the rubber dam. The rubber dam also serves as a vehicle for educating the parents, who can be shown various stages of treatment to the isolated teeth. This increases the pride, which every dentist has, in his work.

Technique

Teeth to be Clamped

This will depend on which teeth are to be restored. When a single surface restoration is planned, only the affected tooth needs to be clamped. When a posterior quadrant is to be isolated, the most distal tooth should be clamped; individual anterior teeth are ligated or isolated by rubber dam inversion into the gingival sulcus, assisted where necessary by wedges (*Fig. 24*). The isolation should include all teeth to be restored and the adjacent teeth when Class 2 lesions exist. Some clinicians prefer to extend isolation to the midline; this requires very little additional time but is seldom necessary in the child, especially since it is difficult to isolate mandibular primary incisors.

Clamp Selection

Each operator develops his own preference for clamps, and a scientific approach to clamp selection has been described (Wiland, 1973). The following winged clamps will suffice in a paedodontic practice:

Ash 14	Second primary molars.
Ivory 14	First and second permanent molars.
Ivory 14A	Partially erupted first and second permanent molars.
Ivory 8A	Narrow (mesiodistally) partially erupted second permanent molars. Second primary molars.
Ivory 2 and 2A	Premolars. First primary molars.

For the vast majority of child patients (about 90 per cent), the Ivory 14A and Ash 14 clamps are used on first permanent and second primary molars respectively. The Ivory 8A clamp will fit both of these teeth (*Fig. 24*). The other clamps are rarely used. Routine use of these clamps improves efficiency and reduces indecision and operating time. Anaesthesia is required both buccally and lingually to place rubber dam clamps on primary and partially erupted young permanent teeth. Topical anaesthesia may suffice although a palatal or long buccal infiltration may be required.

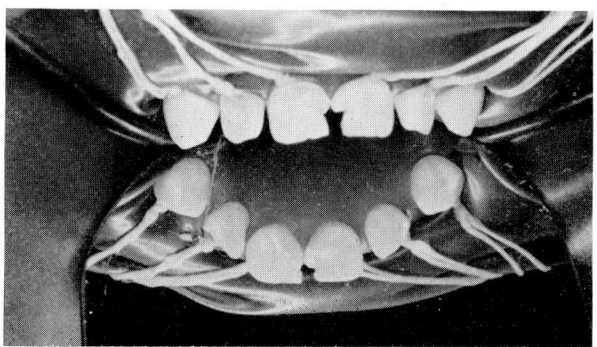

Fig. 27.—Primary anterior teeth isolated by ligation only.

First primary molars and primary canines are difficult to clamp and like primary incisors should be ligated instead of clamped (*Fig. 27*). Winged clamps are recommended since they are essential for Method 1 of application (to be described). Trial fitting of the clamp is recommended until the operator gains experience. Dental floss should be attached to the clamp so that it can be easily retrieved if dislodged.

Punching the Holes

Placement of the holes for the teeth has been well described by Jinks (1966). Alternatively, a stamp for both primary and permanent dentitions can be stencilled on the rubber dam to give the correct position of punch holes for every tooth. Individual variations in tooth position will determine the exact location of the holes.

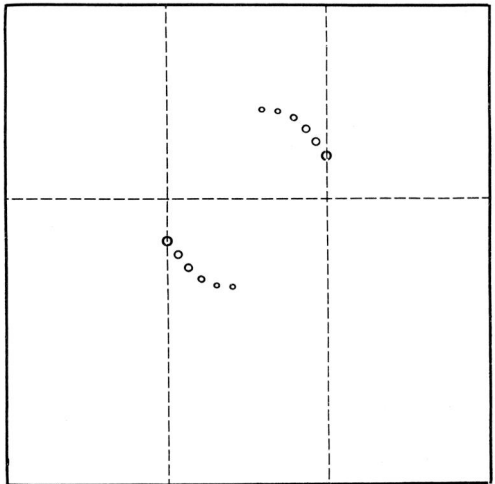

Fig. 28.—Correct location of punch holes for maxillary left and mandibular right quadrants.

The holes are easier to punch when the dam is held under tension by the frame. Permanent molars warrant the largest hole, second primary molars the second largest and so on to the primary incisors, which have the smallest. The distance between punch holes should be 2 mm. Intervals that are too small allow interproximal leakage while too much dam between the holes makes it difficult to pass the dam through the broad and flat primary molar contact areas. *Fig. 28* shows the correct position of the punch holes. Note that the posterior holes are on an angle of 45 degrees. The dam can be mentally divided into four quadrants, right and left, upper and lower, and the holes punched appropriately. Posterior teeth are closest to the horizontal midline and the incisors are closest to the vertical midline. Consideration must be given to any edentulous areas by leaving greater space between punch holes. The trained dental assistant can punch the dam for the appropriate quadrant as indicated on the treatment plan. She can determine which tooth to clamp and therefore which clamp to use by looking at the treatment records and noting the patient's age. All this can and should be done before the patient arrives for his appointment, the rubber dam being incorporated into every operative tray set up. This is the key to efficient use of the rubber dam.

Selection of Materials (Fig. 29)

Young's rubber dam frame★ is recommended since it holds the dam away from the child's face. Its size is commensurate with the dimensions of the child's face. Waxed dental floss is preferred for individual ligatures since it frays less than unwaxed floss on sharp edges. Dark, heavy or extra heavy bodies 5 in × 5 in† rubber dam is recommended. The dark colour provides good contrast and the extra heavy dam best retracts and protects the soft tissues. Winged clamps are preferred (*see* Method 1).

Methods of Application

There are three methods of applying the rubber dam. In all instances the rubber dam is punched beforehand.

METHOD 1: The clamp is placed in the appropriate punch hole in the dam which is already stretched on the frame. The dam can be stretched between thumb and forefinger as described by Jinks (1966) so that its wings are engaged by the rubber dam. The clamp is then placed on the appropriate tooth. The tension on the stretched dam should be eased by releasing the dam from the lower corner of the frame on the side to be clamped. Once the clamp is firmly secured, the rubber is eased off the wings with a plastic instrument; grooves cut in the wings facilitate this (Jinks, 1966) (*Fig. 29b*).

Individual teeth are then ligated. Waxed dental floss passed through the contacts helps retract the dam through the broad flat primary molar contact areas. Primary canines provide good retraction of the dam and these teeth should be ligated first. Open carious lesions sometimes have jagged edges that repeatedly fray the floss, leaving interproximal wedging as an alternative to individual ligation.

The main advantage of this method is that it can be applied singlehandedly. This makes it attractive in areas where dental laws allow the trained dental assistant to place and remove the dam. The technique is quickly learned, is safe, and is recommended for general use.

★ Cottrell & Co., London.
† Hygienic Co. (available from Amalgamated Dental Co., 26 Broadwick St., London).

METHOD 2: This differs only slightly from the above-described method. The clamp can be placed in the dam as before; alternatively, the bow of the clamp only is engaged in the dam, which is held

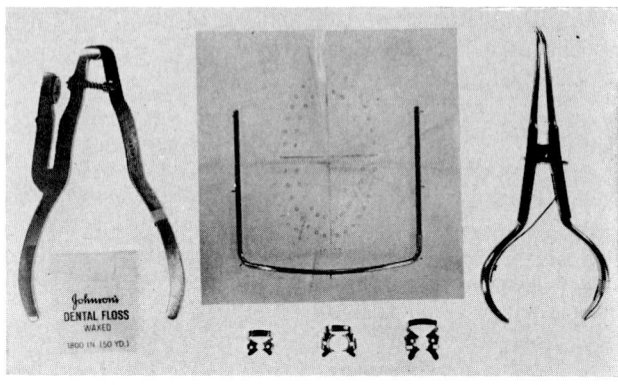

a

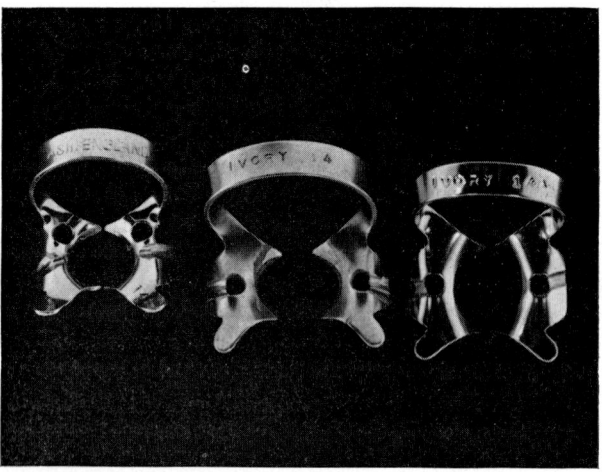

b

Fig. 29.—a, Materials for rubber dam placement: 5 × 5 dark heavy rubber dam, Ivory 14A and Ash 14 clamp (note grooves in wings), Forceps, Young's Frame, Waxed Dental Floss, Plastic. *b*, Ash 14, Ivory 14 and 14A clamps. Note grooves cut in the wing of the clamp to facilitate removal of the rubber.

superior to the clamp. The clamp and dam are placed on the tooth and the frame is applied later. The advantage of this is that the dam is not under any tension when placed. However, Starkey (1957) recommends having a dental assistant hold the upper corners of the dam to improve visibility while placing the clamp.

METHOD 3: This method involves placing the clamp on the appropriate tooth. The rubber dam, already punched, is stretched over the clamp and the frame is then placed. Wingless clamps mean less stretching and therefore less likelihood of tearing of the rubber dam; however, this method is possible with winged clamps also. This can be performed singlehandedly, although it entails the greatest risk of clamp inhalation or ingestion. Should the clamp not be secure or should the child suddenly move while the rubber dam is being stretched, the clamp could come loose and be either inhaled or swallowed (Alexander and Delholm, 1971). For this reason the clamp must have floss attached to it so that it can easily be retrieved if it is dislodged. Therefore this method is not recommended as a first choice, although it may be the only way of isolating a broken down posterior tooth where cheek tissues make visibility a problem if Method 1 is used.

Modifications

Some anterior teeth present problems with individual ligation. Partial eruption and active soft tissues may lead to poor stability of the dam. In these instances the dam can be stretched over a posterior tooth which is then clamped; this secures the dam and permits easier isolation of anterior teeth (*Fig. 30*). Occasionally clamps may be required bilaterally.

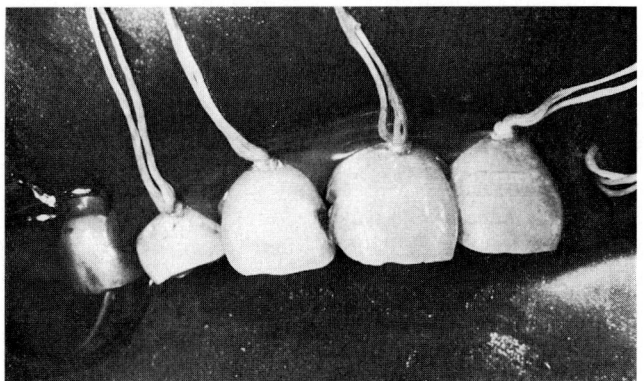

Fig. 30.—Clamp over posterior tooth to secure dam prior to anterior isolation.

Misadventures and Disadvantages

The improperly directed clamp forceps can traumatize the lip of the arch opposite to the one being restored. Improperly placed clamps and ligatures can impinge upon and/or traumatize the gingivae, but this injury is transient. It is also possible to engage either tongue or cheek tissues within the jaws of the clamp, but this can be avoided by sliding an index finger along the buccal sulcus while the clamp is placed. Insecurely placed or poorly selected clamps are prone to be dislodged easily; the dangers of inhalation and ingestion have already been mentioned. Poor retention of the clamp may also be caused by fatigue of the bow of the clamp resulting in loss of springiness. Periodic squeezing the jaws of the clamp can prolong its life. However, worn-out clamps should be discarded. Weakened cusps can conceivably fracture should a clamp suddenly come off a tooth, although this has not been reported in the literature to this author's knowledge.

The rubber dam frame can cause pressure marks on the face but this can easily be avoided by placing a cotton roll under the frame or a large cotton gauze under the dam. Incorrectly punched holes can move the frame and dam unnecessarily high on the face, with the frame coming close to the eyes and the dam covering the nose. The claustrophobic sensation which is sometimes experienced can be eliminated by cutting the dam away from the nostril and, when necessary, cutting a hole in the centre of the rubber to allow an oral airway.

Once the rubber dam is in place stimuli to salivary flow are decreased. If any build-up of saliva occurs which may create a drowning feeling, it can be removed by high-speed suction. Personal experience with saliva ejectors has not been favourable since they tend to irritate the child. Build-up of saliva can also result in leakage should the clamp be incorrectly placed. This often occurs on the lingual surface of partially erupted mandibular molars. The problem is corrected by holding the dam down with finger pressure on the lingual and rolling the clamp buccally and occlusally, allowing the rubber dam to re-adapt to the lingual surface at the same time. The clamp is then allowed to assume its original position.

Patient acceptance of the rubber dam should not be a problem to the experienced paediatric dentist when the child has never received dental care before. Rubber dam placement can be presented as a normal part of operative dentistry, just as is local anaesthesia. It is explained as a tooth raincoat, the clamp being the raincoat's button. When children are correctly managed they come to expect rubber dam application as normal since they know no other way. Routine use of the rubber dam is one of the greatest assets in paediatric operative dentistry, both to the clinician and to the child. Its use eliminates the problems of saliva contamination and interference by soft tissues which contribute to poor amalgam restorations. Clinicians who object to the dam should ask themselves whether they are really happy with the isolation method they are now using. If they are dissatisfied, they may be surprised how easy it is to apply the dam to a single molar. From the easy cases they may progress to isolating quadrants and finally the most difficult teeth, the incisors (Curzon and Barenie, 1973).

COTTON ROLL ISOLATION

Cotton rolls placed in the buccal and lingual sulci can be used as an alternative to the rubber dam. Alternatively, cotton gauze (2 in × 2 in) can be rolled tightly and used. Maxillary teeth are easier to isolate than mandibular teeth since 70 per cent of the saliva is produced by the submandibular gland. Thus a cotton roll placed opposite the parotid duct by the second primary molar, along with a saliva ejector is sufficient isolation for maxillary teeth. Mandibular teeth require cotton rolls in both buccal and lingual sulci;

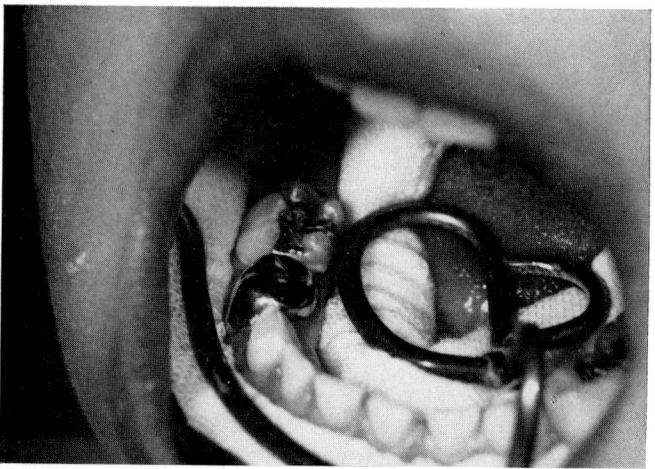

Fig. 31.—Conduit holder stabilizes cotton rolls in buccal and lingual sulci.

in addition, the maxillary buccal sulcus of the appropriate side should be isolated to eliminate parotid saliva. A 6 in cotton roll can be used for both mandibular and maxillary sulci. In addition a saliva ejector with a tongue retractor insert can be useful in the lingual sulcus. The Conduit* holder can be used to hold the cotton rolls in position (*Fig. 31*). The profuse salivation sometimes encountered in the child makes it mandatory to have a supply of spare cotton rolls on hand, as well as proficiency at quick changing to prevent moisture contamination of the restorative material.

* Conduit Co., Boston, Massachusetts.

REFERENCES

ALEXANDER R. E. and DELHOLM J. J. (1971) Rubber dam clamp ingestion, an operative risk: report of case. *J. Am. Dent. Assoc.* **82,** 1387.

CRAGG T. K. (1966) Water evacuation when using rubber dam. *J. Can. Dent. Assoc.* **32,** 402.

CURZON M. E. J. and BARENIE J. T. (1973) A simplified rubber dam technique for children's dentistry. *Br. Dent. J.* **135,** 532.

GROSSMAN L. I. (1971) Prevention in endodontic practice. *J. Am. Dent. Assoc.* **82,** 395.

HEALEY H. J. and PHILLIPS R. W. (1949) A clinical study of amalgam failures. *J. Dent. Res.* **28,** 439.

HEISE A. L. (1971) Time required in rubber dam placement. *J. Dent. Child.* **38,** 116.

JINKS G. M. (1966) Rubber dam technique in pedodontics. *Dent. Clin. North Am.* 327.

STARKEY P. E. (1957) The application of the rubber dam in the pre-school child. *J. Dent. Child.* **24,** 230.

STONER J. E. (1967) Dental caries in deciduous molars. *Br. Dent. J.* **123,** 130.

WILAND L. (1973) An evaluation of rubber dam clamps and a method for their selection. *J. Am. Dent. Assoc.* **87,** 160.

RECOMMENDED READING

CURZON M. E. J. and BARENIE J. T. (1973) A simplified rubber dam technique for children's dentistry. *Br. Dent. J.* **135,** 532.

JINKS G. M. (1966) Rubber dam technique in pedodontics. *Dent. Clin. North Am.* 327.

CHAPTER 6

THE CLASS 1 LESION

DIAGNOSIS

IN the pre-school child Parfitt (1956) found that the occlusal surface of primary molars is attacked by caries more often than any other surface. Furthermore, the depth and inclination of the fissures determine that the second primary molar is affected more often than the first primary molar. For this same reason mandibular teeth are carious more often than their maxillary counterparts. This trend is also seen in the first and second permanent molars (Walsh and Smart, 1948). It is not uncommon for the occlusal surface to become carious within two years of eruption. The above epidemiology should be remembered when examining the child patient.

The following should be available for the diagnostic examination: a sharp explorer, a source of good light, a source of air to dry the tooth, current bite-wing radiographs, and an assessment of the patient's past and projected caries experience. Exploration of a gross lesion is contra-indicated since it is unnecessary in establishing the diagnosis and it may distress the child. This is not the case with the incipient lesion. However, care should be exercised not to apply heavy pressure to a recently erupted permanent molar whose pit and fissure enamel may be incompletely coalesced or immature because of lack of saliva contact.

The grey discoloration that results from the undermining of enamel by caries is best seen on a well illuminated dry tooth. The occlusal lesion may sometimes be observed on a bite-wing radiograph as two radiolucent triangles, one in the enamel and one in the dentine. The bases of the two triangles are coincident at the amelodentinal junction and the apices are towards the fissure and the pulp, respectively. The fissure may extend very close to the amelodentinal junction, which helps account for the rapid onset of occlusal caries after the tooth's eruption into the mouth. Also, the shape of the fissure may defy any attempt at cleansing because its orifice is finer than a toothbrush bristle (Cawson, 1972).

The use of topical fluoride has lulled the clinician into a sense of false security in the diagnosis of Class 1 lesions. Topical fluorides, though least effective on the occlusal surface, seem to have the ability to make the pits and fissures hard and firm to exploration. This can occur after a lesion has reached dentine. Careful examination of bite-wing radiographs may reveal extensive caries involving the dentine that is not observable clinically. In fact, the lesion may progress to the pulp without showing any enamel surface breakdown. Therefore special care should be taken in the diagnosis of occlusal lesions in patients who are regularly receiving topical fluoride; this same dictum applies to patients with pit and fissure sealants. Their use in the prevention of Class 1 lesions will be discussed in Chapter 14.

Another consideration in the diagnosis of Class 1 lesions is the past and projected caries experience of the patient. The astute clinician should always be alert to the possibility of a clinically unobservable but radiographically apparent Class 2 lesion in a tooth with occlusal caries. There is little value in spending an operative visit restoring a Class 1 lesion, only to spend more time six months later replacing it with a Class 2 alloy, when a Class 2 lesion existed from the outset but was undiagnosed. A questionable fissure can be kept under observation if there is no radiographic evidence of a dentinal lesion, the patient's past decay experience is low, and a good prognosis is expected of his home care. However, it is unwise to delay restoring such an area in a child who may be moving to a location without a dentist or whose parents are not highly motivated towards good dental health.

The term 'sticky fissure' is frequently used to describe the occlusal surface; unfortunately, its interpretation can lead to confusion. To say that a fissure is 'sticky' indicates that an explorer will catch in the depths of the fissure. If this is so, the fissure is carious and should be restored. The only exception has already been mentioned, namely the recently erupted tooth whose enamel is not fully mature and whose fissures should not be explored with heavy pressure. The other diagnostic criteria (the grey discoloration, the radiographic appearance and the previous decay experience) also help establish the diagnosis.

THE CLASS 1 CAVITY
GENERAL CONSIDERATIONS

The outline form should include all areas susceptible to further decay; that is, the cavity should be extended for prevention. This usually means including all deep pits and fissures in the preparation so that the margins can be easily finished and can be readily cleansed by the patient. If too many discrete fillings are placed in the occlusal surface, this patchwork restoration is inclined to early breakdown. The actual amount of fissure extension is determined by the anatomy of the fissure, the presence of caries and stain, and the patient's previous caries experience. It is better to err on the side of over-extension of fissure elimination for safety. This does not mean that overdestruction of tooth structure intercuspally is acceptable. When incipient lesions are being treated the preoperative occlusal anatomy seldom requires gross reduction; the maximum intercuspal cavity width should be one-quarter to one-third of the intercuspal width. The buccal and lingual extension of the Class 1 cavity, both mesially and distally, determines the isthmus width of any Class 2 cavity which is subsequently prepared in that tooth; this justifies conservative preparations. A small fissure bur (No. 2L) can be used to prepare the cavity.

Class 1 cavities should be extended at least 0·5 mm pulpally to the amelodentinal junction for the reasons outlined in Chapter 4. Any remaining caries can be removed with round burs run at slow speed. The pulpal floor should be flat wherever possible. The deeper portions of the cavity are lined with a pulp-protecting base, although it is not necessary to replace all carious material with a base. Internal line angles should be rounded; this will normally provide an undercut in the dentine for retention. The cavo-surface margin should be 90 degrees since amalgam alloy is usually the material of choice for restoring Class 1 cavities.

The extension and depth of the cavity will be determined by the amount and location of caries and preoperative occlusal anatomy. Every effort should be made to retain as much well supported enamel as possible. However, when decay has undermined a cusp or wall, a modification must be made by removing that weakened enamel and effectively making the preparation a Class 2 type.

THE FIRST PRIMARY MOLAR

The central pit of first primary molars usually becomes carious before the mesial pit, which decays less frequently. Thus the outline form should be limited to the central pit and its adjacent buccal and lingual developmental grooves and distal triangular fossa (*Fig. 32*). Seldom is it necessary to cross the ridge of enamel joining the

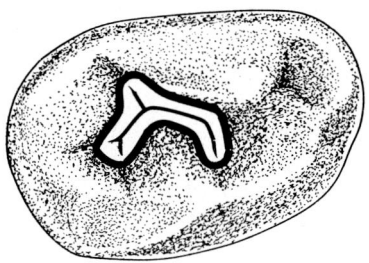

Fig. 32.—Correct cavity outline form in mandibular right first primary molar. It is unnecessary to cross the central ridge.

mesiobuccal and mesiolingual cusp to eliminate caries, in fact it is inadvisable to do so because of the proximity of the mesiobuccal pulp horn. Amalgam alloy should be used for *routine* Class 1 cavities in first primary molars.

The occlusal aspect of the first primary molar may be extensively destroyed at a young age in the nursing bottle mouth syndrome (described in Chapter 1). The young age of the child and the extensive lesions that are seen warrant special consideration which differs from the previously recommended principles. The extent and depth of decay may necessitate a wider outline form and even the use of indirect pulp treatment (Chapter 17) to avoid pulp exposure. When treating these lesions, the clinician must also consider the prognosis for improvement in home care, which is in part determined by the parents' ability to break the child's feeding habit and the child's acquired taste for sugar. If the parent is unsuccessful, the tooth may be subject to further decay. For this reason amalgam alloy is not always the restorative material of choice for Class 1 lesions in the nursing bottle mouth syndrome. Rather a temporary 'treatment filling' is preferred while the indirect pulp treatment is being used and the home care is being assessed.

Resin-bonded zinc oxides or zinc oxide cement to which alloy fillings are added to the powder are suitable intermediate restorative materials; their durability has been clinically proven (Hutchins and Parker, 1972; Weaver et al., 1972). The bland qualities of these materials may eliminate the need for a pulp-protecting base and their ease of manipulation make them attractive for use in the very young child when working time and child cooperation may be at a premium. Also useful in the treatment of the nursing bottle mouth syndrome are fluoride impregnated cements (Jinks, 1963). However, the acidity of this material must be neutralized by a pulp-protecting base such as calcium hydroxide. Its major advantage is the continued release of fluoride to the adjacent enamel in a mouth that has a high caries potential. It is important to inform the parent that treatment fillings have been placed and that they will need replacement later. The term 'treatment filling' is preferred to 'temporary filling' since it implies such fillings have a purpose and serves as a means of educating the parent. The treatment restorations can be replaced after a *minimum* of 6–8 weeks if indirect pulp treatment has been used (*see also* Chapter 17). However, a longer interval (6 months to 1 year) is advisable before replacement, to permit further assessment of the home care. Also the child may mature to the extent that he will accept more extensive treatment.

Sometimes the caries is so extensive that the whole occlusal surface is destroyed. In such instances, direct pulp therapy followed by a stainless-steel crown may be the treatment of choice.

SECOND PRIMARY AND FIRST PERMANENT MOLARS

These teeth are considered together because of their almost identical anatomy. The outline form should include the fissures throughout the occlusal surface (*Figs. 33, 34,* and *35*). However, the intercuspal dimensions of the cavity should be kept small, as previously described.

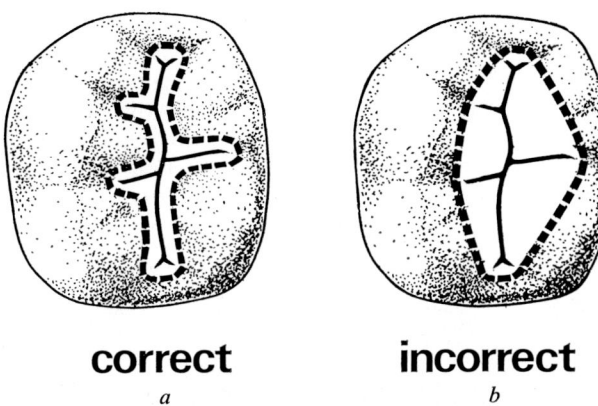

correct   incorrect

a   *b*

Fig. 33.—*a,* Correct cavity outline form for minimal Class 1 lesion in mandibular first permanent molar. Note extension into fissures and maintenance of intercuspal width. *b,* Incorrect cavity outline form for minimal Class 1 lesion in mandibular first permanent molar. Excessive destruction of tooth will result in weakening of cusps if ever a Class 2 restoration is placed in this tooth.

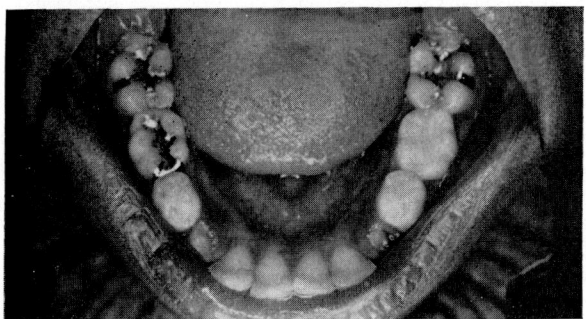

Fig. 34.—Completed occlusobuccal restorations in mandibular first permanent molars.

a. MANDIBULAR: The danger areas for underextension and development of recurrent caries seem to be at the extremities of the lingual and buccal fissures. It will be necessary in some instances to extend the cavity preparation to include a poorly supported, a carious, or pre-carious buccal or lingual fissure. This would make an occluso-buccal or occlusolingual cavity (*Fig. 34*). Stain, active caries, and deep fissures are deciding factors in the need for such extension buccally. It is not universally necessary; it is better that the fissure remain intact, with separate occlusal and buccal restorations being placed, if necessary. The undermining effect on the lingual wall by caries is the reason for including a mandibular lingual extension. The cavity walls buccally and lingually should be straight and either parallel or converging occlusally with square external line angles. The extensions should be cut 0·5 mm into the dentine and should extend gingivally to include the buccal developmental pit. Retention grooves can be placed at the amelodentinal junction. The 'isthmus' area where the buccal or lingual extension meets the occlusal section should be rounded or bevelled to increase the bulk of the alloy in this area, which is subject to heavy masticatory forces during lateral movements.

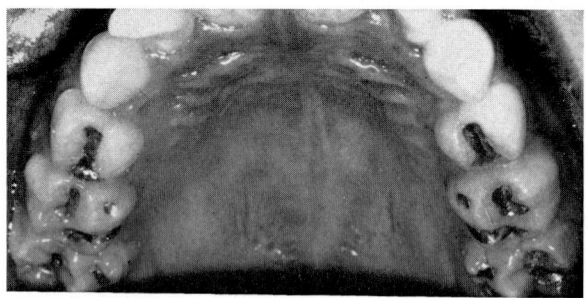

Fig. 35.—Completed occlusal and occlusolingual restorations in second primary molars.

b. MAXILLARY: Carious attack is usually limited to the following areas: the central pit, the distal pit, the lingual pit and the groove separating the fifth cusp (Cusp of Carabelli) from the mesiolingual cusp. Therefore it is seldom clinically necessary to cross the oblique ridge joining mesiolingual and distobuccal cusps when treating small lesions (*Fig. 35*); this should be done only when the oblique ridge is undermined by caries.

The depth of the lingual development groove and its continuity with the distal pit and distal development groove frequently necessitate the placement of an occlusolingual restoration in maxillary molars. Inclusion of the lingual developmental groove and lingual pit can be regarded as extension for prevention, just as with the mandibular buccal extension. The outline and depth of this lingual extension are similar to those of the buccal extension seen in the mandibular molar. Occasionally an accessory groove runs from the lingual developmental groove to the groove separating the Cusp of

Carabelli and mesiolingual cusp; when this fissure is carious or pre-carious it may have to be included in the cavity preparation as 'extension for prevention'. The width of the lingual extension should be minimal with alloy bulk being compensated for by deepening the cavity. The reason for this is that excessive tooth removal would weaken the distolingual and mesiolingual cusps should a Class 2 lesion ever require restoration subsequently. Straight cavity margins at the buccal and lingual extensions with square external line angles are easy to prepare and they also facilitate finishing of the restoration.

It is seldom necessary to place a matrix band to help condense the alloy; direct condensation is advised. A common fault is to underpack and overcarve at the junction of the occlusal and lingual extensions (or buccal in mandibular teeth).

THE SECOND PERMANENT MOLAR

The principles outlined for first permanent molars apply also for the second permanent molars. The occlusal anatomy differs, particularly in the maxillary arch when the distolingual cusp may be absent or rudimentary. The central developmental groove may extend distally across a very flat oblique ridge joining up with the distal pit and distal developmental groove. Also, the absence of a distolingual cusp may eliminate the lingual developmental groove. Since cavity design should be related to the occlusal anatomy, it may be unnecessary to include a lingual extension in the cavity design. Two separate occlusal pits (mesially and distally) may require separate occlusal cavities. However, the presence of an extended central developmental groove may require that the outline form encompass both central and distal pits, crossing a rudimentary or absent oblique ridge.

The mandibular second permanent molar sometimes presents a unique problem. This tooth may become carious very shortly after eruption and the caries seems to spread very rapidly. Questionable occlusal fissures in mandibular second permanent molars should be restored. To add to the problem, the tooth may be only partially erupted, the distal aspect being covered by an operculum of tissue that persists for as long as a year following initial eruption into the oral cavity. *Figs. 25* and *26* (*see* Chapter 5) demonstrate the use of the rubber dam to solve the problem of partial eruption. The extensive caries that is sometimes seen may require indirect pulp treatment (Chapter 17) to avoid pulp exposure.

DEVELOPMENTAL PITS

These can occur in four areas:

1. Midway down the mesiobuccal developmental groove in mandibular second primary, first and second permanent molars.

2. Midway down the lingual developmental groove in maxillary second primary, first and second permanent molars.

3. Between the fifth cusp (Cusp of Carabelli) and the mesiolingual cusp of second primary and first permanent molars.

4. The lingual pit in maxillary permanent incisors and, rarely, in maxillary permanent canines; the permanent lateral incisor is most frequently affected.

The developmental pit and any accessory developmental groove should be included in the outline form. Other requirements for cavity preparation have already been mentioned. As noted in the previous sections, it may be necessary to include the developmental pit in a lingual or buccal extension from the occlusal cavity in second primary and permanent molars. This should not be done if the lingual and mesiobuccal developmental grooves are neither stained nor considered pre-carious.

Amalgam alloy is preferred for restoring posterior developmental pits, while the operator can choose between silicate, resin, and alloy for the lingual pits of lateral incisors. A lingual pit and an accessory lingual cusp on a maxillary permanent lateral incisor represent just one step towards a dens in dente. Caries in this area may lead to a non-vital pulp in a tooth with an open apex, the endodontic treatment of which is neither straightforward nor associated with a good prognosis. These pits should often be restored as a prophylactic measure; sealants can also be considered for this area. A maxillary anterior radiograph at age 6 years may alert the astute paediatric dentist to deep developmental pits on maxillary permanent lateral incisors.

Increased awareness and effectiveness of preventive dentistry in all facets may result in a resurgence in the use of gold foil as a restorative material. The ideal indication would be for the restoration of these minimal developmental pits in an otherwise caries-free, well maintained mouth.

REFERENCES

CAWSON R. A. (1972) *Essentials of Dental Surgery and Pathology*, 2nd ed. London, Churchill, p. 14.

HUTCHINS D. W. and PARKER W. A. (1972) Indirect pulp capping: Clinical evaluation using polymethyl methacrylate reinforced zinc oxide–eugenol cement. *J. Dent. Child.* 39, 55.

JINKS G. M. (1963) Fluoride-impregnated cements and their effect on the activity of interproximal caries. *J. Dent. Child.* 30, 87.

PARFITT G. J. (1956) Conditions influencing the incidence of occlusal and interstitial caries in children. *J. Dent. Child.* 23, 31.

WALSH J. P. and SMART R. S. (1948) Relative susceptibility of tooth surfaces to dental caries and other comparative studies. *N.Z. Dent. J.* 44, 17.

WEAVER R. G., JOHNSON B. E., CVAR J. F. and McCUNE R. J. (1972) Clinical evaluation of intermediate restorative materials. *J. Dent. Child.* **39,** 189.

CHAPTER 7

THE CLASS 2 LESION

DIAGNOSIS (PRIMARY TEETH)

THE Class 2 lesion occurs after primary molar contacts have been established. For this reason occlusal lesions are more prevalent than interproximal lesions in the very young child (under 4) prior to the establishment of primary molar contacts; this pattern is reversed in older children prior to the eruption of permanent molars (Parfitt, 1956). It has been estimated that 70–80 per cent of the primary molar lesions restored by the paediatric dentist will be of the Class 2 type (McDonald, 1974). This is probably explained by the fact that the child's first dental visit occurs well after the primary molars have established closed contacts.

Incipient primary molar Class 2 lesions can be diagnosed only with bite-wing radiographs. The flat broad elliptical primary molar contact areas defy clinical exploration. Once primary molar contacts have been established, the taking of bite-wings should not be delayed in the hope of detecting the lesion clinically, either by exploration or by observation of grey discoloration of the marginal ridge. It has been shown that the pulp will frequently become exposed during excavation of primary molar Class 2 lesions where the marginal ridge is broken down (Stoner, 1967). Also grey discoloration of the marginal ridge indicates an already extensive lesion. In fact, the rapid spread of primary molar interproximal lesions encourages the repetition of bite-wings at 6-month intervals.

Early diagnosis of the Class 2 lesion enables the clinician to prepare a cavity of conservative extension and dimensions; it is hoped that the well-supported margins will permit the restoration to endure for the life of the tooth. This concept of early diagnosis and restoration is in agreement with the histological finding of carious involvement of the dentine in primary molars which exhibit radiographic interproximal lesions confined to enamel (Dwyer et al., 1973). Accordingly, any enamel interproximal radiolucency in primary molars can be considered in need of restoration.

It is also clinically important that a recognizable Class 2 lesion on one primary molar is associated with some carious involvement of the adjacent surface of the adjacent tooth. This is explained by the fact that the plaque whose metabolism was responsible for the one definite lesion is in close proximity to the other tooth. Although no lesion may be evident radiographically, direct clinical observation when the adjacent Class 2 cavity is prepared will reveal demineralization. Because of the thin primary molar enamel and close proximity of pulp horns to the amelodentinal junction, there may be rapid involvement of the pulp by caries in untreated Class 2 lesions. Therefore there is every justification to treat such areas with Class 2 restorations. Although this may seem a drastic measure, the alternative of topical fluoride application to such demineralized areas has produced disappointing results, in the author's experience. Invariably a Class 2 restoration is required within one year of restoring the adjacent primary molar. This requires another visit for the child, another administration of anaesthetic, and further inconvenience to the parent; all could be avoided by providing simultaneous Class 2 restorations of the adjacent primary molars.

It is also significant that primary molar interproximal lesions are frequently seen in all quadrants of the mouth simultaneously. If they are not seen, they may become evident within a short time (McDonald, 1974). This finding should encourage the clinician to maintain the highest possible standard of radiography; bite-wing radiographs which do not open contacts must be retaken. The clinician must also recognize the location and nature of interproximal lesions on radiographs. The lesion will appear as a radiolucent triangle in enamel whose apex points toward the amelodentinal junction and whose base is at or just below the contact area. If the lesion has progressed to dentine, a second radiolucent triangle will be seen whose base is at the amelodentinal junction and whose apex is toward the pulp. Critical analysis of bite-wing radiographs, including when necessary the use of a magnifying glass and comparison with previous radiographs, is essential to the early diagnosis of Class 2 lesions.

THE CLASS 2 CAVITY

This section will be divided into three units:
1. The incipient lesion where the cavity dimensions are not determined by caries—primary molars.
2. The large lesion where the cavity dimensions will be determined by caries—primary molars.
3. Permanent molar preparations.

Cavity preparations will be discussed in relation to the use of amalgam as the restorative material.

The Class 2 cavity is made up of an occlusal lock (or keyway) and an interproximal box which join at the isthmus. A small plain cut tapered fissure bur (No. 2L)* or pear shaped bur (No. 2L)† in the high speed can be used for the major part of the preparation.

---

* No. 2L = No. 170L American.
† No. 2L = No. 330L American.

1. The Incipient Lesion—Primary Molars

The *occlusal lock* has the same outline form as the Class 1 cavity (*Fig. 36*). That is, the margins are placed in readily cleansed areas and all carious, stained and pre-carious fissures are included in the preparation. The criteria used for determining whether to cross an oblique or central ridge have been described in Chapter 6. Minimum cavity depth is 0·5 mm pulpal to the amelodentinal junction; the pulpal floor should be flat. If any caries remains it can be removed with slowly revolving round burs or excavators. Deep portions of the cavity should be lined with a pulp-protecting base (such as a hard setting calcium hydroxide) although it is unnecessary to line out

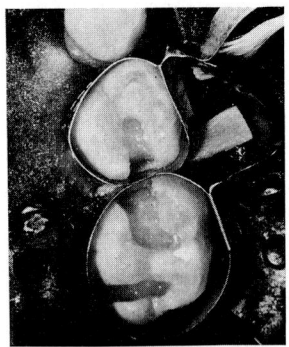

Fig. 36. Completed Class 2 maxillary primary molar cavity preparations. Banded and wedged ready for amalgam.

to ideal cavity dimensions. Indeed this may be undesirable since it may leave insufficient bulk of alloy for strength. Internal line angles should be rounded to relieve the stresses of mastication (Lampshire, 1955); they also provide mechanical undercut for retention.

The *margins of the interproximal box* should extend into self-cleansing areas (*Fig. 36*). The broad, flat, elliptical, gingivally-located primary molar contact areas dictate that the gingival floor of the interproximal box be wide so that the gingivobuccal and gingivolingual margins are self-cleansing. However, the occlusal convergence of buccal and lingual walls determines that the occlusal width of the proximal box should be less than the gingival width. The same small fissure bur (No. 2L) that was used to prepare the occlusal lock is placed at the amelodentinal junction adjacent to the marginal ridge. Using a pendulum action, the bur is taken gingivally through to the interproximal lesion; the farther gingival the bur, the wider is the arc of the pendulum. In this way the walls of the proximal box will diverge from occlusal to gingival so that they almost parallel the respective external tooth surface (*Fig. 37*).

Overextension of the buccolingual width of the box at the occlusal aspect results in poor support of the proximal walls and in turn to marginal deterioration. When the proximal box walls are being prepared parallel to the respective external tooth structure, the clinician may be concentrating on the gingival position of the bur while the opposite proximal wall is being overextended by the inclination of the bur. The operator is then tempted to correct

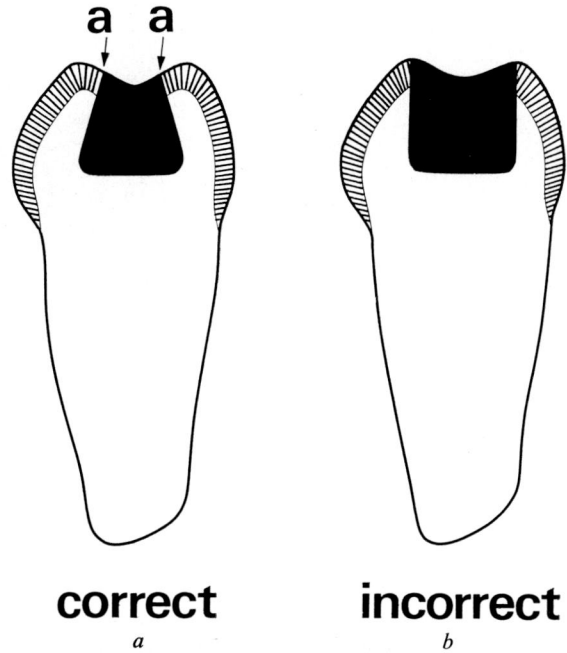

correct   **incorrect**

a   *b*

Fig. 37.—*a*, Mesiodistal view of correct Class 2 primary molar preparation. The walls of the proximal box parallel the external surfaces. Areas a are easily overextended by improper use of burs. *b*, Incorrect Class 2 primary molar preparation: mesiodistal view. Overextension of the occlusal width of the proximal box weakens the cusps and leaves both enamel and amalgam poorly supported.

the error by further extension. Often the enamel rods are un-supported at the proximobuccal and proximolingual margins (*Fig. 37*); this will eventually result in failure of the restoration (Castaldi, 1957; McRae et al., 1962). Commonly the failure occurs at the distobuccal margin of mandibular first primary molars.

Another common error occurs when the direction of the walls of the proximal box and occlusal lock are considered from an occlusal view (*Fig. 38*). Because of the narrow occlusal table, the narrow isthmus width, and the minimal extension of the box at the occlusal aspect, the walls of the proximal box should not flare widely to the embrasure. Rather, the walls of the proximal box should meet the occlusal walls in a straight line so that no points of weakness are incorporated in the preparation. If the walls of the box are converged in the imagination towards the opposite embrasure, they should meet at the opposite marginal ridge (*see Fig. 38a*). Flared proximal walls result in inadequately supported enamel, leading to subsequent marginal deterioration (*Fig. 38d*).

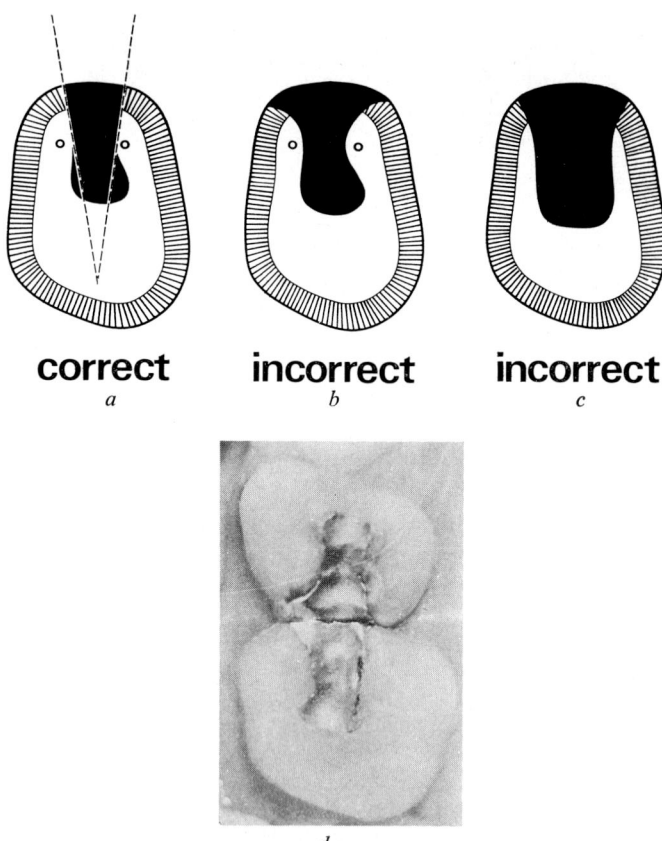

Fig. 38.—Occlusal view of Class 2 primary molar preparations. *a*, Correct diagram demonstrates absence of flaring or proximal box walls. Imaginary extensions of the walls meet at the opposite marginal ridge. *b*, Widely flaring walls of proximal box cannot parallel enamel rods, predisposing the restoration to failure. *c*, Wide isthmus results in weakening of cusps and possible pulp exposure if the cavity floor is taken too deep. *d*, Marginal deterioration resulting from poorly supported proximal walls. 0=pulp horn.

72

Critical analysis of *Fig. 38b, c* reveals that the widely flared and overextended margins cannot parallel the enamel rods, predisposing to amalgam failure. When these problems are encountered, limited increase in isthmus width and further refinement of the proximal walls may result in well supported walls. More often, the weakened proximal wall will have to be reduced and overlaid with amalgam. When gross flaring of both proximal walls occurs in the pre-school child, use of the stainless-steel crown should be seriously considered. Though this may seem drastic, it is preferred to placing an amalgam restoration which will have to be replaced.

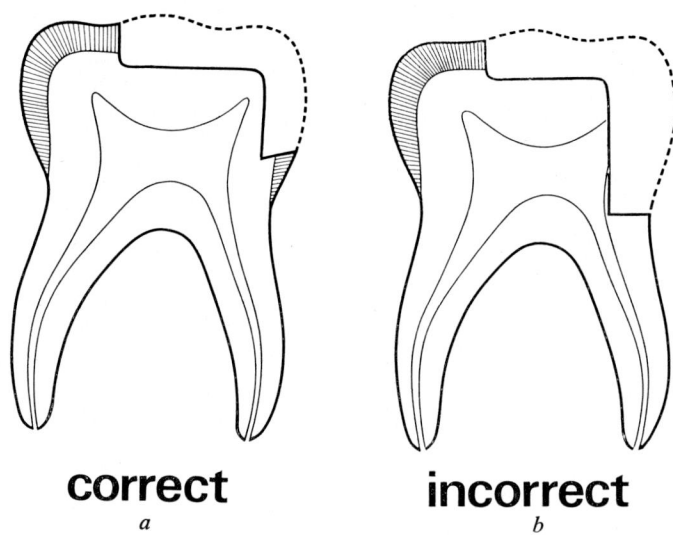

correct

a

incorrect

b

Fig. 39.—a, Line diagram depicting cross-sectional view of primary molar cavity preparation in buccolingual plane. Note rounded axiopulpal line angle, minimum cavity depth and occlusal inclination of the floor of proximal box. *b,* Line diagram depicting incorrect Class 2 primary molar preparation in buccolingual plane. The floor of the interproximal box is taken too far gingivally: when it is widened the axial wall exposes the pulp.

The gingival floor of the proximal box is placed just beneath the free margin of the gingiva so that it is self-cleansing. When the depth of the lesion requires that the floor be taken farther gingivally great care must be exercised so as not to expose the pulp. The farther gingival the floor of the box, the narrower it becomes because of the cervical bulge of enamel and normally bulbous crowns of primary molars (*see also Chapter* 3). The clinician may be tempted to widen the gingival seat, but unfortunately this can be done only at the expense of moving the axial wall pulpally, often to expose a pulp horn (*see Fig. 39b*).

The occlusal inclination of primary molar enamel rods encourages the same inclination of the floor of the interproximal box (*Figs. 39a, 40*). While loose enamel rods should be removed from the gingival seat, no attempt should be made to use a gingival margin trimmer as is conventionally done for permanent teeth. Its use would leave a poorly supported restoration. The correct inclination can be obtained by using a small inverted cone bur (No. 2)* with a slightly occlusal angulation. Alternatively a gingival margin trimmer can be used in the opposite manner, i.e , mesial trimmer for distal proximal box. A fissure bur is contra-indicated since angulation of the bur would move the axial wall unnecessarily close to the pulp.

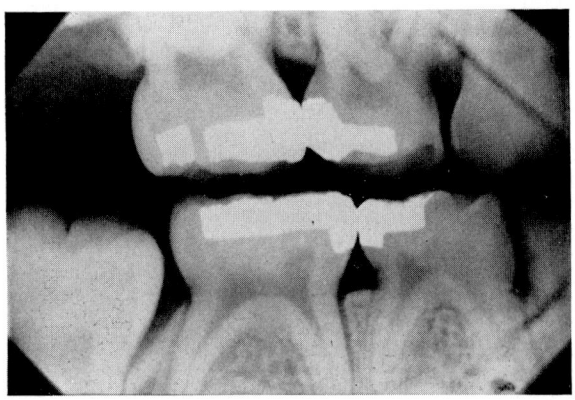

Fig. 40.—Bite-wing radiograph demonstrates Class 2 alloys in adjacent primary molars. Note minimal depth, extension of proximal box into a self-cleansing area gingivally, occlusal inclination of cervical seat and good contour.

The isthmus is at the junction of occlusal lock and interproximal box. In the 1950s Lampshire (1955) recommended a wide isthmus to provide bulk of alloy at a point of weakness, so preventing fracture (*Fig. 41*). Current trends (Law et al., 1966; McDonald, 1974) are to narrow this isthmus and obtain the bulk of alloy by making the cavity deeper. Ideally, the isthmus width should not exceed one-third of the intercuspal width in primary molars. However, the axiopulpal line angle must be either rounded, tunnelled, or grooved to provide sufficient bulk at this weak isthmus area. While the student may be fearful of exposing the pulp horns by laying a groove or tunnel along the axiopulpal line angle, it should be re-emphasized that the pulp horns are located beneath the cusps. Thus, provided the isthmus width is conservative, there is no danger

---

* No. 2 English = No. 35 American.

of exposure; the danger arises as the isthmus width increases. A No. 2L fissure bur* is used to round the axiopulpal line angle. This bur is later used to place retention grooves and refine the proximal box walls.

The trend towards narrower and deeper preparations is supported on two grounds. First, the preparation is less destructive of sound tooth structure. Second, at the isthmus area amalgam is three times stronger when it is placed in depth rather than in width (Davies and

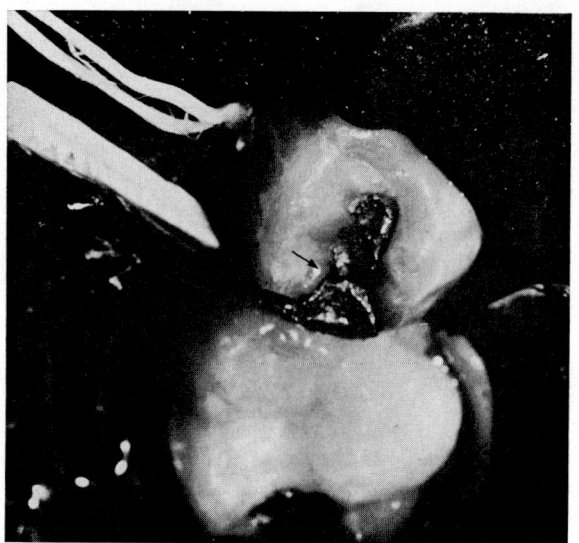

Fig. 41.—Fractured isthmus. (*From: Current Therapy in Dentistry,* Vol. 6 (1977) St Louis, C. V. Mosby Co.)

King, 1961). A contributing factor to isthmus fracture is trauma from the opposing cusp. Routine selective grinding of the opposing tooth will permit more effective bulk of alloy. This grinding should occur before and not after the occlusion of the alloy has been checked. Isthmus fracture probably occurs in the immediate post-operative period (first 24 hours) since the child is likely to follow postoperative instructions less rigidly than the adult. Thus it is wise not only to routinely grind the opposing tooth but also to dismiss the child with a cotton roll between the teeth. The parent is given a supply so that they can be changed at home. This helps remind the child not to bite on his new restorations, and keeps him from unknowingly traumatizing anaesthetized tissues.

---

* No. 2L Tapered fissure = No. 170L American.

External Line Angles

Opinions differ on the desirability of rounded or sharp *external line angles* for the proximal box. The main disadvantage of sharp angles is the tendency for incomplete condensation of amalgam, and subsequent failure of the restoration. It has been proved that the

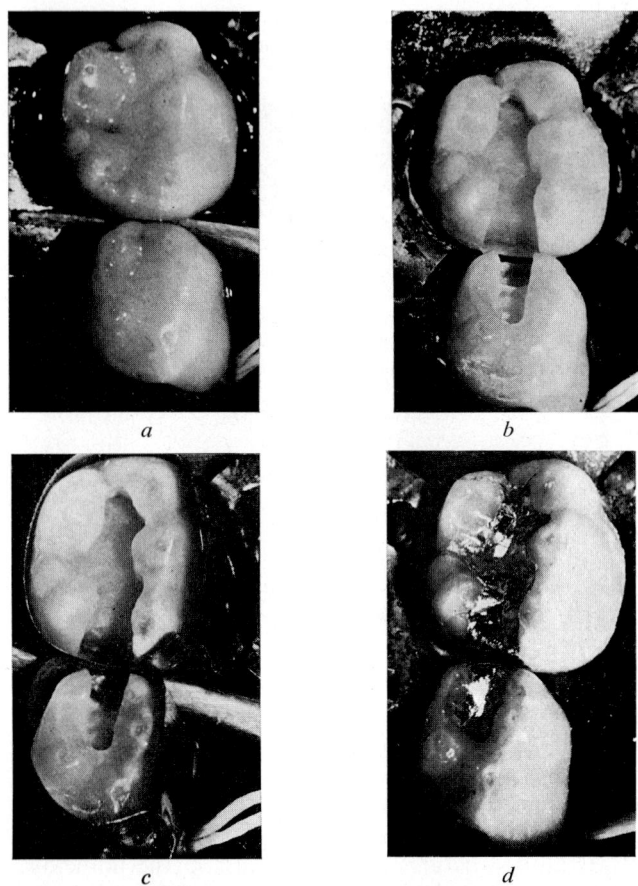

a *b*

c *d*

Fig. 42.—a, Preoperative. *b.* Cavity preparations. *c,* Wedged matrices. *d,* Completed restorations. (*From: Current Therapy in Dentistry,* Vol. 6. (1977) St Louis, C. V. Mosby Co.)

ability to condense amalgam into a line angle decreases as the angle becomes more acute (Azar et al., 1968; Heim, 1962). However, awareness of this, the correct use of specially designed condensers, and the routine use of mechanical condensation of amalgam can overcome this disadvantage. An advantage of rounded external line angles is the ease with which amalgam can be condensed. Also, a long plain-cut, pear-shaped bur* can be used to simultaneously prepare the walls of the proximal box, the rounded external line angles and the rounded internal line angles of the occlusal lock (McDonald, 1974). The major difficulty with rounded external line angles is the inability of the clinician to evaluate them. From a practical standpoint many clinicians find that sharp external line angles are both easier to produce and easier to evaluate. On this basis they can be recommended; also there is no *clinical* proof that restorations placed with rounded external line angles are superior to those with sharp line angles. In other words, the clinician has freedom of choice; this author finds the sharper angles easier to produce.

Retention

Retention of the restoration results from the mechanical undercut obtained by the rounded internal line angles of the occlusal lock and the diverging walls of the interproximal box. It is important that retention of the interproximal box and the occlusal lock be independent of one another since each may be subjected to different displacement forces. Additional retention can be obtained by placing a U-shaped retention groove along the amelodentinal junction of the proximal box. A No. 2L* plain cut fissure bur is used and the grooves are limited to the dentine. These grooves do not contribute to marginal deterioration (Mathewson et al., 1974). There should be little danger of pulp exposure if they are placed at the amelodentinal junction. When placed along the gingival floor at the amelodentinal junction, the retention groove encourages an occlusal inclination of gingival seat (*Figs. 39, 40*).

Finishing the Cavity

Final refinement of the cavity walls is made with hatchets and the No. 2L plain cut fissure bur. The tungsten carbide plain cut fissure bur is used to round the axiopulpal line angles; it also produces a smooth finish to Class 2 cavity walls (Grieve, 1968). The occlusal enamel support of the occlusal lock and interproximal box should be tested with chisels. This is especially important because most failures occur at the proximal margins.

Further Considerations

When interproximal lesions occur both mesially and distally on the same tooth, it must be determined whether separate Class 2 cavities are indicated or whether an MOD restoration would be preferable.

* No. 3L Pear (English) = No. 331L American.
* No. 2L plain cut tapered fissure bur = No. 170L American.

The occlusal anatomy and extent of occlusal decay are the determining factors. In mandibular second primary and maxillary first primary molars, an MOD restoration is indicated to eliminate the danger areas on the occlusal surface. In the maxillary second and mandibular first primary molar, the oblique ridge and central ridge, respectively, encourage the placement of two two-surface restorations. Extension across these ridges to place an MOD is indicated only when caries undermines them or when retention is in doubt.

2. The Large Lesion—Primary Molars

Unless the primary molar Class 2 lesion is diagnosed at the incipient stage from accurate bite-wing radiographs, the lesion will progress to undermine the marginal ridge. Eventually this will break down to present the clinician with a large Class 2 lesion closely approximating the pulp (Stoner, 1967). Because of the broad gingivally located primary molar contact areas, undiagnosed and/or untreated Class 2 lesions will undermine the proximobuccal and proximolingual cusps before the marginal ridge finally breaks down. Using conventional Class 2 cavity design in these large lesions invites subsequent failure since it will be impossible to maintain adequate support proximobuccally and proximolingually. Widely flaring walls (*Fig. 38b*) from a narrow isthmus cannot be prevented.

Therefore the clinician must look beyond conventional cavity preparations. Castaldi (1957) and MacRae et al. (1962) recommended reduction of a weakened cusp and overlaying it with amalgam. This recommendation was made after analysis of primary molar Class 2 amalgams revealed proximal marginal deterioration as the main cause of failure. This was most frequently seen in mandibular primary molars at the distobuccal margin. Because of this finding, overlay of the distobuccal cusp can be strongly recommended in mandibular first primary molars whenever cavity dimensions exceed those of the minimal preparation. In fact the projected failure rate of the modified preparation drops to 5 per cent from 29 per cent in mandibular first primary molars (MacRae et al., 1962). Rotations of primary molars can also weaken a proximal cusp even when an incipient lesion is prepared. This cuspal weakening is due to the breaking of a different contact area to leave the interproximal margins self-cleansing.

In making the recommended modification, the weakened cusp should be reduced to the level of the pulpal floor of the occlusal lock. The minimum amount of overlaid alloy should be one-third of the clinical crown height. The weakened cusp should be reduced in a mesiodistal direction no more than one-third of the crown's mesiodistal length. When these criteria are used there should be no danger

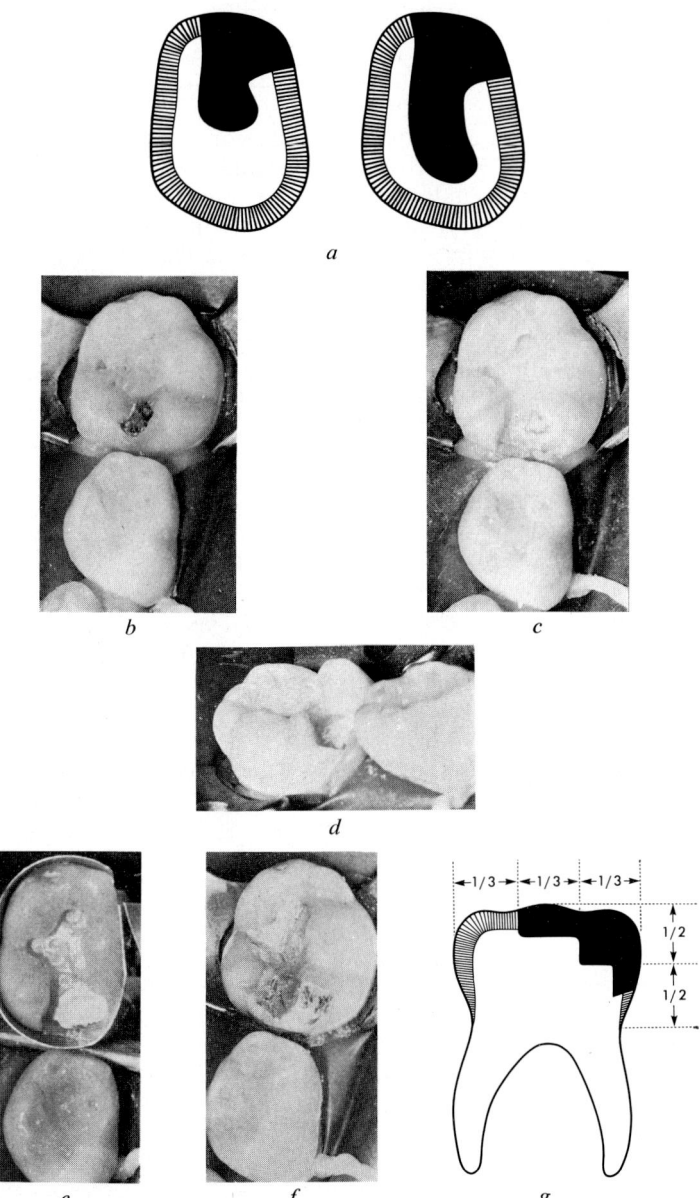

Fig. 43.—*a*, Line diagram shows that overlaid cusp leaves well-supported enamel at the margins. *b*, Preoperative—note open contact. *c*, Modified Class 2 preparation—occlusal view. *d*, Modified Class 2 preparation—buccal view. *e*, Wedged matrix and lining. *f*, Completed restoration. *g*, Line diagram—buccal view.

79

of exposing the pulp. External line angles should be sharp and preferably 90 degrees (*Fig. 43*). Special care should be taken when checking the occlusion of the completed restoration; adjustment of the opposing tooth is strongly recommended since the buccal cusps of mandibular teeth are liable to masticatory forces particularly in lateral excursions. Retentive pins are contra-indicated because of possible inadvertent pulp exposure. However, retention grooves placed at the amelodentinal junction are recommended. Additional retention can be obtained by extending the occlusal lock across the oblique ridge in maxillary second primary molars and across the central ridge in mandibular first primary molars. No attempt should be made to overlay more than one weakened cusp.

Alternative treatments for the large Class 2 primary molar lesion are the Willett inlay, cast gold crowns and the stainless-steel crown.

Primary Molar Class 2 Amalgam Failures

The frequency of failure in multisurface primary molar amalgam restorations is alarmingly high (MacRae et al., 1962; Graff, 1975). In mandibular first primary molars, the distobuccal margin was defective in 29 per cent of teeth evaluated after one year (MacRae et al., 1962). Braff (1975) found that only about 12 per cent of multisurface amalgam restorations lasted over four years without the need for further care. Of the remaining 88 per cent, the majority required replacement; this reflects a need for a critical review of our attention to detail in restorative procedures.

The common failures are:
1. Marginal deterioration at the proximal margins.
2. Isthmus fracture (accounts for less than 2 per cent; Law et al., 1966).
3. Recurrent caries.
4. Inadvertent pulp exposure.

1. *Marginal deterioration* is due to inadequate enamel support and faulty manipulation of, and selection of, the restorative material (*see Fig. 38d*). The means of ensuring adequate proximal wall support by conservative cavity preparation and cusp overlay have been described. Although marginal discrepancy usually becomes apparent several months or even years following restoration, the clinician may sometimes be faced with this discrepancy immediately after the matrix is removed. The amalgam has probably been insufficiently carved prior to matrix removal; 'ditching' (marginal discrepancy) at this early stage may also be indicative of faulty cavity design. Ideally the faulty cavity preparation should be modified; when child cooperation is not endangered and time permits, this can be done immediately. From an economic standpoint to the clinician and to the parent and child in terms of invested time,

such an action may be unjustifiable if a second visit is required and the marginal discrepancy is minimal. Horizontal reduction of the affected area with an abrasive green stone can often eliminate the deficiency. This is recommended when the child's cooperation is reduced by fatigue.

Severe discrepancies occur when the marginal ridge is removed together with the matrix band or when the child bites down hard before the restoration has been carved. Attempts to add amalgam should be discouraged since the strength of the bond with the existing amalgam is less than desirable. Rather, the restoration should be removed in the partially set state and replaced using a new matrix. Such action should be deferred to another appointment when the child is fatigued or when the day's appointment schedule does not permit sufficient time for this.

Marginal deterioration that occurs years after the placement of the restoration may be due to clinical variation in the material's performance or to wear from occlusal interference. The first problem will be discussed in Chapter 12. The latter problem can be minimized by using articulating paper prior to cavity preparation. In this manner the margins can be placed away from occlusal interference. At recall appointments, the occlusion can be rearticulated and the restorations repolished where necessary to eliminate occlusal interference.

2. *Isthmus fracture* can be avoided by providing sufficient effective bulk of amalgam at the axiopulpal line angle. Grooving of the latter increases amalgam bulk, while grinding the opposing cusp reduces the trauma from occlusion. The fractured isthmus will be apparent clinically (*Fig. 41*); when the interproximal part of the restoration is devoid of retention it may be displaced, giving the radiographic appearance of an overhang. Ingress of saliva, bacteria, and food encourage the development of recurrent caries. It is not uncommon to see a very deep lesion closely approximating the pulp after isthmus fracture; direct pulp therapy is often required.

3. *Recurrent caries* can occur after isthmus fracture, as indicated earlier. Inadequate extension of the interproximal margins into a self-cleansing area also encourages development of recurrent caries. This also occurs at the gingivolabial and gingivolingual line angles of the proximal box when the amalgam is improperly condensed.

4. *Inadvertent pulp exposure* occurs because of deepening of the occlusal or axial wall beyond the limits of the lesion. Frequently the pulp horn is exposed at the axial wall; the mesiobuccal pulp horn in primary molars is commonly closest to the surface and special care should be exercised when preparing this area. The distance between pulp horn and external enamel surface may be as little as 2 mm. The effects of inadvertent pulp exposure may not

become apparent until the child's recall examination, when a fistula may be seen; alternatively, radiographic internal or external resorption are observed. This assumes, of course, that any base which was placed was not successful in direct pulp capping. Once this has occurred, the tooth can be saved only with pulpectomy procedures; otherwise it must be extracted (*see* Chapter 17). Either action does little to enhance the image of the profession or the individual dentist. When this repeatedly occurs, it is not surprising for parents to develop the attitude that primary teeth cannot be filled and as a result for children to be denied the benefits of regular care.

3. *The Permanent Molar*

Current trends in permanent molar preparations have been described by Gilmore (1964). The tendency towards narrower and deeper cavity preparations is more conservative of sound tooth structure. Principles of cavity design already described for primary molars also apply to permanent molars. The following variations are recommended, however.

The occlusal lock should be as narrow as possible, commensurate with the philosophy of extension for prevention. Intercuspal cavity

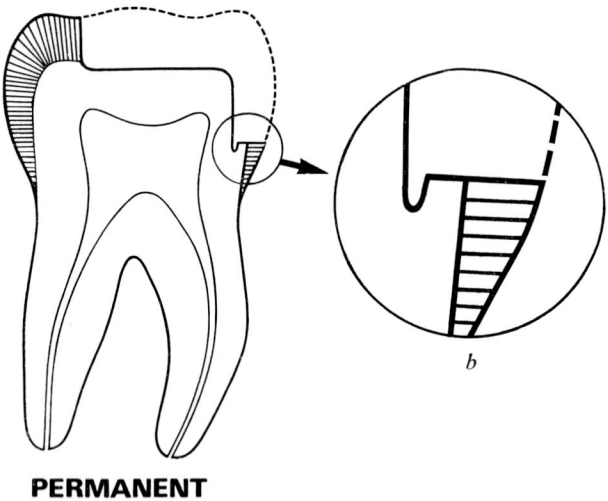

PERMANENT

a

Fig. 44.—*a*, Line diagram depicting Class 2 permanent molar preparation in buccolingual plane. Note rounded axiopulpal line angle, inclination of the proximal box floor, and retention groove. *b*, Enlarged view of floor of proximal box. Note that when a margin trimmer is used to bevel the floor, the enamel rods are supported by dentine.

width of the occlusal lock should be minimal with eradication of susceptible pits and fissures. Minimal cavity depth is 0·5 mm into dentine; it may be advisable to deepen this to provide more bulk of amalgam in depth due to the minimal cavity width. The isthmus should not exceed one-fourth of the intercuspal dimensions. The axial wall should meet the pulpal floor of the occlusal lock at 90 degrees, the axiopulpal line angle being rounded to relieve the stresses of mastication. The margins of the interproximal box should be just self-cleansing to allow passage of an explorer between the adjacent tooth and the cavity margins. The gingival seat of the proximal box must be prepared with a gingival margin trimmer to ensure that all weakened enamel is removed (*Fig. 44*). Retention grooves are mandatory for these 'modern' type preparations to ensure independent retention of occlusal lock and proximal box. It should be re-emphasized that these retention grooves do not contribute to marginal deterioration.

The clinician should be extremely careful to avoid unnecessary overextension of minimal lesions. Although any restoration placed in a young child's permanent molar has a potential lifetime of use ahead of it, clinical experience shows the need for replacing restorations due to marginal deterioration. Each time a restoration has to be replaced the danger of further tooth destruction exists. This should encourage a conservative approach in young children.

REFERENCES

AZAR E. S., WELK D. A., STIBBS G. D. and HODSON J. T. (1968) Quantitative evaluation of the adaptation of dental amalgam into line angles. *J. Dent. Res.* **47**, 533.

BRAFF M. H. (1975) A comparison between stainless steel crowns and multi-surface amalgams. *J. Dent. Child* **42**, 474.

CASTALDI C. R. (1957) Analysis of some operative procedures currently being used in paedodontics. *J. Can. Dent. Assoc.* **23**, 377.

DAVIES G. N. and KING R. M. (1961) *Dentistry for the Pre-school Child.* London, E. & S. Livingstone, p. 237.

DWYER D. M., BERMAN D. S. and SILVERSTONE L. M. (1973) A study of approximal caries lesions in primary molars. *J. Int. Assoc. Dent. Child.* **4**, 41.

GILMORE H. W. (1964) New concepts for the amalgam restoration. *Practical Dental Monographs* **5**, Nov.

GRIEVE A. R. (1968) Finishing cavity margins. *Br. Dent. J.* **125**, 12.

HEIM R. L. (1962) Condensation of silver amalgam with rounded and acute retentive grooves. *J. Dent. Child.* **29**, 140.

LAMPSHIRE E. L. (1955) Evaluation of cavity preparations in primary molars. *J. Dent. Child.* **22**, 3.

LAW D. B., SIM J. M. and SIMON J. F. (1966) A new look at Class II restorations in primary molars. *Dent. Clin. North Am.* 341.

McDonald R. E. (1974) *Dentistry for the Child and Adolescent.* St. Louis, C. V. Mosby, p. 191.

MacRae P. D., Zacherl W. and Castaldi C. R. (1962) Study of defects in Class II dental amalgam restorations in deciduous molars. *J. Can. Dent. Assoc.* **28,** 491.

Mathewson R. J., Retzloff A. E. and Porter D. R. (1974) Marginal failure of amalgam in deciduous teeth: a two-year report. *J. Am. Dent. Assoc.* **88,** 134.

Parfitt G. J. (1956) Conditions influencing the incidence of occlusal and interstitial caries in children. *J. Dent. Child.* **23,** 31.

Stoner J. E. (1967) Dental caries in deciduous molars *Br. Dent. J.* **123,** 130.

RECOMMENDED READING

Castaldi C. R. (1957) Analysis of some operative procedures currently being used in paedodontics. *J. Can. Dent. Assoc.* **23,** 377.

Kennedy D. B. (1977) Cavity preparations in primary teeth. In: *Current Therapy in Dentistry,* Vol. 6. St Louis, C. V. Mosby Co., pp. 473–485

CHAPTER 8

THE CLASS 3 LESION

DIAGNOSIS

THE most common site for a Class 3 lesion in the primary dentition is the mesial surface of the primary incisors. The maxillary arch is affected more than the mandibular. In the 18–39 month age group, the mesial surfaces of both primary central and lateral incisors are more frequently carious than the distal surfaces. This predilection for the mesial surfaces occurs in both the maxillary and the mandibular arch (Hennon et al., 1969). The distal surface of the primary canine is commonly affected in the mixed dentition. Not surprisingly, this lesion occurs when the primary canine and first primary molar have closed contact areas. Thus the presence of this lesion is in part determined by the absence of a primate space;* in the mandibular arch the eruption of the first permanent molars may obliterate the primate space. Any occlusal changes that occur result in the Class 3 lesion occurring to a lesser degree on the mesial surface of the primary canine than on the distal.

The Class 3 lesion is often diagnosed by clinical means alone, particularly when the contact areas are open or when the lesion is larger than incipient. The bite-wing radiograph is invaluable in the diagnosis of incipient Class 3 lesions in primary canines when posterior contacts are closed. Bite-wing radiographs for pre-school children should include the posterior arch from primary canine to developing first permanent molar. This enables the practitioner to see all interproximal contact areas, as well as any developing abnormalities in first permanent molar eruption. Likewise the clinical diagnosis of Class 3 lesions in primary incisors may be supplemented by a maxillary anterior occlusal radiograph which can also determine the presence of any abnormality in the developing permanent incisors. The Class 3 lesion may be accompanied by an adjacent Class 5 lesion on the same tooth. This is commonly seen on the maxillary primary incisors in the nursing bottle mouth syndrome. Here the Class 3 and Class 5 lesions often blend into one to produce a circumferential pattern of decay. The untreated Class 3 lesion will progress to undermine the incisal edge. This occurs at a faster rate in the primary than in the permanent dentition because of the relatively small incisogingival height of the primary incisor clinical crown. In effect, the Class 3 lesion has now progressed to a Class 4 lesion and will be discussed in Chapter 9.

---

* Primate Space—*See* Glossary.

THE CLASS 3 CAVITY—PRIMARY ANTERIORS

When the contact areas are open and the lesion is incipient the cavity can be prepared directly; therefore there is no need for a dovetail lock to improve access and retention. The outline form should be triangular, with the base of the triangle at the gingival aspect of the cavity. The buccal and lingual cavity walls should parallel the respective external surfaces of the tooth to meet at the apex of the triangle. A small inverted cone bur (No. 2*) is suitable for preparing the cavity. The gingival cavity wall should incline slightly occlusally, thereby paralleling the enamel rod/prism structure. This also provides an undercut for mechanical retention. The incisal aspect of the cavity should not be undercut since this will undermine incisal enamel which is later subject to occlusal wear. The primary canines frequently exhibit gross wear, especially when premature contacts may encourage a lateral shift to produce a posterior crossbite. Cavity depth should be 0·5 mm pulpal to the amelodentinal junction. Retention grooves can be placed along the amelodentinal junction with a No. 2L tapered fissure bur run at slow speed; alternatively, retention pits can be placed at the buccogingival and linguogingival internal point angles with the No. 2L tapered fissure bur.

More often than not, a lock or dovetail will be required to facilitate access to the carious lesion and to aid in the retention of the restoration. This lock should be placed only in primary, and not in permanent anteriors. It is most commonly required in the primary canines, particularly when the contact area is closed and the lesion is larger than incipient. The dovetail should be placed in the middle one-third of the tooth at a depth of 0·5 mm into the dentine (*Fig. 45*). The incisal one-third of the tooth is avoided because of the anticipated wear, while the gingival one-third is avoided since plaque retention may be encouraged by restorations and gingival irritation is to be avoided whenever possible.

The interproximal area of the cavity should be shaped like the letter 'C' when observed directly. The open end of the 'C' meets the retentive lock (*Fig. 45*). In some ways the cavity is similar to the Class 2 lying on its side. The width and location of the lock are partly determined by the extent and position of the caries. The inclination of the incisal and gingival enamel walls should be towards the incisal, paralleling the enamel rods. This recommendation applies to the walls of both the retentive lock and the interproximal area. A retention groove can be placed along the amelodentinal junction of the gingival wall with a 700 or No. 2L fissure bur.

---

* A No. 2L tapered fissure bur can also be used. English No. 2 inverted cone = No. 35 American. No. 2L tapered fissure bur = No. 170L American.

Retention points can also be placed as described earlier, although these are seldom necessary when a lock is placed.

The lock need extend only to the middle of the tooth and should be dovetail-shaped to provide resistance to lateral displacement of the restoration. Because of ease of access and the minimal aesthetic

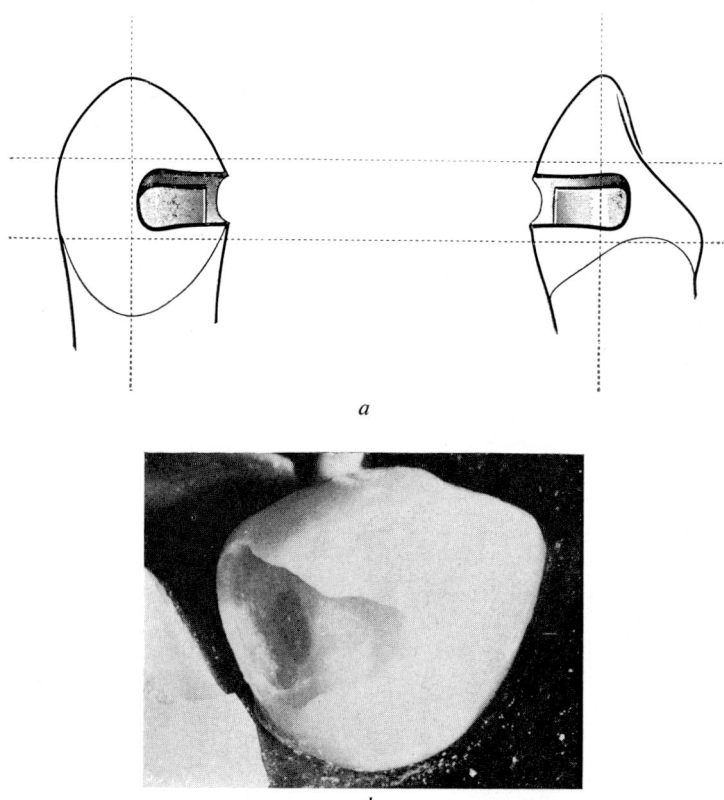

a

b

Fig. 45.—*a*, Primary canine Class 3 preparation with retentive lock: view from the buccal and the interproximal. The lock is in the middle one-third of the tooth and does not extend across the midline. Note the incisal inclination of the enamel walls. *b*, Large distolingual Class 3 preparation in maxillary primary canine.

requirements of the restoration, the lock is placed on the labial surface in the mandibular primary anteriors. For aesthetic reasons, it is commonly placed on the lingual surface in the maxillary anteriors. Also, because of the location of caries it often develops that less sound tooth structure is destroyed by the lingually placed maxillary dovetail.

Deviation from this set pattern is dictated by the presence of both a Class 3 and a Class 5 lesion on the same tooth. In this instance, the Class 5 cavity becomes the retentive lock. It may be necessary when both mesial and distal lesions occur on the same tooth to form a common retentive dovetail.

The Class 3 cavity can be restored with amalgam alloy or resin. The final choice of restorative material is governed first by aesthetics, then by the anticipated longevity of the tooth and finally by operator preference. Amalgam alloy, though difficult to condense in a small cavity, can be so highly polished that it need not be unaesthetic at the front of the child's mouth; it can pass as a fleck of saliva. The low pH of silicates and unfavourable pulp response make them unacceptable for use in the primary and young permanent dentition. Almost ideal colour matching and biological compatibility can be achieved with simple direct filling resins or composites. They are often the material of choice since they provide good retention, minimum tooth destruction, and maximum tooth support.

REFERENCE

HENNON D. K., STOOKEY G. K. and MUHLER J. C. (1969) Prevalence and distribution of dental caries in pre-school children. *J. Am. Dent. Assoc.* **79**, 1405.

RECOMMENDED READING

ROCHE J. R. (1970) In: *Current Therapy in Dentistry*, Vol. 4. St Louis, C. V. Mosby Co., p. 540.

CHAPTER 9

THE CLASS 4 LESION

DIAGNOSIS

THE most common site for the Class 4 lesion is the mesio-incisal edge of the maxillary primary central incisor, followed in frequency by the mesio-incisal corner of the maxillary primary lateral incisor. The small vertical height of the primary incisor crown, which is further reduced by attrition, may account for the rapid spread of a Class 3 to Class 4 lesion. The disto-incisal corners of the maxillary primary central and lateral incisors seldom appear to be carious in the same frequency and degree as the mesio-incisal corners (Hennon et al., 1969). Mandibular primary incisors and primary canines (either maxillary or mandibular) are less common sites for Class 4 lesions. No doubt the anatomical shape of the primary canine excludes this tooth from the possibility of a Class 4 lesion. Loss of incisal corners also occurs in young permanent incisors as a result of trauma.

The diagnosis of the Class 4 lesion should present no problem since the lesion is obvious. Since there is always the possibility that the lesion has progressed close to the pulp, the preoperative evaluation should include an assessment of the pulp status (Chapter 16). A preoperative radiograph will indicate the presence of any resorption (internal and external) which can either be pathological or physiological. The anticipated longevity of the tooth can be determined by the child's age and the radiographic extent of physiological root resorption. Prolonged investment of time in the comprehensive restorative treatment of Class 4 lesions is not justified if the tooth will exfoliate within 18 months.

Parental attitudes towards dental health should be evaluated. It may be that heroic efforts to save extensively broken down primary incisors are contra-indicated because of parental apathy in appointment keeping, poor performance of the child's oral hygiene, and a lack of concern for dental health. In such instances the extraction of these teeth may be required; failure to perform any treatment will eventually result in acute or chronic abscess formation and increase the likelihood of hypoplastic or hypocalcified defects occurring on the developing permanent incisors. Should the parents subsequently become more dentally aware and the child become concerned about aesthetics, a partial denture can be fabricated at a later date. This should be deferred until a good response to preventive care has been obtained.

Sometimes one or two maxillary primary incisors, often the centrals, may be non-vital while the remainder are vital but also extensively carious. Should the non-vital incisors be unsuitable candidates for pulp therapy and require removal, the remaining incisors should also be considered for extraction. Indeed, pulp therapy may be desirable in some instances since the pulp chamber can be used for retention (*see* section on anterior crowns). In these cases sufficient time should be allowed so that the pulp therapy can be performed within the appropriate appointment.

TREATMENT

For many years paediatric dentists have sought the ideal treatment of the Class 4 lesion. This indicates that there are a few hard and fast rules to be followed and also explains the many different treatment techniques that have been recommended, none of which is ideal. The main problems in restorative treatment are:

1. That insufficient tooth is left, following caries removal, to retain a restoration; and

2. That the patients selected for treatment are very young since the teeth to be restored can be maintained in the mouth over several years; the child's age may result in working conditions being less than ideal.

The following possibilities of treatment exist:

Discing.

The Class 4 Cavity.

Orthodontic Bands.

Anterior Crowns.

Discing

Discing of the interproximal area is done to remove superficial caries and make the area self-cleansing, or at least more readily cleansed. It is hoped that any remaining caries will arrest subsequently (*Figs. 46, 47*). The size and anatomy of the primary anterior pulp imposes limitations on the extent of the discing that can be performed. Preoperative radiographs give the clinician a guide for tooth reduction. Sandpaper discs are recommended since they remove tooth surface more slowly and probably generate less heat than lightning strips or metal discs; they are also less traumatic to the soft tissues, should the lips and tongue be improperly retracted. The exact angulation of the disc is dictated by the site of the lesion. After discing, the incisal edge must be no wider than the maximum gingival mesiodistal width so that the area is self-cleansing. The end result should be a parallel-sided or tapered tooth, narrowest at the incisal edge. Closed contacts should be opened by the discing in the hope of preventing recurrence of the lesion.

It is seldom possible to remove all decay by discing; to do so may expose the pulp. Therefore the oral environment must be changed so that the remaining caries will arrest. Topical fluoride has been shown to arrest incipient lesions (Muhler et al., 1967; Hyde, 1973). Silverstone (1971) has also demonstrated *in vitro* the phenomenon of enamel remineralization after fluoride application. The pulpal response to stannous fluoride applied to open cavities is minimal (Evans and Massler, 1968). In fact, 10 per cent stannous fluoride has been recommended by Nordstrom et al. (1974) as one method that is effective in indirect pulp treatment; it can arrest the progress of deep lesions and prevent pulp exposure.

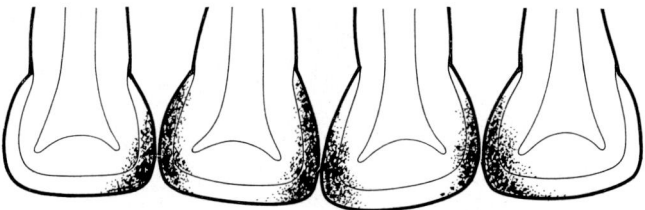

Fig. 46.—Diagram depicting maxillary primary incisor suitable for discing. The lesions have not reached the pulp.

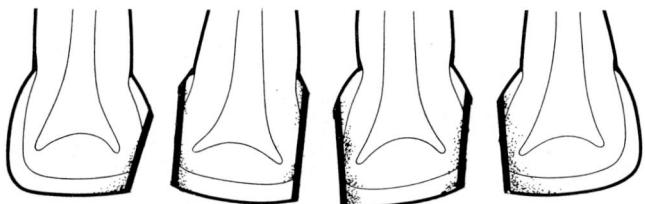

Fig. 47.—Diagram of primary incisors following discing. Note the tapered appearance, breaking of contact areas, incomplete removal of caries, and self-cleansing appearance.

The teeth should be polished smooth after discing; then 10 per cent stannous fluoride (freshly mixed) should be applied. Alternatively, 1·23 per cent acidulated phosphate fluoride can be used. At subsequent recall visits, success is judged by hardening of the disced surfaces to exploration; frequently these surfaces are stained dark brown or black (*Fig. 48*). Since the discing is usually done without the rubber dam, a cotton roll should be held lingual to the incisors to prevent the sour-tasting stannous fluoride from reaching the taste buds. There is no evidence to support the use of a topical application of silver nitrate to arrest the remaining caries. Its effect on the pulp is potentially harmful (Klein and Knutson, 1942) and therefore its use is strongly condemned.

91

The Class 4 lesion is often accompanied by a Class 5 lesion on the same tooth with the two lesions merging. In such instances the ideal treatment may consist of a Class 4 restoration or a crown. However, the dental age of the patient and anticipated longevity of

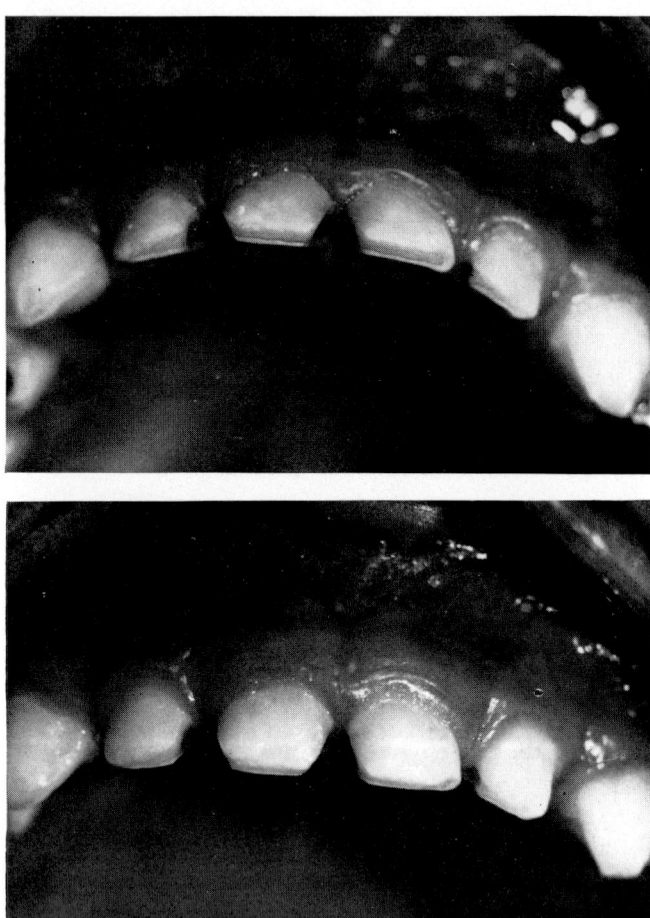

Fig. 48.—Clinical view of disced maxillary primary central incisors.

the tooth may encourage the operator to perform a compromise treatment consisting of a Class 5 restoration and a self-cleansing interproximal slice. Since the Class 5 lesion cannot be made self-cleansing, it must be conventionally restored as described in Chapter 10. The Class 5 cavity must exhibit resistance to displacement in the direction of the interproximal slice. Where the two lesions meet, the Class 5 cavity will in effect have no cavity wall or margin; the restorative material should be made flush with the slice made by the discing.

The attraction of discing is the simplicity of the procedure and the resulting reduction in clinical time required of both the dentist and the child. The success of the treatment will mainly depend on the parent's ability to remove plaque from the mouth and to change the child's diet by reducing the frequency of intake of fermentable carbohydrates. Parental instruction in oral hygiene techniques and nutritional counselling are thus important parts of the treatment. The application of topical fluoride alone is not an adequate method of prevention.

In favour of discing is the fact that space loss does not occur in the incisor region of uncrowded mouths from loss of interproximal contacts once the primary canines are fully erupted into occlusion (usually at age 3 years). Discing of small Class 4 lesions is therefore most appropriate in the 4-, 5-, and 6-year-old children who can expect to lose these teeth within two years. It should not be used when caries has progressed to the pulp.

The major disadvantage of discing is the poor aesthetic result; the narrow tapering teeth have a fang-like appearance that the child's peers may be quick to notice and ridicule. It is arguable that the preoperative appearance was equally unaesthetic. This same argument involving aesthetics is used against stannous fluoride on the ground that it will cause staining (Hyde and Muhler, 1963). There is no doubt that some children suffer psychological trauma as a result of discing and would benefit from a more aesthetic treatment. The clinician must also realize that parents may feel extreme guilt for allowing their children's teeth to reach this state; they are frequently most appreciative of an aesthetic treatment for unsightly Class 4 lesions. Therefore, each child should be carefully evaluated preoperatively to determine the best treatment for that child, as well as for the individual tooth.

The Class 4 Cavity

Doyle (1967) reported favourable results in treating Class 4 lesions in primary incisors with Sevriton* resin (*Figs. 49–52*). The cavity preparation included an interproximal slice and labial and lingual retentive dovetails, as in the Class 3 primary anterior cavity. The retentive dovetails are located in the middle one-third of the tooth, extending up to but not across the midline. These should be placed

---

* Sevriton Simplified—Amalgamated Dental Co., 26 Broadwick St., London.

to a depth of 0·5 mm pulpal to the amelodentinal junction with a small inverted cone bur (No. 2).* Obviously they should include any Class 5 lesion that may be present, in which case the position of the lock will be determined by the location of the Class 5 lesion. When both interproximal areas are carious, the retentive locks should extend across the midline and serve both lesions.

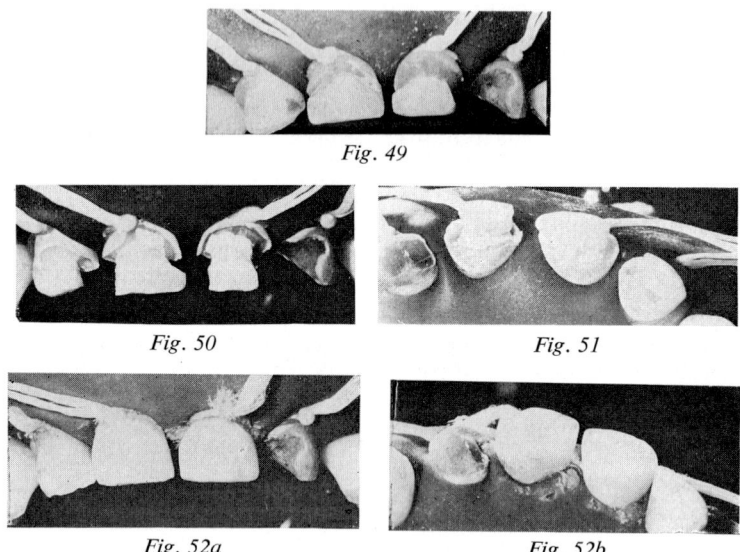

Fig. 49

Fig. 50   *Fig. 51*

Fig. 52a   *Fig. 52b*

Figs. 49–52.—Class 4 preparations. *Fig. 49.*—Preoperative. *Fig. 50.*—Mesial incisal B|; distal incisal mesial A|; mesial incisal distal incisal |A; buccal view. Preparations lined. *Fig. 51.*—Lingual view. *Fig. 52.*—Completed restorations. *a*, Buccal view. *b*, Lingual view.

The carious lesion is partially eliminated by an interproximal slice. This leaves a finite labial and lingual margin. At the gingival aspect of the slice there should be a definite interproximal shoulder or gingival seat rather than a chamfer; this will facilitate finishing of the restoration. Any remaining caries can be removed with a slow running No. 2 round bur. A calcium hydroxide pulp protecting base should be placed in the deepest parts of the cavity. Eugenol-containing bases are not used since the resin will be discoloured by the eugenol. Most calcium hydroxide bases are white and tend to show through the translucent resin to spoil the appearance of the finished restoration. Therefore the base should be avoided on the labial surface whenever possible.

---

* English No. 2 inverted cone = No. 35 American.

Doyle (1967) recommended Sevriton resin, using the Nealon bead paint-on technique, as the restorative material of choice. Wedged celluloid strips are used as matrices after the resin has been applied to the retentive lock (*Fig. 53*). The incremental addition of Sevriton resin reduces both polymerization shrinkage and exothermia from the setting reaction. This is less injurious to the vital pulp than bulk packing of Sevriton. The improved coefficient of thermal expansion and increased abrasion resistance of composite resins, compared to Sevriton, make them an attractive alternative restorative material. Placement and finishing of the restoration are discussed in Chapter 12.

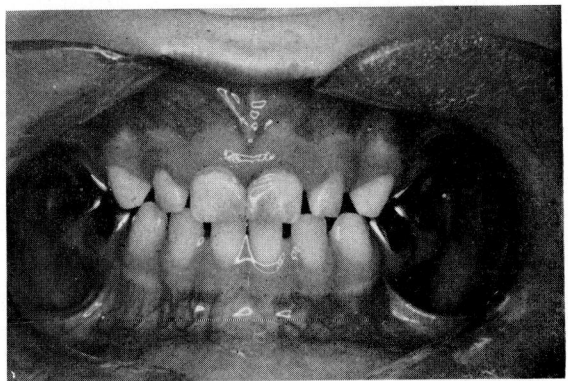

Fig. 53.—Completed Class 4 restorations in Sevriton after one year. Some discoloration has occurred.

The initial postoperative appearance may be impressive but staining, marginal deterioration and discoloration are to be expected after the first year (*Fig. 53*). The Doyle type preparation is most suitable for the small Class 4 lesion in a cooperative 3- or 4-year-old whose parents have demonstrated their interest in dental health by improving the child's oral environment during treatment. It can also be used in infants (under 3 years) in selected instances. The anteriors should be treated only after completing posterior restorations because of the importance of the primary molars in maintaining arch length. In the primary dentition aesthetic restorations are secondary in importance to the maintenance of arch length.

Orthodontic Bands

McConville and Tonn (1967) recommended using orthodontic bands for restoring extensively decayed primary incisors with Class 3 and Class 4 lesions. A strip of 3/16 by 0·0020 orthodontic band* can be

---

* Alternatively, Ash Siqueland Band material—Amalgamated Dental Co., 26 Broadwick St., London.

trimmed with scissors so that it is no wider than the clinical crown. The band is drawn tight with the anterior band forming plier or a 110 plier;* the excess band material is on the labial aspect of the tooth. The band is spot welded and the excess cut. The remaining tag of band material is folded over and spot welded. Any rough edges are smoothed with a stone. Preformed orthodontic bands† can also be used; they preclude the need for a spot welder which is required for the custom-made band. The decay is then removed with a slow running round bur; a base and cavity varnish are placed, and the band is cemented with zinc phosphate cement or a fast setting resin hardened zinc oxide.

It is easier to fabricate the band before removing the caries since more tooth structure is present. Also, such a procedure is atraumatic for the very young child and it can be used as a stepping stone in behaviour management before introducing the handpiece which may be necessary for caries removal. The orthodontic band is often used to retain a pulp-protecting dressing when indirect pulp treatment (Chapter 17) is being performed and tooth destruction is severe.

The disadvantages of this technique are many. The aesthetic result is poor although the final restoration after indirect pulp treatment may be an improvement. Furthermore, the band margins, however well adapted, are sites for increased bacteria retention (Sakamaki and Bahn, 1969); the band is therefore an aggravating factor in further carious development and in gingival disease. Severe tooth destruction may leave little remaining sound tooth for adequate retention. Loss of the band does little to enhance parental confidence, particularly when there is the danger of band ingestion or inhalation. Successful treatment of the very young child, who may suffer from the ravages of nursing bottle mouth, is essential if parental attitudes towards dental health are to improve.

Despite these disadvantages, the temporary and semi-permanent restoration of Class 3 and Class 4 lesions in primary incisors with orthodontic bands has a definite place in paediatric operative dentistry. Its major role is in the initial treatment of primary anteriors affected by the nursing bottle mouth syndrome; the band is used to retain a pulp-protecting dressing during indirect pulp treatment. Careful preoperative evaluation will result in the use of this technique only when sufficient tooth is left to ensure adequate retention of the band and when pulp vitality can be maintained by indirect pulp treatment.

---

* Unitek Band Forming Plier or 110 plier, Unitek Corporation, Monrovia, California, available from Orthomax Ltd., Queens House, Queens Road, Bradford, Yorks., England.
† Preformed Bands, Unitek Corporation.

Anterior Crown

Severe tooth destruction, the anticipated longevity of the tooth, and a strong desire by the parents to save the teeth encourage the use of primary anterior crowns. Primary incisors with loss of mesial and distal incisal corners, as well as circumferential Class 5 lesions such as may occur in nursing bottle mouth, are most suitable candidates for crowning. Other indications are children with disfiguring hypoplasias. Before the advent of the polycarbonate crown, the stainless-steel crown was used exclusively (*see* Chapter 12) although a cured acrylic crown has also been recommended (Sherman et al., 1966).

The *polycarbonate crown** is a preformed tooth-coloured crown whose dimensions approximate those of the tooth they are designed to replace. It is more aesthetic than the steel crown but cannot be contoured; rather, it has to be trimmed in bulk as with any temporary acrylic crown. These crowns come in different sizes and are hollowed to facilitate fitting and cementing. Often the crown's labiolingual dimensions exceed those of the tooth.

Recent advances include appropriately sized primary incisor celluloid crown forms† which can be used in conjunction with composite resin; retention can be obtained by mechanical undercuts and enhanced by acid etching. Improvements in the use of open-faced stainless steel crowns have also been reported.

JACKET CROWN—VITAL TEETH

The following single-visit technique is recommended. Whenever possible, the tooth's preoperative mesiodistal width is measured with callipers and a crown or crown form of the same mesiodistal width is selected. Tooth preparation is very similar to the preparation for a permanent tooth jacket crown. The tooth must be reduced on all surfaces to make room for placement of the crown. Most of this tooth reduction will probably occur automatically during the removal of caries. The plain-cut No. 2L tapered fissure bur‡ can be used to perform the remaining minimal crown preparations on the interproximal, labial and incisal surfaces; a diamond stone is used for lingual reduction. A small circumferential shoulder should be cut, as with a permanent anterior crown preparation, so that the margins of the crown will fit in the gingival crevice. Mechanical retention should be provided as much as possible by undercuts. Any remaining caries should be removed.

---

* Polycarbonate crowns—Unitek Corporation, Monrovia, California. Available from Orthomax Ltd., Queens House, Queens Road, Bradford, Yorks., England.
† Unitek Co.
‡ No. 2L = No. 170L American.

Should an exposure be encountered, appropriate pulp therapy can be performed before the crown is placed. If there is no exposure, the deep areas of the preparation should be covered by a base. Any remaining undercuts should be eliminated with a hard-setting calcium hydroxide (e.g. Dycal) or resin; the incremental use of simple unfilled resin (e.g. Sevriton) reduces the heat of setting reaction and resulting pulp insult.

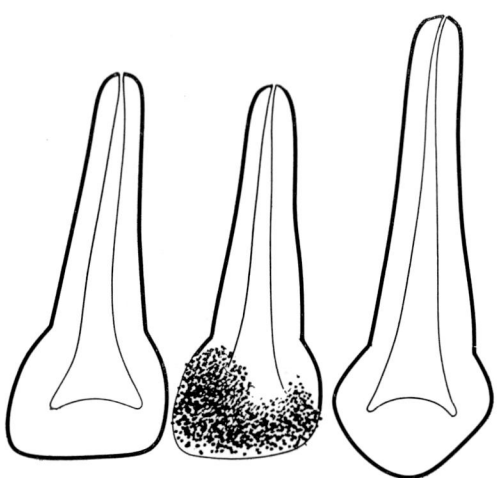

Fig. 54.—Gross carious destruction of primary incisor.

The crown should be trial fitted and trimmed with a stone until the crown approximates the gingival shoulder. The polycarbonate crown can be cemented using Sevriton resin as a cementing medium; the simple resin bonding to the resin crown, as well as its low film thickness, enhances retention (Kopel and Batterman, 1976). Once polymerization is complete, final gingival margin trimming is performed with a tapered diamond bur.

Doyle (1979) reports a modification to the technique to minimize the potential for postoperative failure from abrasion. In his preparation the incisal edge is not reduced. After caries removal, placement of lining and acid etching a preformed resin crown* is cemented using a simple resin. The crown is finished as before. Doyle feels that the abrasion resistance is increased because of the enamel incisal edge.

The exothermic setting reaction of resin may be detrimental to the vital untreated pulp. This explains the need for coverage of dentine by a base and the incremental use of Sevriton to eliminate

---

* Medidenta, 39–23 62nd St., Woodside, New York 11377.

undercuts prior to cementation with Sevriton. However, the possibility of this adverse pulp reaction prompts some to use a bland cementing medium, (e.g. zinc oxide), in preference to Sevriton. This alternative cementing technique can be used provided the operator realizes that the retention of the crown will be reduced since there is no bonding of cement to the crown. This has been demonstrated in laboratory tests (Kopel and Batterman, 1976). Also, the gingival adaptation is dependent on cement rather than on resin. Composite

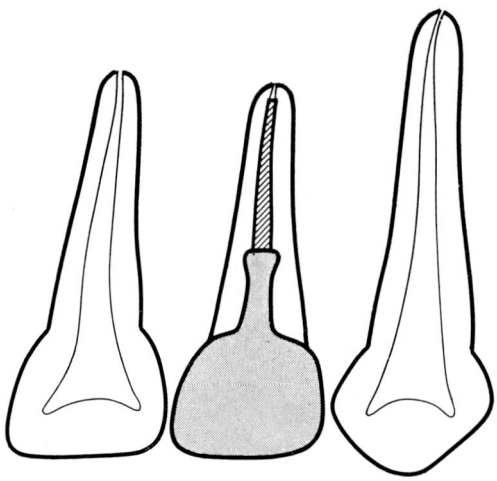

Fig. 55.—Pulpectomy performed and a resin post crown replaced.

resins of low viscosity and low film thickness may provide a more suitable means of cementing polycarbonate crowns. Priming of the polycarbonate crown with methyl methacrylate monomer or a methyl methacrylate monomer and powder syrup produces a bond with the composite; this has greater resistance to displacement forces under laboratory conditions (Nitkin et al., 1977). The occlusion should be checked with articulating paper since the preformed polycarbonate crowns frequently need reduction on the lingual surface.

POST CROWN—NON-VITAL TEETH
(Figs. 54–57)

Sometimes, because of the site of the carious lesion along with attrition, virtually no tooth structure is left to retain a crown. After caries removal there may be a small supragingival stump remaining; it is not surprising to find that the pulp is cariously exposed. Often

99

extraction will be indicated; however, a successful alternative treatment is pulp treatment and a post crown. A high level pulpotomy or pulpectomy should be performed. Depending on preoperative pulp status, this pulp therapy is performed in one or two visits (Chapter 17). The root-filling material is placed, and the pulp chamber up to and just apical to the cemento-enamel junction is used for retention. Resin is placed in the pulp chamber and built up to act as a post and core. Celluloid crown forms should be trimmed so that their margins are subgingival. Relief holes can be placed at the incisal corners to allow expression of resin during placement.

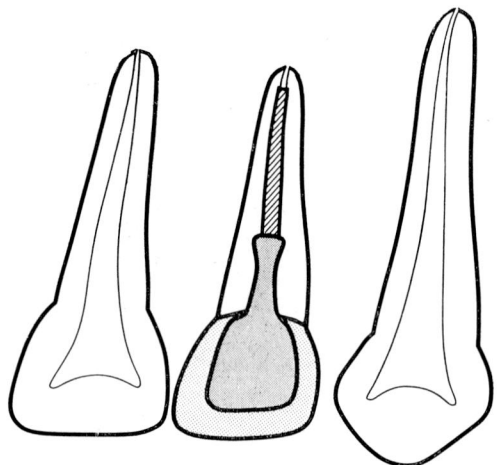

Fig. 56.—Jacket crown (polycarbonate) fitted over resin post and core.

Retention can be enhanced by acid etching all available enamel. Because of difficulty in retaining primary anterior crowns, the resin should overlap the enamel surface in a feather edge rather than meeting at a butt-joint. In this manner more etched enamel is available to the resin. In some instances it will be necessary to accept a subgingival flash of resin in the interest of retention.

Once this is set a crown preparation can be made and a polycarbonate crown is fitted as described before. The aesthetics, shape, and retention of the resin post and core prior to crown preparation may be most impressive. Indeed, this result may eliminate the need for crown preparation and fitting. Personal experience with Sevriton and Adaptic post crowns on non-vital primary incisors has been most favourable (*Fig. 57*). Pin reinforcement of the resin post and core can be provided with orthodontic wire. Non-vital primary

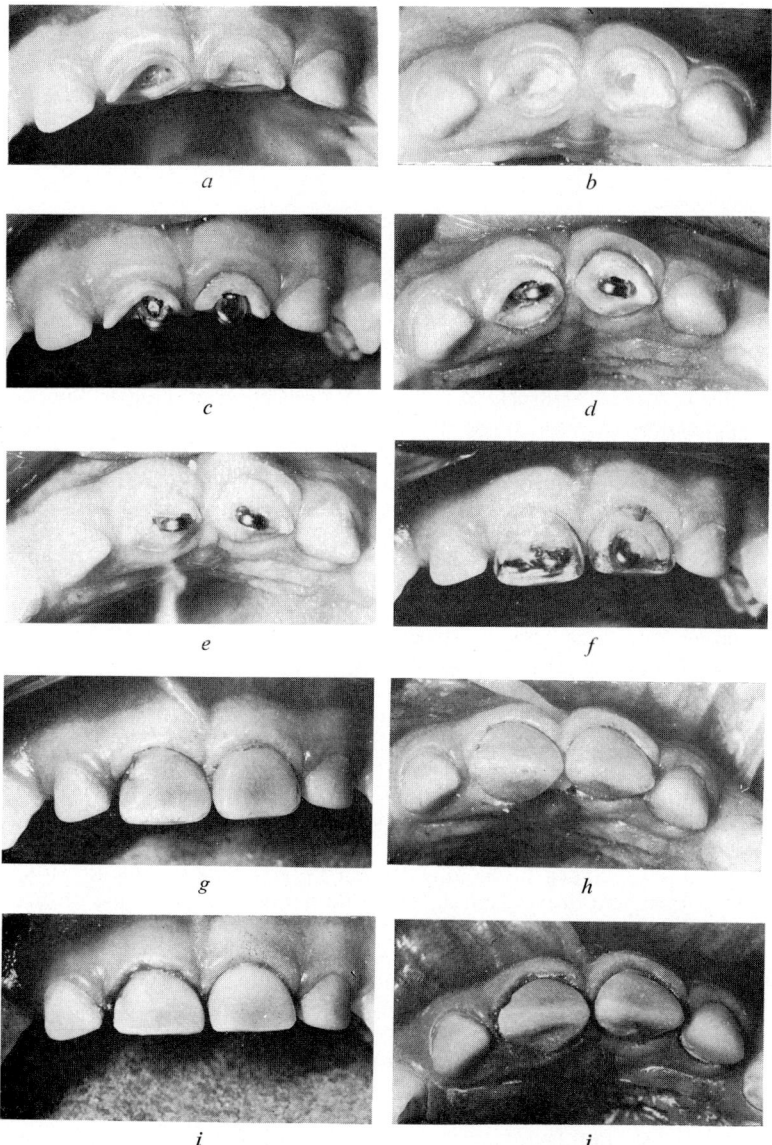

Fig. 57.—Composite post crowns with wire reinforced post in
<u>a</u>|<u>a</u>. <u>b</u>|<u>b</u> have jacket crowns placed. *a*, Preoperative. *b*, After
pulpectomy. *c*, Wire in canal. *d*, Occlusal view. Wire in canal.
e, Post cemented in canal with composite. *f*, Unitek celluloid
crown forms. *g*, Composite placed. Buccal view. *h*, Composite
placed. Occlusal view. *i*, Finished restorations. Buccal view. *j*,
Finished restoration. Occlusal view.

101

incisors treated in this way may exfoliate prematurely; the problems associated with resorption of primary teeth treated by pulpectomy and root-canal filling are described in Chapter 17. However, it should be emphasized that the post part of the post crown rarely represents a problem in resorption because of its relatively coronal position.

REFERENCES

DOYLE W. A. (1967) Esthetic restoration of deciduous incisors: a new Class 4 preparation. *J. Am. Dent. Assoc.* **74**, 82.

DOYLE W. A. (1979) A new preparation for primary anterior jackets. *Pediatr. Dent.* **1**, 38.

EVANS J. A. and MASSLER M. (1968) Non-reaction of pulp to fluoride application. *J. Dent. Child.* **35**, 91.

HENNON D. K., STOOKEY G. K. and MUHLER J. C. (1969) Prevalence and distribution of dental caries in pre-school children. *J. Am. Dent. Assoc.* **79**, 1405.

HYDE E. J. (1973) Caries-inhibiting action of three different topically-applied agents on the incipient lesions in newly-erupted teeth. Results after 24 months. *J. Can. Dent. Assoc.* **39**, 189.

HYDE E. J. and MUHLER J. C. (1963) Pigmentation of teeth treated with stannous fluoride and its association with caries incidence and oral hygiene. *J. Can. Dent. Assoc.* **29**, 514.

KLEIN H. and KNUTSON J. W. (1942) Studies on dental caries. XIII. Effect of ammoniacal silver nitrate on caries in the first permanent molar. *J. Am. Dent. Assoc.* **29**, 1420.

KOPEL H. M. and BATTERMAN S. C. (1976) The retentive ability of various cementing agents for polycarbonate crowns. *J. Dent. Child.* **43**, 333.

McCONVILLE R. S. and TONN E. M. (1967) A method of restoring deciduous anterior teeth. *J. Am. Dent. Assoc.* **75**, 617.

MUHLER J. C., SPEAR L. B. jun., BIXLER D. and STOOKEY G. K. (1967) The arrestment of incipient dental caries in adults after the use of three different forms of SnF$_2$ therapy: results after 30 months. *J. Am. Dent. Assoc.* **75**, 1402.

NITKIN D. A., ROSENBERG N. M., and YAARA A. M. (1977) An improved technique for the retention of polycarbonate crowns. *J. Dent. Child.* **44**, 108.

NORDSTROM D. O., WEI S. H. Y. and JOHNSON R. (1974) Use of stannous fluoride for indirect pulp capping. *J. Am. Dent. Assoc.* **88**, 997.

SAKAMAKI S. T. and BAHN A. N. (1969) Effect of orthodontic banding on localized oral lactobacilli. *J. Dent. Res.* **47**, 275.

SHERMAN G. jun., BUGG J. L. jun. and CARRUTH K. R. (1966) Restoration of primary incisors with acrylic jacket crowns—One appointment procedure. *J. Dent. Child.* **33**, 182.

SILVERSTONE L. M. (1971) The effect of topical application of calcifying fluids on human dental enamel *in vitro*. *J. Int. Assoc. Dent. Child.* **2**, 39.

RECOMMENDED READING

DOYLE W. A. (1967) Esthetic restoration of deciduous incisors: a new Class IV preparation. *J. Am. Dent. Assoc.* **74,** 82.

MINK J. R. and HILL C. J. (1973) Crowns for anterior primary teeth. *Dent. Clin. North Am.* **17:1,** 85.

SNAWDER K. D. (1977) Dental caries and related problems in the nursing child. In: *Current Therapy in Dentistry*, Vol. 6. St Louis, C. V. Mosby Co.

STEWART R. E., LUKE L. S. and PIKE A. R. (1974) Preformed polycarbonate crowns for the restoration of anterior teeth. *J. Am. Dent. Assoc.* **88,** 103.

CHAPTER 10

THE CLASS 5 LESION

DIAGNOSIS

THE Class 5 lesion is considered separately from those lesions that appear in developmental pits, which were discussed in Chapter 6. It occurs on the gingival one-third of the tooth and its aetiology can be directly linked with poor oral hygiene, since this area is accessible to the toothbrush; indeed, it is probably the only lesion that can be prevented by toothbrushing alone. Dietary habits, such as mint sucking and gum chewing, can also be an aetiological factor. The initial decalcification is caused by the breakdown of sucrose-containing foods, held in close proximity to the buccal surfaces of the posterior teeth for long periods.

Diagnosis of Class 5 lesions should present no problem since they are clinically obvious to exploration. However, if the practitioner examines the patient in too hasty a manner he may fail to diagnose cervical caries in those areas that require retraction of soft tissues to improve access and visibility. Such areas are the buccal surfaces of maxillary molars and the lingual surfaces of mandibular molars.

Class 5 lesions are more prevalent in the more distally positioned teeth; therefore the first primary molars are affected less than second primary and first and second permanent molars. The most likely reason for this is the better accessibility to the toothbrush of anterior teeth. Also food debris from the distobuccal surface of the maxillary first and second permanent molars may be retained due to inactive tongue and cheek muscles. Further, the first permanent molar erupts at a time when parental control of the child's dietary habits is diminished now that the child is of school age. Hennon et al. (1969) found that decay in primary canines was most often located on the buccal surfaces in the 18–39 month age groups. It could be that a neonatal hypoplastic defect commonly seen on the buccal surface of mandibular primary canines acts as an area for plaque retention and subsequent caries development in these young children whose oral hygiene is often neglected. Furthermore, many parents do not realize the need to brush the teeth of infants.

CONSIDERATIONS IN TREATMENT

The treatment of these lesions needs to be discussed in broader terms than a mere description of the design of the Class 5 cavity. This is because the Class 5 lesion, particularly when it occurs in all quadrants of the mouth simultaneously, is almost pathognomonic of a severe dietary and/or oral hygiene problem. This history and any projected changes in patient behaviour must be taken into consideration when operative treatment is performed.

Regular examination and preventive care, including topical fluoride application, should permit the practitioner to diagnose the lesion in its early stages. At this time the initial decalcification may present as a white chalkiness or brown stain limited to the enamel. When the patient is a regular attender with a low past decay experience and there is no other decay in the offending teeth, it is appropriate to scale the decalcified areas, polish the surface smooth, and apply topical fluoride to arrest the incipient lesion. However, if the lesion extends to the dentine, a Class 5 cavity should be prepared. At the same time vigorous attempts should be made to improve the oral home care. Disclosing tablets and solutions can demonstrate the plaque to both child and parents. Toothbrushing instruction should be given, followed by an assessment of the child's ability to brush that area. With young children, particularly those of pre-school age, it is necessary for the parent to perform the brushing (Starkey, 1961; McClure, 1966). Children under 7 years do not have the manual dexterity to use a toothbrush correctly; and their parents should be instructed in the scrub-brush method, which is most effective for plaque removal in the primary dentition (Sangnes et al., 1972).

When gingival decalcification is occurring in many areas, a fluoride mouth rinse should be recommended. However, this is appropriate only for children of school age who can rinse effectively. The parent and child should be warned of the severity of the problem. Such multiple decalcified areas should be re-evaluated earlier than the normal six-month recall period. This conservative approach is justified on the basis that the patient has been and will continue to be a regular attender. In that case the decalcification can be interpreted as the result of a lapse in oral hygiene and dietary habits. Alterations in the child's daily toothbrushing routine can easily be caused by such things as parental illness or breakdown of the marriage, while an increase in the eating of sweets may be attributed to the child's introduction to the sweet shop by his newly acquired school friends.

The treatment of multiple areas of gingival decalcification in a new patient must also allow for any other caries present. Since access to the Class 5 lesion can be as difficult for the operator as it is for the child's toothbrush, it is more difficult to place an excellent restoration and there is less chance of the restoration being well cleansed. The longevity of a Class 5 restoration is thus put in doubt, and the patient's dental age must be considered to determine if the Class 5 lesion could be better treated by a method other than cavity preparation and restoration. A pre-school child who presents with extensive gingival decalcification may have Class 2 lesions in the same teeth. The operator may place both Class 2 and Class 5 restorations in the primary molars of this pre-school child and expect them to last more than six years until the premolars erupt. This approach may result in disappointment if the restorations fail. Perhaps the child's oral hygiene and diet have not improved or the Class 2 cavity design has encouraged marginal deterioration (*see also* Chapter 7); this is most likely to occur in mandibular first primary molars (Castaldi, 1957; MacRae et al., 1962). Much time could have been saved for both patient and practitioner if a stainless-steel crown had been placed initially.

The orthodontic implications of cervical caries in the first permanent molar must be considered by the practitioner. When extensive lesions are present close to the eruption time of these teeth, their longevity is in question. If a malocclusion would be best treated by extractions, teeth with a poor long-term prognosis should always be considered as possible choices for extraction. Orthodontic extraction of the first permanent molars may be considered for a child with a Class 1 skeletal base, an Angle's Class 1 molar relationship, a full complement of permanent teeth, none of which are developing ectopically, and minimal crowding (Tulley and Campbell, 1970). Such a serious and far-reaching decision should be made in conjunction with an orthodontist. Treatment planning in relation to the first permanent molar has been well described (Crabb and Rock, 1971). Unfortunately, removing four permanent molars under general anaesthesia is often more attractive to the busy practitioner than managing a difficult child while placing extensive restorations or stainless-steel crowns. However, the apparently easy route may not be in the child's best dental or emotional interests. Each child must be carefully evaluated and treatment must be performed in the best interests of the child, and not for the convenience of the dentist.

THE CLASS 5 CAVITY

Once cavity preparation has been undertaken, every effort should be made to place a restoration which will be long-lasting. Rubber dam application is strongly recommended, mainly because of the improved access afforded. Outline form should be limited to the carious lesion and any adjacent decalcified areas. Decalcified areas and carious defects occurring 2 mm apart should be included in the same cavity outline as extension for prevention, rather than as separate lesions. The Class 5 cavity may be kidney-shaped; a gently curved outline form is as acceptable as a square, sharp outline form at the mesial and distal margins. The No. 2 inverted cone bur* can be used to cut the cavity 0·5 mm into the dentine.

Dentinal undercuts for mechanical retention will be placed if the inverted cone bur is used. Any remaining caries can be removed with a slow running round No. 2 bur; a pulp protecting base should be used in deep areas of the cavity. Additional retention can be obtained by placing small retention pits with the No. 2L plain cut fissure bur† at the mesial and distal gingival-pulpal point angles. The gingival enamel margin should follow a regular curve parallel to the gingival attachment unless the lesion extends subgingivally. The margins should be trimmed with hatchets to ensure that no enamel unsupported by dentine remains. This is especially important because of the possible decalcification adjacent to the lesion.

Amalgam alloy is the material of choice when improvement in oral hygiene and dietary habits is expected. Since that will not always be the case, a fluoride-impregnated cement is recommended as a semi-permanent restoration (Jinks, 1963) (*see* Chapter 12). It will normally last at least two years and in many instances considerably longer. An advantage of this semi-permanent restoration is the continued fluoride release, which outweighs the dissolution that occurs with time. This fluoride release is most beneficial to margins that are both susceptible to further caries and finished somewhat less than perfectly due to difficult access. With time, age, and increased eruption, there may be improvements in the access, oral hygiene, and dietary habits, and the restoration can then be replaced with amalgam alloy.

REFERENCES

CASTALDI C. R. (1957) Analysis of some operative procedures currently being used in paedodontics. *J. Can. Dent. Assoc.* 23, 377.

CRABB J. J. and ROCK W. P. (1971) Treatment planning in relation to the first permanent molar. *Br. Dent. J.* 131, 396.

HENNON D. K., STOOKEY G. K. and MUHLER J. C. (1969) Prevalence and distribution of dental caries in pre-school children. *J. Am. Dent. Assoc.* 79, 1405.

JINKS G. M. (1963) Fluoride-impregnated cements and their effect on the activity of interproximal caries. *J. Dent. Child.* 30, 87.

MACRAE P. D., ZACHERL W. and CASTALDI C. R. (1962) Study of defects in Class II dental amalgam restorations in deciduous molars. *J. Can. Dent. Assoc.* 28, 491.

MCCLURE D. B. (1966) A comparison of toothbrushing techniques for the pre-school child. *J. Dent. Child.* 33, 205.

---

* No. 2 inverted cone bur = No. 35 American.

† No. 2L plain cut fissure bur = No. 170L American.

SANGNES G., ZACHRISSON B. and GJERMO P. (1972) Effectiveness of vertical and horizontal brushing techniques in plaque removal. *J. Dent. Child.* **39**, 94.

STARKEY P. E. (1961) Instructions to parents for brushing the child's teeth. *J. Dent. Child.* **28**, 42.

TULLEY W. J. and CAMPBELL A. C. (1970) *A Manual of Practical Orthodontics*, 3rd ed. Bristol, John Wright, pp. 101–108.

RECOMMENDED READING

CRABB J. J. and ROCK W. P. (1971) Treatment planning in relation to the first permanent molar. *Br. Dent. J.* **131**, 396.

JINKS G. M. (1963) Fluoride-impregnated cements and their effect on the activity of interproximal caries. *J. Dent. Child.* **30**, 87.

CHAPTER 11

MATRICES

JUSTIFICATION FOR USE

RESTORATION of the primary dentition prevents space loss by maintaining arch length; carious teeth should thus be restored to their original dimensions and contour whenever possible. Restorations should be provided whose contour discourages the retention of food debris, materia alba and plaque so that they will not be detrimental to gingival health or encourage recurrent caries. To fulfil these objectives, a well adapted and contoured matrix must be used when restoring Class 2, 3 and 4 cavities. This recommendation applies both to permanent and temporary restorations, since the requirements are the same.

Maintaining correct arch length by properly contoured interproximal restorations is especially important in the young child since tooth movement accompanies the transition from primary to permanent dentition. The first permanent molars often erupt into a cusp-to-cusp relationship; this occlusion may then change to an Angle Class I by differential mesial migration, either at the expense of the mandibular primate space,* if present, or when the primary molars are lost (Baume, 1950). There is more leeway space† in the mandibular than in the maxillary arch since the mandibular second primary molar is larger mesiodistally than its maxillary counterpart. When the primary molars are lost, this small discrepancy allows the mandibular first permanent molar to migrate farther mesially than its maxillary counterpart; hence an Angle Class I relationship is obtained. Undercontoured maxillary Class 2 restorations may permit early mesial migration of the maxillary first permanent molar from a cusp-to-cusp relationship into an Angle Class 2 before any mandibular leeway space has been used; steep cuspal inclines may then prevent any spontaneous alteration of this iatrogenic malocclusion (Davey, 1967).

Undercontoured interproximal restorations with either flat or open contacts encourage retention of food debris, materia alba, and plaque. Also, restorations with overhanging margins may deprive the gingivae of mechanical stimulation, besides providing an area for plaque retention. Nothing is more discouraging than to see an iatrogenic gingivitis in an otherwise healthy mouth, when the cause is related to improper use of matrices.

* Primate Space—*see* Glossary.
† Leeway Space—*see* Glossary.

MATRICES FOR PRIMARY MOLARS

The matrix band must be compatible with the size of the primary molar and the child's oral environment. It must have good adaptation to the interproximal margins of the cavity, enough stability to withstand the pressures of condensation, and retention to resist any effort of the child to dislodge it. Although it is impossible to

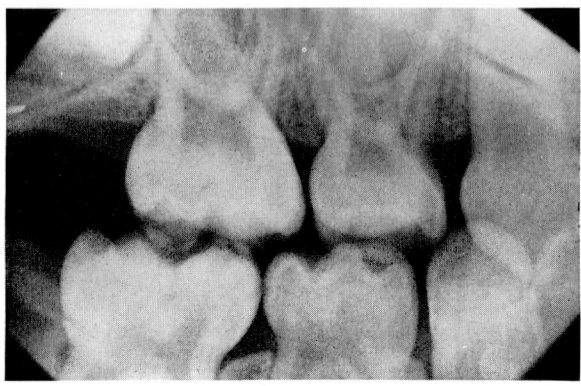

a

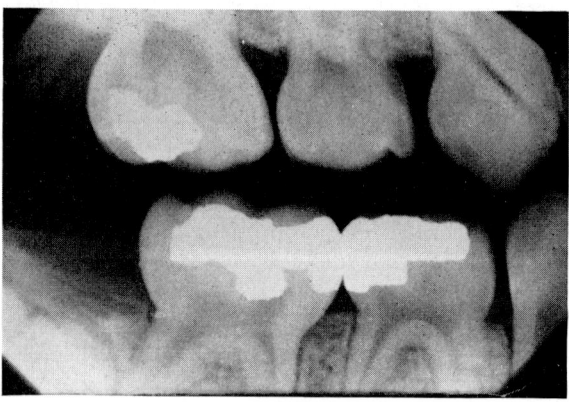

b

Fig. 58.—*a*, Preoperative bite-wing of a 3-year-old. *b*, Postoperative bite-wing demonstrating correct interproximal contour of Class 2 amalgam restorations. The distobuccal cusp on the first primary molar has been overlayed in amalgam.

reproduce interproximal contour precisely, the best results are obtained when the matrix is contoured, wedged, and supported (Phillips et al., 1956). The ideal interproximal contour is shown in *Figs. 58, 59*; there should be smooth contour and a positive contact with the adjacent tooth.

WEDGING

A wedge must be used with any of the matrices to be described so that a cervical overhang of restorative material is avoided (Phillips et al., 1956). The correctly placed wedge improves the cervical adaptation of the band to the cavity walls and stabilizes the band to the extent that composition support is often unnecessary. The

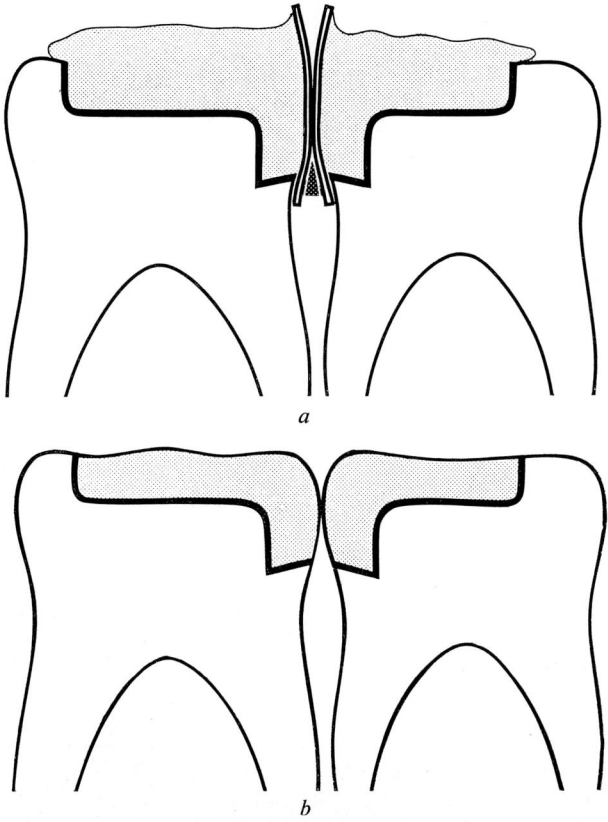

Fig. 59.—a, Line diagram depicting correctly wedged matrices for adjacent Class 2 primary molar restorations. *b*, Line diagram depicting correct interproximal contour of adjacent Class 2 primary molar restorations.

wedge can be inserted from either the lingual or the buccal, depending on ease of access; occasionally both a buccally and lingually placed wedge are necessary to obtain good adaptation. Pressure is recommended to spring the teeth slightly apart and thus help ensure a tight contact following wedge removal. The thickness of band material must be compensated for by using heavy condensation

111

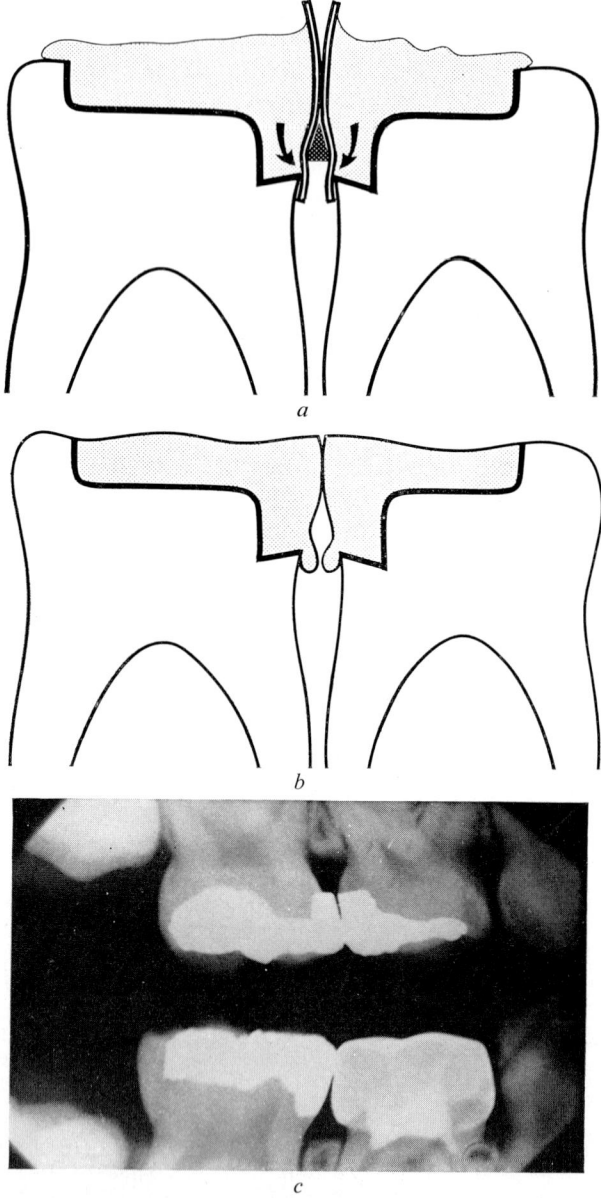

Fig. 60.—a, Incorrect location of wedge for adjacent Class 2 restorations. *b*, This results in a flat contour and gingival overhang. Note also the undercarved marginal ridge area. *c*, Bite-wing demonstrates flat contour of D and an overhang on E, resulting from improperly wedged matrices. Note also the undercarved marginal ridge.

112

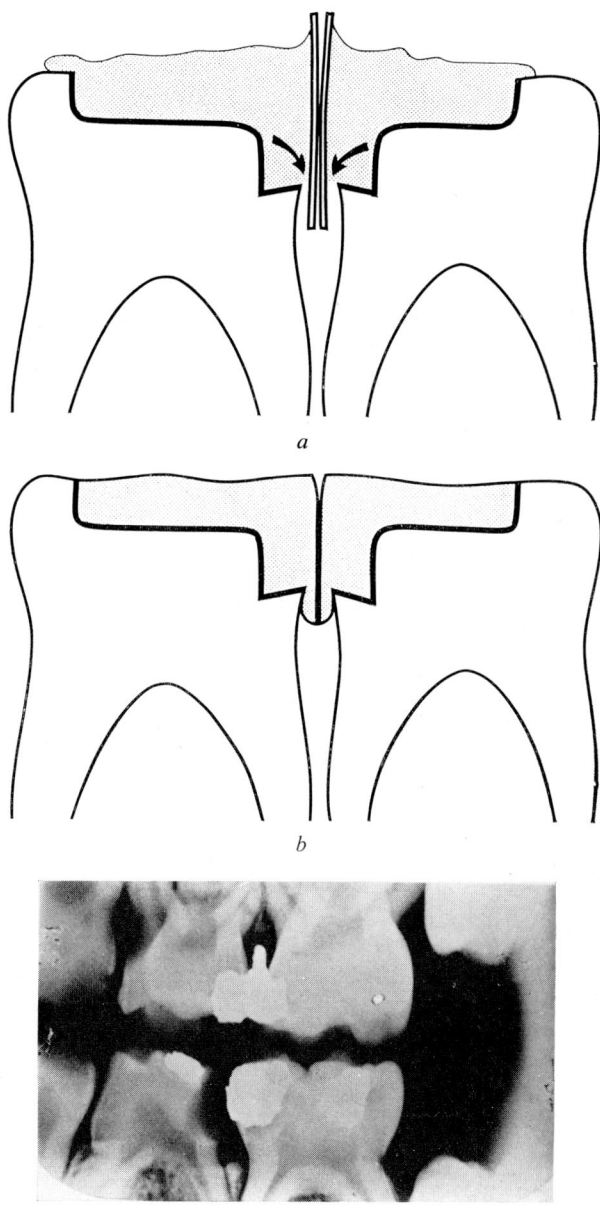

Fig. 61.—a, Failure to use a wedge in adjacent Class 2 primary molars invites the production of an overhang. *b*, Resulting overhang. *c*, Bite-wing demonstrates gross overhang from failure to use a wedge or carve the interproximal area.

113

pressures and separation by positive wedge placement. If the wedge is placed too far occlusally, a flat contact may result with an over-hang gingivally (*Fig. 60*). Failure to use any wedge invariably results in a gingival overhang (*Fig. 61*). The Wizard wedge (Slim Jim Size)* is compatible with the size and anatomy of primary molars.

Adequate anaesthesia is required to place a matrix and wedge effectively and painlessly. Local anaesthesia will probably have been used for cavity preparation. In addition, routinely used

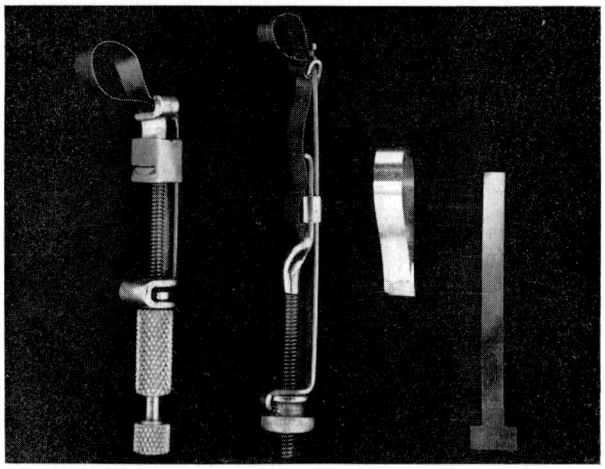

Fig. 62.—Available matrices for primary molars. *Right to left:* T band, Custom-made orthodontic band, Child-size Siqueland, Child-size Tofflemire.

palatal and long buccal anaesthesia (in upper and lower arch, respectively) assures the operator that all procedures can be per-formed painlessly. Topical anaesthesia can be used as an alternative.

The following posterior matrices are commonly used:
1. T Band.
2. Custom-made Orthodontic Band.
3. Tofflemire or Siqueland (*Fig. 62*).

1. *T Band*

The T band can be purchased prepunched in different sizes† or can be custom-made from strips of brass or German silver alloy.‡ The

---

* Wizard Wedges—Wm. Getz Corporation, Chicago, Illinois, U.S.A. Available from Amalgamated Dental Co., 26 Broadwick St., London.
† P.N. Conduit Inc., Action, Massachusetts, U.S.A. Dr. Levitt's T Band—Claudius Ash Co. Ltd., London.
‡ Claudius Ash Co. Ltd., London.

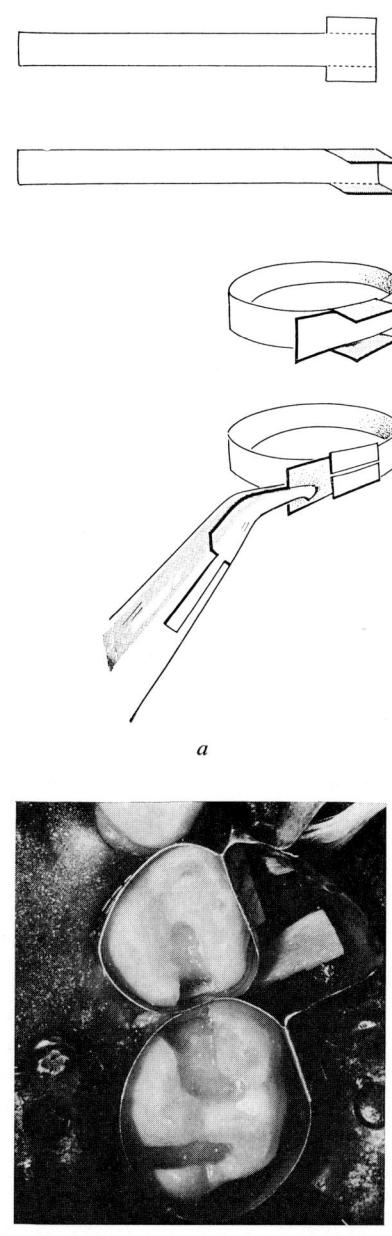

a

b

Fig. 63.—a, T band formation. *b*, T bands placed on adjacent primary molars.

115

band is fabricated either before or after cavity preparation; a T-shaped metal band is cut with the proportion shown in *Fig. 63*. The short arms of the T are folded over to form a loop; the free end is passed through the loop, ensuring that it is on the buccal side of the band, and freely sliding. The band is placed on the tooth so that it passes below the level of the gingival seat of the proximal box. The 110 plier* applied to the free arm tightens the band; at the same time, finger pressure stabilizes it. Once tightened, the band's dimensions are maintained by bending the free sliding arm back on itself; the folded-over short arms of the T act as a fulcrum. This can be done either inside or outside the mouth. Excess band material is then cut with scissors. The band can also be tightened on a trial and error basis out of the mouth; this need not require the use of a 110 plier, but necessitates more attempts at reinsertion.

The band is cut if it impinges on the gingivae; this commonly occurs on the lingual surface of first primary molars. It is then contoured with a 114 or 137 plier out of the mouth. After reinsertion, it is wedged and checked for adaptation and retention before placement of the restoration. The T band is often difficult to use either because of insufficient anaesthesia or inadequate contouring and wedging.

In removing the T band, the loop is first undone and the wedge removed so that the band is loose. The band is then cut close to the marginal ridge, and the remaining interproximal band material is grasped with the 110 plier or locking cotton tweezers and withdrawn in a buccolingual direction, sliding it through the contact area. A condenser can be used to lightly hold the marginal ridge area. It will be very difficult to remove the band occlusally if it has been properly contoured; occlusal withdrawal invites marginal ridge fracture. The brass prepunched T band is recommended over all others for routine use in paedodontics by the general practitioner because of its ease of use.

2. *Custom-made Orthodontic Band*

This is similar in size and shape to the T band, and can be prepared either before or after cavity preparation. A one and one-half inch long strip of 3/16 by 0·0020 orthodontic steel band material is spot welded to form a loop larger than the average sized primary molar. This loop is placed on the tooth; where necessary a tight contact can be sprung open by a wedge to allow the loop to be placed. A posterior band-forming plier† is placed on the buccal side over the

---

* 110 Plier—Unitek Corporation, Monrovia, California, U.S.A. Available from Orthomax Ltd., Queens House, Queens Road, Bradford, Yorks., England.
† Unitek Band Forming Plier (Double Beak Posterior) No. 800-105, Unitek Corporation, Monrovia, California, U.S.A.

top edge and under the lower edge of the band material; by acti-
vating the plier, the band is drawn tightly against the tooth. The
(Howe) 110 plier can also be used to draw the loop tight. It is
removed and spot welded to maintain this accurately adapted
contour; alternatively, the free ends can be riveted with the 141
plier* (McDonald, 1974). Excess band material, which may impinge
on buccal tissues, is cut with scissors away from the second spot
weld.

Following cavity preparation the band is tried on the tooth and
contoured if necessary with a 114 or 137 plier. A wedge, used to
ensure adequate gingival fit of the band, also assists in stability. To
remove the band after placement and finishing of the restoration, a
plastic instrument (e.g. Hollenbach carver) is passed between the
tooth and band material on the buccal side close to the spot weld.
While the band is stabilized with finger pressure, the spot weld is
broken by drawing the instrument buccally. The importance of
using the correct amount of spot welding to join the band is now
evident; this is best achieved on a trial and error basis. The wedge
is removed, and as with the T band, the band is withdrawn in a
buccolingual direction.

A major disadvantage of the custom-made orthodontic band is
the expense of a spot welder. Those in exclusive paedodontic practice
are encouraged to use this method routinely since the spot welder
may also be used for stainless-steel crowns, emergency treatment of
fractured incisors, and minor tooth movement. Bands of different
sizes can be fabricated on a die by a trained dental assistant, and
the appropriate size can then be selected. This minimizes clinical
time.

3. *Tofflemire or Siqueland*

These can also be used for the primary dentition, although narrow
sized band material† (5 mm compared to 6 mm) is recommended to
prevent excessive gingival trauma and to improve retention of the
matrix. The main advantage of these bands and retainers is that
the clinician may feel proficient with them since they are commonly
used for adults. An advantage of the Tofflemire is that, as with the
T band and custom-made orthodontic bands, the band material can
be removed in a buccolingual direction. The Tofflemire will also
require wedging; this may not always be the case with the Siqueland
retainer, although wedging is recommended whenever possible.

These advantages are outweighed on several counts. First, the
Siqueland has to be removed occlusally, which invites marginal

---

* S. S. White Company, London.
† Tofflemire—narrow size band material, Wm. Getz Corporation, Chicago,
Illinois, U.S.A. Siqueland Narrow Retainer with 5 mm band material—
Amalgamated Dental Co., 26 Broadwick St., London.

ridge fracture, as described earlier. Second, compared to the T band and custom-made orthodontic band, there is additional bulk in the child's mouth, which may rest against lip, cheek and tongue. The additional tactile stimuli increase salivation; also the retaining arms may annoy the child so that he will dislodge the band, often just when the alloy is to be inserted. Both of these disadvantages are eliminated when the rubber dam is in place. Third, the retainer part of these matrices is bulky in the child's small mouth. Also, since the matrices may impinge on a rubber dam clamp, the clamp sometimes has to be removed and replaced by the matrix band, which then serves to retract the rubber dam (Jinks, 1966).

GENERAL CONSIDERATIONS

Final selection of matrix band must be left to the individual practitioner. Whichever band he selects, he should use a mirror and an explorer to test the marginal adaptation of the band to the cavity walls before inserting the restoration (*Fig. 64*). Any discrepancies should be corrected before the restoration is placed, unless those areas can be adequately contoured postoperatively.

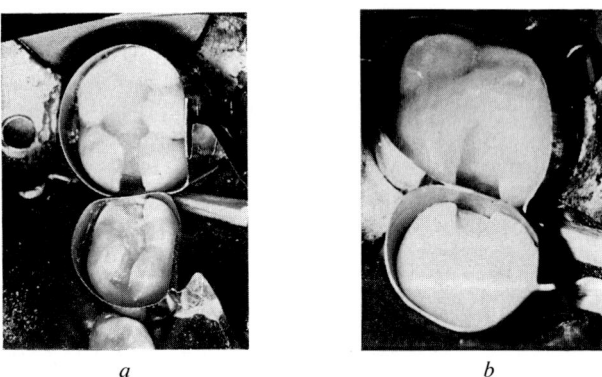

a   *b*

Fig. 64.—a, T bands. *b*, Spot welded orthodontic bands.

Some clinicians recommend placement of adjacent Class 2 restorations at separate visits to obtain the best interproximal contour. However, there is no evidence to contradict placing two adjacent Class 2 restorations in primary teeth at the same appointment, provided each restoration is supported by its own matrix. In fact, such treatment may remove the need for a second visit by the patient and a second injection for that particular quadrant. When adjacent interproximal lesions are restored at the same visit, the alloy should be condensed alternately in the interproximal boxes

(Hill, 1973). This prevents one restoration from being over-contoured and the other undercontoured.

Unfortunately, not all Class 2 lesions lend themselves to ideal cavity preparation; adjacent deep interproximal lesions which have been untreated for some time have contact areas that are very deep gingivally since space loss has already occurred. Since matrix application is difficult in these instances, floss should be passed between the adjacent bands before the wedge is inserted. After the alloy has been placed and the wedge and band removed, the floss can dispose of any overhanging gingival excess before the alloy is set. Rubber dam will also retract the papillae so that postoperative carving is occasionally possible. Alternatively, a gold knife or curette can be used once the alloy is set.

ANTERIOR MATRICES

Where alloy is used, as in Class 3 distal cavities in primary canines, a wedged metal matrix is essential to provide strength to resist amalgam condensation. A flat straight piece of band material* about 20 mm long is recommended. It should be looped around the

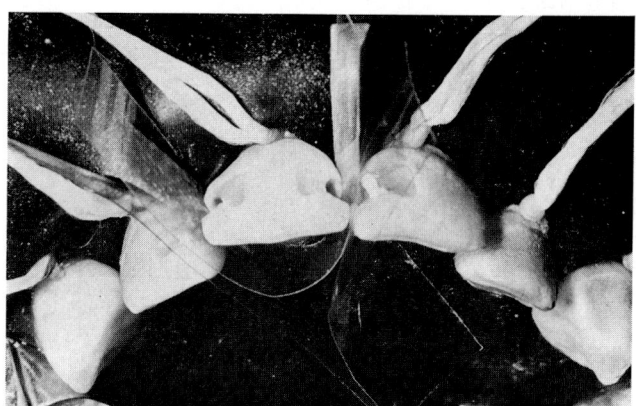

Fig. 65.—Wedged celluloid matrices.

tooth to be treated and the tooth adjacent to the lesion so that the band appears S-shaped when viewed from the occlusal. In this way, there will be access for condensation of the restorative material and good support of the band to prevent displacement during condensation.

---

* 5 mm Dentatus Matrix Band, A. B. Dentatus, Hagerstein, Sweden or Siqueland Matrix Band—Child Size, Amalgamated Dental Co., 26 Broadwick St., London.

A wedged celluloid matrix is advised for Class 3 cavities when resin is used (*Fig.* 65). One advantage is that the operator can see through the translucent matrix to determine whether the resin is adequately condensed and contoured. Furthermore, no loose remnants of metal can be deposited within the resin if celluloid is used.

Class 4 cavities present a special problem because the incisal edge requires replacement. A wedged celluloid matrix is one alternative; however, there will be an excess of material incisally, which will require additional finishing. The other alternative requires considerably more preparation, but affords support for the incisal edge; therefore, less finishing is required and a better surface of the restoration is achieved, particularly if composites are used. This method involves the fabrication of an open-faced celluloid crown which may need wedging for support, or an open-faced stainless-steel crown. The buccal surface of each crown is open to permit access for placement of the restorative material.

REFERENCES

BAUME L. J. (1950) Physiological tooth migration and its significance for the development of occlusion. 1. The biogenetic course of the deciduous dentition. *J. Dent. Res.* **29**, 123.

DAVEY K. W. (1967) Effect of premature loss of primary molars on the anteroposterior position of maxillary first permanent molars and other maxillary teeth. *J. Dent. Child.* **34**, 383.

HILL C. J. (1973) Approximating Class II amalgam restorations for primary molars. *Dent. Clin. North Am.* **17:1**, 77.

JINKS G. M. (1966) Rubber dam technique in pedodontics. *Dent. Clin. North Am.* 327.

MCDONALD R. E. (1974) *Dentistry for the Child and Adolescent.* St. Louis, C. V. Mosby Co., p. 200.

PHILLIPS R. W., CASTALDI C. R., RINARD J. R. and CLARK R. J. (1956) Proximal contour of Class II amalgam restorations made with various matrix band techniques. *J. Am. Dent. Assoc.* **53**, 391.

RECOMMENDED READING

HILL C. J. (1973) Approximating Class II amalgam restorations for primary molars. *Dent. Clin. North Am.* **17:1**, 77.

CHAPTER 12

DENTAL MATERIALS

THIS chapter supplements previous chapters on cavity preparation and matrices. It is by no means complete in its description of dental materials. No attempt will be made to discuss in detail the physical and chemical properties; rather, their use will be justified and described as they relate to paediatric operative dentistry.

FLUORIDE
(IN PAEDIATRIC OPERATIVE DENTISTRY)

Teeth or quadrants of teeth isolated during operative dentistry should be polished with a fluoride prophylaxis paste and should also receive a topical fluoride application. These and other ways of using fluoride in operative dentistry are described in this chapter and in Chapter 14. The fluoride solution is best applied as soon as cavity preparations are complete, so that adjacent interproximal surfaces are protected. The margins of the restoration also require protection, and fluoride, either in solution or in the form of paste or both, should be applied to the completed restorations. This is supplementary to the normal applications every six months.

Another possible means of increasing topical fluoride exposure is to use a fluoride rinse as the mouthwash. Because of the dangers of fluoride overdosage, this should be used only in those children who are old enough to expectorate. One potential advantage of using the fluoride rinse is based on the fact that those children who require the most visits for operative dentistry are the ones who require the most preventive care; and they will be receiving the additional fluoride exposure.

PULP-PROTECTING BASES

A base is recommended in those cavities where removal of caries leaves the pulpal floor and/or axial wall of the cavity in close proximity to the pulp. The main purpose of the base is to minimize thermal insult to the pulp through the restorative material. Such a base may help stimulate the formation of secondary dentine as in indirect pulp treatment (Chapters 15 and 17). These recommendations apply both to primary and permanent teeth. Contrary to previously accepted teaching, there is evidence to indicate that deep lesions in primary teeth benefit from pulp-protecting bases (Kerkhove et al., 1967; Traubman, 1967; Geller et al., 1971).

121

The small dimensions of primary molar cavity preparations require that a thin layer of base be used which can not only withstand the condensation pressures of amalgam but also leave sufficient room for the restorative material. A hard-setting calcium hydroxide base (e.g. Dycal*) fulfils these requirements; pure calcium hydroxide powder mixed with water or saline is not recommended since it does not adequately withstand condensation. This also applies to zinc oxide, even though it is effective in stimulating secondary dentine formation (Kerkhove et al., 1967). On the other hand, resin-bonded zinc oxides (e.g. Kalzinol,† Timurex‡) can be recommended, although the handling properties of Dycal are in this author's opinion superior. Zinc phosphate cements are contra-indicated because of the acidity which may adversely affect the pulp.

The decision to place a pulp-protecting base must lie with the individual practitioner. Although the pulp may have already responded to the carious lesion by laying down secondary dentine, this should not discourage the placement of a base which may stimulate further pulp protection. As a rule, whenever the pink outline of the pulp shows through the cavity walls a base is mandatory; this applies also to dark-stained dentine left in the depths of the cavity. However, it is unnecessary to line out the cavity to ideal dimensions; a minimum of 0·5 mm of Dycal is recommended. Enamel walls must be free from the base. Additional bulk of restorative material is provided by the deeper cavities and this is advantageous in Class 2 cavities.

VARNISHES

Varnishes are synthetic or natural resins in a chloroform solvent (e.g. Copalite).

The purposes of the varnish are (in order of importance):

1. To reduce marginal microleakage.

2. To minimize ion diffusion.

3. To protect the pulp by sealing dentinal tubules against acid penetration.

The dye penetration study of Going (1964) demonstrated that Copalite reduces marginal microleakage around amalgam alloy restorations. This is especially important in the immediate post-insertion period, before any amalgam breakdown products fill the marginal discrepancy that always exists between enamel wall and restorative material. The staining within the enamel which occurs close to the margins of amalgam alloy restorations is caused by ion diffusion (particularly of silver and tin) from amalgam to tooth;

---

* Dycal—Amalgamated Dental Co., 26 Broadwick St., London.
† Kalzinol—Amalgamated Dental Co., 26 Broadwick St., London.
‡ Timurex Cement—Interstate Dental Co. Inc., New York.

this is minimized by varnish. The pulp-protecting properties of a varnish are negligible when compared to Dycal; certainly they are no substitute for pulp-protecting bases. However, if a zinc phosphate cement is required as well as a calcium hydroxide base, varnish should be applied before the zinc phosphate cement base is placed, to minimize acid penetration. Varnishes are applied to the floor and walls of the cavity by a fine cotton pellet or a camel hair paintbrush. As the chloroform evaporates, the resin contracts and leaves small voids. Reapplication after a 20-second evaporation period is indicated to fill these voids. It is impossible to avoid coating the enamel walls with varnish. However, this is of no clinical significance since the varnish thickness is 4 microns and one purpose is to reduce marginal microleakage around amalgam restorations.

Varnishes are recommended prior to amalgam restorations and cementation of crowns on vital teeth. They should not be used prior to any resin restoration (either simple or composite) since polymerization is altered and the resin is softened. Some commercially available products incorporate fluoride within the varnish. In the absence of any clinical studies known to this author, the incorporation of fluoride into the varnish must be considered as empirical. Presumably it is hoped that the fluoride will prevent or minimize recurrent decay.

CEMENTS

Cement bases can be used to:
1. Line out large cavities in young permanent teeth.
2. Cover pulp dressings prior to amalgam placement.
3. Cement crowns.

In cavity preparations (indications 1 and 2) the zinc phosphate cement is used to provide resistance to condensation of amalgam alloy. It can be used to partially fill very large cavities in young permanent teeth where a calcium hydroxide pulp-protecting base has already been placed. The dimensions of the cavity may require so much amalgam alloy to be placed that it would be impossible to fill it before the alloy had set. A thick mix of zinc phosphate cement is recommended for such cavity preparations since this reduces the amount of free acid.

Zinc phosphate cement or resin-bonded zinc oxides are recommended for cementing stainless-steel crowns. When the pulp is vital the deep areas of the preparation should be covered with Dycal; a varnish should also be used prior to cementing stainless-steel crowns on vital teeth. This is unnecessary if pulp therapy has been performed. Cementation of crowns is described in Chapters 9 and 12.

INTERMEDIATE RESTORATIVE MATERIALS

These materials are required to hold medications adjacent to the pulp between appointments. They are also needed in the indirect pulp treatment of deep carious lesions (Chapter 17). Their ability to seal the tooth and prevent leakage is most important in avoiding contamination of the pulp; since the material must withstand occlusal forces and whenever possible restore the tooth to correct contour and function, a matrix band is essential. If necessary, the material should be supported by an orthodontic band to ensure retention. The concept that a temporary restoration need not be as meticulously placed as a permanent one is dangerous since the ability of the temporary restoration to prevent leakage is most important.

Of these materials, the most commonly used are cements, zinc oxides (resin-bonded), zinc oxides, and gutta-percha. In clinical evaluations of indirect pulp treatment in primary and young permanent teeth (Hutchins and Parker, 1972; Weaver et al., 1972), reinforced resin-bonded zinc oxides have produced the best results for periods up to two years.

Cements: In addition to routine use as cement bases, these materials can be reinforced by adding amalgam filings to the powder. Such reinforced zinc phosphate cement proved to be a satisfactory intermediate material in teeth treated by indirect pulp treatment (Weaver et al., 1972); of course a calcium hydroxide protecting base is required initially, followed by varnish in these vital teeth.

Fluoride-impregnated cements (Jinks, 1963) can also be used as a temporary dressing or intermediate restorative material. Sodium silicofluoride powder is added to the phosphate cement powder before mixing. Amalgam filings can also be added to increase radiopacity. Jinks (1963) feels that one advantage of this cement is constant fluoride release from the material. He feels that this may benefit other teeth, in addition to the immediately adjacent enamel. This may be of immense value in patients who have multiple lesions and poor oral hygiene, and who are candidates for indirect pulp treatment. This material is also useful in treating Class 5 lesions (*see* Chapter 10).

Resin-bonded zinc oxides: Of the various commercially available products, IRM* has been clinically proven to be superior (Hutchins and Parker, 1972; Weaver et al., 1972). Ninety-five per cent of teeth treated by IRM were satisfactory after 18 months (Weaver et al., 1972). When chipping of the restoration from the margins did occur, usually enamel and not dentine was exposed (Hutchins and

---

* Intermediate Restorative Material—L. D. Caulk Co., Milwaukee, Wisconsin, available from Amalgamated Dental Co., 26 Broadwick St., London.

Parker, 1972). One advantage of IRM is its colour (white, blue or pink): the parent can be instructed to check periodically for the material's presence in those teeth where retention is in doubt. Other resin-bonded zinc oxides (e.g. Kalzinol, Timurex) can also be used.

Zinc oxides: These are ideal temporary restorations over the short term since they are non-injurious to the vital unexposed pulp and have good marginal seal initially. However, their crushing strength is low and this, in conjunction with a tendency to dissolve in the mouth, makes them unsuitable for periods exceeding two weeks. Furthermore the smell and taste of the eugenol are distressing to some children. Their routine use cannot be recommended in view of the improved properties of resin-bonded zinc oxides.

Gutta-percha: Although this material is biologically inert, its sealing ability is poor. This results in a material which is unsuitable for the retention of direct pulp medicaments; the ingress of saliva results in bacterial contamination which increases the chances of failure of vital pulp therapy (Hargreaves, 1969).

SILICATES

Silicate restorations are contra-indicated for routine use in primary and young permanent teeth because of the pulp irritation that results from the material's acidity and exothermia on setting. Their ability to cause pulp death in permanent teeth has been documented (Kaye, 1968). However, the enamel adjacent to silicate restorations rarely decays, even in caries-active patients, since the silicate restoration continually releases fluoride. This occurs even in the presence of the marginal deterioration, erosion and staining that are always seen with silicate restorations. It may therefore be a treatment possibility to use silicate restorations in the anterior teeth of caries-active patients who have failed to respond to preventive recommendations. However, almost all exposed dentine should be covered by a pulp-protecting base before a silicate restoration is placed. Cavity varnishes are not recommended since they inhibit fluoride uptake in adjacent enamel. Rubber dam should be used and the restoration left undisturbed during setting. It is covered with varnish for a minimum of 24 hours before finishing. Silicate restorations are not strong enough for use in Class 4 cavities.

RESINS

Acrylic resins are either simple (unfilled), such as Sevriton, composite (filled), such as Adaptic, or modified composites, a group which includes adhesives using acid conditioners and accelerators of polymerization. Fissure sealants (discussed in Chapter 14) belong to this third group. Improved retention and reduced microleakage can be obtained by the routine use of acid etching.

125

The simple, unfilled resins have been superseded in recent years by the development of composite resins. The composites are similar in composition to simple resins but exhibit improved qualities, particularly of increased hardness, reduced coefficient of thermal expansion, and improved abrasion resistance, which are partly attributable to the quartz filler. These tooth-coloured restorative materials are indicated in the anterior teeth for aesthetics. Commercial manufacturers have also recommended composite resins for the restoration of Class 1 and 2 cavities in posterior permanent teeth where aesthetics is of concern. Their use and manipulation will be described.

Simple Unfilled Resins

These can be used for the restoration of Class 3, 4 and 5 cavities in primary anterior teeth (incisors and canines). Despite their having some poor physical properties, the reader should not condemn simple unfilled resins, particularly since they have been clinically proven in primary incisors (Doyle, 1967). The material can be applied in bulk (bulk-packing) or incrementally (Nealon-Bead paint-on method). Bulk packing is contra-indicated for several reasons: the exothermia from setting irritates the pulp; it is difficult to condense the material into undercut areas of the preparation; the contour of the restoration is more difficult to control; and polymerization shrinkage is increased. These disadvantages do not apply to the Nealon-Bead method of application, which is preferred.

Application: Nealon-Bead method (for Sevriton).

After cavity preparation and acid etching, cavity seal should be applied; this primer increases the flow and wettability of the resin. Excess primer may cause a white line around the restoration, however. The monomer (liquid) and polymer (powder) are placed in separate clean dappen dishes. A fine camel hair paintbrush is dipped in monomer first, then polymer, and small increments are successively added to the preparation. The resin should be kept as moist as possible initially to help increase flow into undercut areas, which should be filled first. The restoration is then built up to correct contour using a wedged celluloid matrix as described in Chapter 10. Overfilling is desirable to compensate for polymerization shrinkage. After each increment is applied, the brush must be cleaned with gauze to prevent contamination of the monomer.

Finishing: During final polymerization, the resin is covered with protective film and left undisturbed until completely polymerized according to the manufacturer's recommendations. Sandpaper discs are used to contour accessible labial, lingual and incisal surfaces while linen strips refine the interproximal surface. Interproximal flashes of resin extending beyond the preparation are removed either

126

with a scalpel (No. 12 blade), a gold knife, or a curette. Vertical and horizontal lines simulating perikymata can be made within the resin with a large round bur run at slow speed; these help break up the reflected light and improve the aesthetics. During finishing procedures, heat is to be avoided; the use of low speeds and lubricant such as petroleum jelly are recommended.

Composites

Composite resins were quickly accepted by the dental profession because of dissatisfaction with silicates and simple unfilled resins. This acceptance occurred in the absence of clinical proof of the composite's ability to withstand the insults of the oral cavity. Their durability in the mouth over the short term (up to three years) has only recently been demonstrated (Phillips et al., 1971, 1973; Ribbons and Pearson, 1973).

Application: There are too many different types of composite resin, including the adhesives, for a description of their individual properties, advantages, or methods of application to be included here. However, even though composites are considered to be non-irritating to the pulp, the use of calcium hydroxide pulp-protecting bases is recommended in all teeth. Cavity varnishes are not recommended since they may alter resin polymerization. The materials should be manipulated according to the manufacturer's instructions. Frequently the materials supplied include an etching kit, a bonding agent consisting of a sealant-type unfilled resin, and the composite material. After etching, the bonding agent is placed with a paint-brush followed quickly by the composite. Elimination of air bubbles from the mix and insertion of the materials before polymerization require a well organized approach by the dental team. Generally they are bulk packed, Class 3 and 4 restorations being supported by a celluloid matrix. The use of rubber gingival stimulators or specially designed commercially available plastic or agate instruments is helpful to condense the material into the depths of the preparation; a pressure syringe can be used to inject the material into the cavity preparation. Metal instruments are not recommended since the composite may be stained by loose metal fragments. The material should be left undisturbed during polymerization. As with all restorative materials, the best results can be expected when the material is placed free of contamination using the rubber dam.

Finishing: Unlike silicate restoration, composite resins can usually be finished within five minutes of placing the restoration. Because the matrix (polymer) and filler of the composite resin have different hardness and abrasion resistance, any finishing will tend to produce a matt finish because of differential wear. Therefore every effort should be made during placement of the restoration to reproduce tooth contour accurately so that finishing is minimized.

Gross excess can be reduced with twelve-bladed tungsten carbide finishing burs run under water coolant at high speed. Small thin flashes of material can be fractured off using sharp tungsten carbide tipped hand instruments (e.g. gold knife, hatchets). White stones lubricated with petroleum jelly can be used to finish the restoration. Polishing with pumice or dark rubber cups is not recommended because of potential staining of the matt surface. Undoubtedly the best surface is produced when finishing is kept to a minimum.

Use in Class 2 Restorations: Mack (1970) described a technique for restoring conventially cut Class 2 primary molar preparations with Adaptic. Since then the use of Adaptic in permanent tooth Class 2 restorations has been evaluated (Ribbons and Pearson, 1973; Phillips et al., 1971, 1973). The results of these studies in *permanent teeth* indicate that Adaptic is not inferior to amalgam alloy over the first two years. Although Adaptic did demonstrate a change in anatomical form in many teeth, there was no appreciable difference between amalgam and Adaptic Class 2 restorations in extent of isthmus fracture, marginal deterioration, and recurrent caries. However, there was a change in colour match in 60 per cent of the Adaptic restorations. Three-year results are almost identical (Phillips et al., 1973). From these results, Adaptic can be recommended for restoration of Class 2 permanent tooth preparations in those areas where aesthetics is a primary consideration and lack of occlusal form is of minimal clinical significance.

The marginal deterioration that occurs with amalgam may have prompted Mack (1970) to use Adaptic, but it is interesting that since his 1970 paper, he has discontinued its routine use (Mack, 1973). He indicates that when marginal deterioration occurs with Adaptic the spread of recurrent caries is fast and quickly involves the pulp; by comparison, the breakdown products of amalgam tend to fill any void and perhaps retard the rate of recurrent caries. Personal observation of many Class 2 primary molar Adaptic restorations supports Mack's opinion (1973). A further complication of Adaptic Class 2 restorations is the material's lack of radio-opacity, which makes subsequent evaluation of recurrent caries even more difficult. Therefore, at present, composites cannot be recommended for restoring Class 2 primary molar preparations. Indeed, a two-year clinical study (Tonn and Ryge, 1978) of a carveable composite and a fine cut amalgam alloy in primary molar Class 2 cavity preparations indicated the superiority of amalgam. As with the permanent teeth, the failures of composite were loss of anatomic form and marginal staining.

128

Clinical Technique: As in all Class 2 restorations, the material must be supported by a wedged matrix (*see* Chapter 11). Ribbons et al. (1971) describe a modification of this which facilitates finishing. A preoperative acrylic splint is made by adapting a thin roll of acrylic dough to the occlusal surfaces of the teeth to be restored and the adjacent teeth. When the lesion is large, contour is established by inlay wax; a lubricant on the occlusal surfaces prevents sticking. This acrylic occlusal splint is used after the composite has been inserted into the wedged matrixed cavity to reproduce correct contour and hence minimize finishing.

Great care must be taken to ensure correct interproximal contour of the restoration since radiographic evaluation is impossible because of the material's radiolucency. Only minor alterations can be made in the gingival areas of the completed restoration; small flashes can be removed with a gold knife but major discrepancies defy alteration. Furthermore, unlike amalgam, composite cannot be condensed to ensure a tight positive contact postoperatively. Positive pressure from the wedge is therefore essential to spring the teeth apart and compensate for the thickness of matrix band. During application of the composite it is imperative that no voids be incorporated between cavity and restoration. This is difficult to ensure since the sticky texture of the composite tends to pull away from the cavity walls. Finishing of the set restoration is the same as described for anterior teeth. Interproximal adaptation and contour of the set restoration are checked with unwaxed dental floss; any fraying indicates an overhang which must be removed.

AMALGAM

Amalgam alloy is the most commonly used restorative material. Its coefficient of expansion, thermal conductivity, compressive and tensile strengths, biological compatibility, failure to dissolve, ease of manipulation and low cost are some of its advantages. Its significant disadvantages are the metallic appearance when used in the anterior part of the mouth and its seemingly inevitable marginal deterioration. However, the by-products of the amalgam breakdown are beneficial because they fill the alloy-tooth interface. This may account for the material's longevity in many teeth. Its time-proven qualities make it the material of choice for restoring all posterior cavities (unless a crown is indicated) and anterior teeth where aesthetics is of secondary importance.

Selection of Alloy

The practitioner is well aware of the variety of commercially available alloys and the claims of improved qualities made by their manufacturers. However, while most of these claims are well documented in laboratory research, few have been subjected to rigorous clinical testing *in vivo*. Although the practitioner will develop a personal preference for a particular material, he should be careful to select one that has been approved by a national testing body, e.g. British Standards Institute or American Dental Association Council on Dental Materials.

Three basic amalgam compositions have been used: fine cut alloys, spherical alloys, and high copper content alloys.

Fine Cut Alloy. Small fine cut alloy particles have the advantage of higher strength, a smoother finished surface and easier manipulation than those prepared from large grained alloy filings. Because of the smaller surface area, it is easier to obtain a homogeneous mix. Zinc-free alloys are preferred since moisture contamination with zinc results in excessive expansion; this in turn leads to marginal deterioration, corrosion and secondary caries. Irrespective of the zinc content, the best properties of the material are obtained when it is condensed in a moisture-free environment.

Spherical Alloys. These alloys are prepared from spherical alloy particles; logically there is more complete amalgamation around all of the particles. The initial strength after one hour is 25 per cent higher than with conventional alloys (Basker and Wilson, 1971); this is important because in the immediate postoperative period the child patient is less likely to be able to follow the recommendations of avoiding biting on his new filling. Also, spherical alloys are superior to lathe cut alloys in marginal strength (Koran and Asgar, 1967). Further advantages of spherical alloy are the improved adaptation into line angles and the reduced expansion on setting.

Undoubtedly the major advantage of spherical alloy is its insensitivity to alterations in manipulation. While this property, which is attributed to the microstructure of the material, can hide inconsistencies and imperfections in clinical technique, it is dangerous since it discourages the clinician from paying sufficient attention to detail in material handling. Compared to lathe cut alloys, it feels wet and offers little resistance to condensation pressure. This is significant in Class 2 preparations where the establishment of a positive contact point postoperatively is partially dependent upon condensation pressure. Therefore greater care must be used when preparing the matrix band in teeth restored with spherical alloy (Phillips, 1973).

Despite these properties, the final test is in the mouth over an extended time period. Since a minimum of two years is required to demonstrate clinical variations in alloy performance (Mahler et al., 1973), studies covering shorter periods are less meaningful. Weaver et al. (1970) reported that after three years, restorations of spherical and conventional filling alloy were identical in clinical performance.

High Copper Content Alloys. These are characterized by a low creep value (laboratory test) and improved clinical performance as shown by reduced marginal breakdown and gross fracture. Clinical studies correlate to laboratory data in that those amalgam alloys that show improved marginal integrity also exhibit low creep values. These alloys are designed to reduce or eliminate the gamma-2 phase of the amalgam alloy setting reaction, which is shown here as:

$$Ag_3Sn + Hg \rightarrow Ag_3Sn + Ag_2Hg_3 + Sn_8Hg$$
$$\text{(gamma) (gamma-1) (gamma-2)}$$

(from Phillips, 1973).

The gamma-2 phase is the weakest portion of the hardened amalgam. The oxidation occurs mainly at the gamma-2 phase, which in turn leads to corrosion and subsequent marginal failure. Therefore, reducing or eliminating this phase may minimize marginal deterioration. The gamma-2 phase can be reduced by the addition of copper to the alloy. Dispersalloy, a high copper content alloy, has been shown clinically to have less marginal failure in both primary (Mathewson et al., 1974) and permanent teeth (Mahler et al., 1973, Osborne et al., 1976) than the fine cut alloys. These studies spanned 2–4 years and therefore are clinically very significant.

The practitioner is encouraged to investigate the manipulative qualities of different alloys until he finds a material that suits him. Since 56 per cent of amalgam failures are attributed to improper cavity design and a further 40 per cent to faulty manipulation of material (Healey and Phillips, 1949), the individual selection of alloy must be kept in proper perspective. Careful attention to details of cavity preparation and manipulation of the amalgam as well as the choice of amalgam will prevent amalgam failure (*Fig. 66*).

Mercury–Alloy Ratio

For maximum strength, the completed restoration should contain as little mercury as possible. There is a serious loss of strength when the mercury content exceeds 56 per cent; ideally it should be 50 per cent or less (Eames, 1959). This can be achieved in one of two ways:

1. Start with as little mercury as possible—close to a 1:1 ratio of mercury to alloy. Such ratios are available commercially in the capsulated forms. One problem with these is the tendency towards incomplete amalgamation because of the low initial mercury content.

2. Start with more mercury than alloy—approximately an 8:5 ratio. This encourages complete amalgamation. However, the excess mercury must be removed prior to and during condensation to bring the final ratio back as close as possible to 1:1.

131

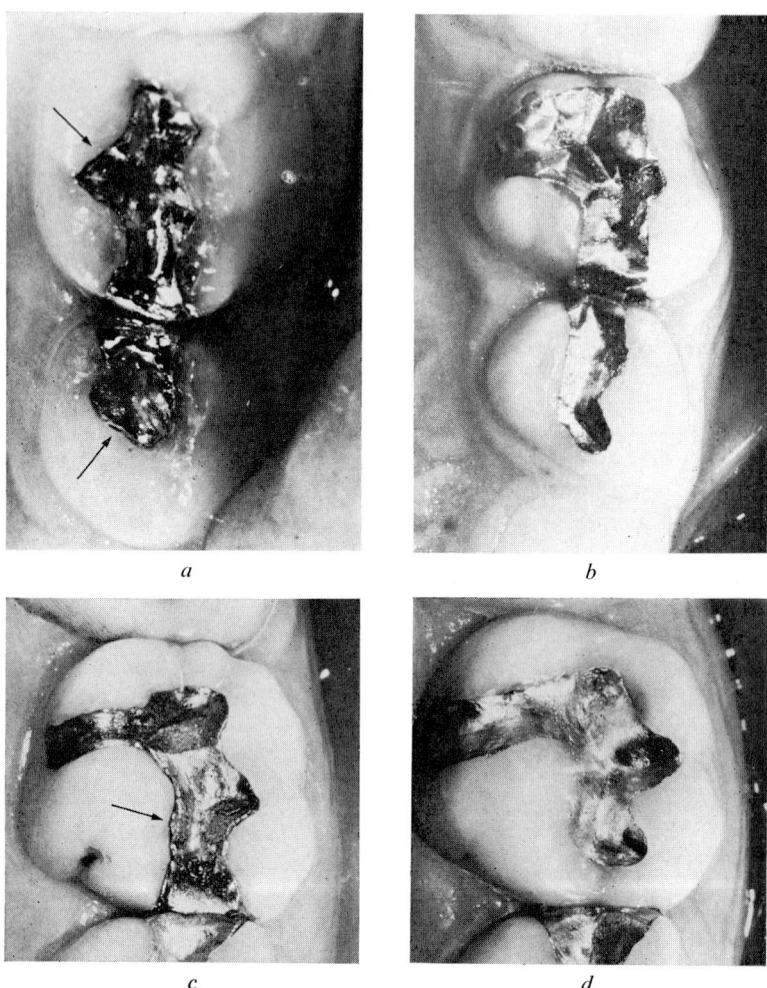

a   *b*

c   *d*

Fig. 66.—Clinical comparison of fine cut and high copper content of amalgam alloys. After 3 years. Marginal breakdown shown with arrows. *a*, Primary fine cut—3½ years. *b*, Primary dispersalloy —3½ years. *c*, Permanent fine cut—4 years. *d*, Permanent dispersalloy—4 years (*c* and *d* are same patient).

Trituration

This is the mixing of mercury and alloy. The significant variation is the trituration time which determines:

1. The thoroughness of the mix.
2. The strength.
3. The expansion.

Undertrituration decreases the thoroughness of the mix and its strength, and increases expansion on setting. Overtrituration increases amalgam contraction—it should be remembered that the use of mechanical condensers run at high speed will effectively lengthen the trituration time. Trituration can be performed by hand using a pestle and mortar or mechanically; the convenience and standard results of the latter method are preferred.

Condensation

The aims of condensation are to adapt the amalgam as closely as possible to the walls of the cavity, at the same time bringing excess mercury to the surface. The cavity is deliberately overfilled so that the mercury-rich superficial layer can be removed by carving. The least accessible parts of the preparation should be filled first so that condensation in these areas can be carried out thoroughly. As each increment of material is added, it should be thoroughly condensed before adding further increments to ensure that the residual mercury content is kept low.

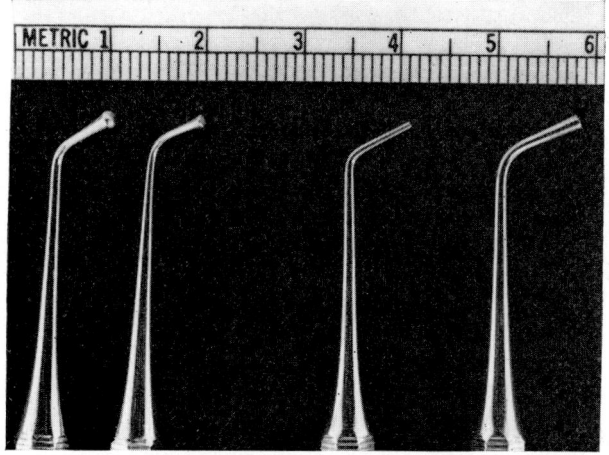

Fig. 67.—Appropriate sized and shaped condensers for conservative preparations in primary and young permanent teeth.

The size and shape of the condensers must conform to the cavity preparation. Round-ended condensers are recommended if the external line angles of Class 2 preparations are also rounded, while flat-ended condensers are used for sharp-angled preparations (*Fig. 67*). Condensation pressure is greater per unit area when small instruments are used; these also comply to the narrow dimensions of cavity preparations in primary and young permanent teeth.

133

Heavy condensation pressure is essential to obtain good adaptation and expression of excess mercury. This is possible either with hand or mechanical condensers, although proper hand condensation is fatiguing and therefore subject to human error and variability. Mechanical condensation is preferred since, like mechanical trituration, the finished results are more standardized. However, the sensation of mechanical condensation is unpleasant for the child and must be explained in terms that can be understood. Such an explanation as, 'This is a woodpecker and it's going to tap on your tooth, feel it on your finger first', is usually sufficient. Also, mechanical condensers run at high speeds effectively lengthen the trituration time, which results in contraction on setting.

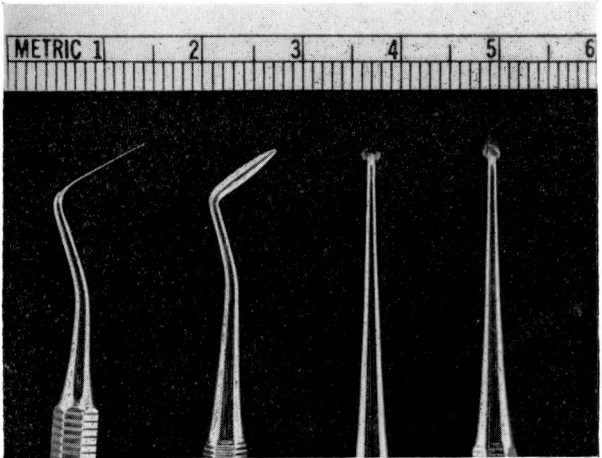

Fig. 68.—Appropriate sized carvers for primary and young permanent teeth. *From left to right:* Hollenbach × 2, Discoid, Cleoid. (Available from Amalgamated Dental, Broadwick Street, London.)

The condensation should be completed as quickly as possible. Once amalgam has started to set for 3 minutes, it should be discarded. If partially set alloy is used, excess mercury cannot be expressed from it. This means that the residual mercury content is too high, resulting in reduced strength and a greater tendency to corrosion, marginal breakdown and secondary caries (McDonald, 1974).

Carving

The purpose of carving is to reproduce anatomy and eliminate flashes or overhanging margins of amalgam. Reproduction of anatomy restores the tooth to correct contour and function. Flashes of amalgam are liable to fracture leading subsequently to marginal

134

deterioration and secondary caries. Although it is often said that the carving of primary tooth restorations should not be too elaborate, this attitude is dangerous since failure to accurately carve all accessory grooves in the occlusal surface will result in overhanging flashes of amalgam in these grooves.

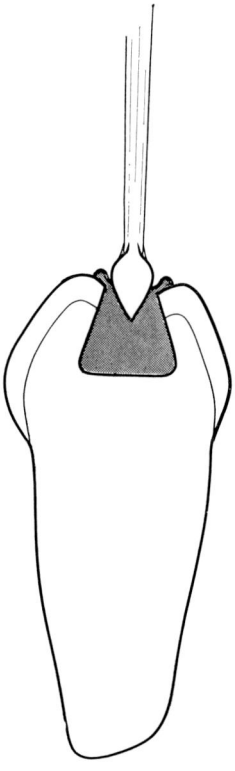

Fig. 69.—Use of cleoid to define occlusal grooves. This is the first step in the carving sequence.

Knowledge of tooth morphology and selection of appropriately-sized instruments (*Fig. 68*) greatly facilitate carving. Because of the shallow depth of primary molar preparations, carving should not be too deep since this would impinge on bulk of alloy. A cleiod-discoid instrument is recommended for carving the occlusal surface. The diamond-shaped cleiod end is used. The carving sequence is shown diagrammatically in *Figs. 69–71*. The depth of the fissure is emphasized initially using a vertical inclination. Because the instrument is small, there is no danger of exposing the margins. In fact, this

135

procedure makes the margins easier to see and carve (*Fig. 70*). The same instrument is used with a more horizontal inclination to refine the margins of the restoration. The instrument should always be drawn from enamel to alloy in this procedure. Finally, any accessory grooves are refined to eliminate flashes.

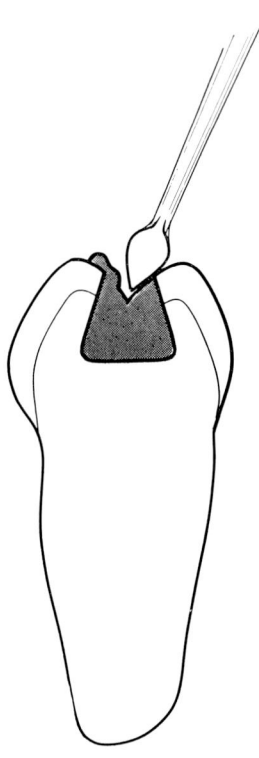

Fig. 70.—The margin is carved with a more horizontal inclination of the cleoid: the second step.

The Hollenbach or Wards carver (No. 1) is recommended for carving Class 3 and 5 restorations and the interproximal part of Class 2 restorations. The instrument is laid flush with the appropriate enamel surface to smooth Class 3 and 5 restorations. These restorations are easily overcarved, leaving a depression. This should be avoided; rather, the carved restoration should be left slightly proud to allow for further removal during the polishing procedure.

Class 2 restorations should be carved as thoroughly as possible before the matrix is removed. A common error is failure

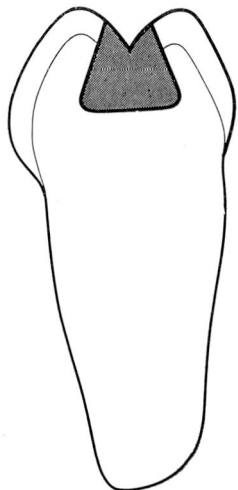

Fig. 71.—Complete restoration.

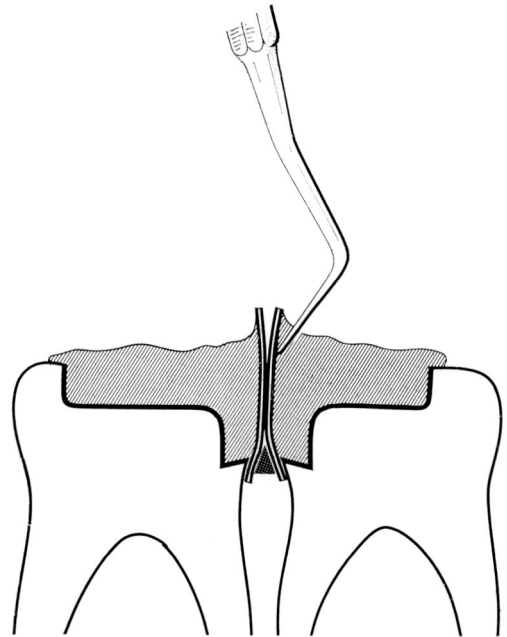

Fig. 72.—Use of a Hollenbach or Wards carver on the marginal ridge. This area must be carved before the matrix is removed to prevent fracture.

137

to carve the marginal ridge area, which is essential so that a smooth interproximal contour is maintained (*see* Chapter 11). (*Fig. 72.*) Failure to carve this area will also result in fracture of the ridge when the matrix is removed. The rounded discoid end of the cleoid-discoid carver can be used to obtain a smooth-rounded marginal ridge area after the matrix is removed.

The carvability of amalgam alloy is partially dependent on its stage of setting. For convenience, the busy practitioner may start to carve as soon as condensation is complete. At this time the alloy is often too 'wet' to carve, resulting in smearing of the alloy into accessory grooves and production of flashes. Waiting for a couple of minutes allows the material to set a little more so that its carvability improves. This waiting time need not be unproductive since other patients will require local anaesthesia and parents will need to be greeted or given reassurance and educational information. The best time to carve alloy is when it peels away and makes a squeaking noise.

Burnishing the margins of partially set amalgam has been a controversial topic. It can be done by running hand instruments over the interface or by lightly polishing the carved partially set material to produce a smooth, scratch-free surface. Clinical evaluation, supported by laboratory data, indicates that this does not predispose the restoration to breakdown. Rather, it reveals discrepancies in carving technique and flashes of amalgam that require removal. Provided excess heat is avoided, which would result in bringing mercury to the surface, burnishing can be recommended.

Polishing

This should be delayed at least 24 hours, or better still a week, to avoid having a mercury-rich outer layer of alloy (Phillips, 1974). Finishing burs which are used to smooth over the surface, should be run at slow speed and always from enamel to amalgam. What is required is a bur which will simultaneously apply equal pressure to both enamel and alloy. Barrel or pear-shaped finishing burs fulfil this requirement. Flame-shaped burs are not recommended since they produce deep grooves in the restoration. Round burs are contra-indicated since their shape tends to cause a depression at the margin. Overzealous use of finishing burs can undo meticulous carving and ruin accurately finished margins.

The depths of the grooves are polished by burnishing a cleoid into them. The accessible interproximal surfaces are refined by slowly revolving fine sandpaper discs; these have the same ability as finishing burs to ruin the contour of the restoration. Scratches are removed from the surface with bristle brushes or rubber cups and a fine grained pumice. Final lustre is achieved with a rubber cup and zinc oxide powder or amalgloss. Commercially available rubber cups of varying abrasiveness can also be used. Heat should be avoided since this brings mercury to the surface. A smooth, scratch-free, polished restoration is less likely to retain food debris and resists tarnishing and corrosion better.

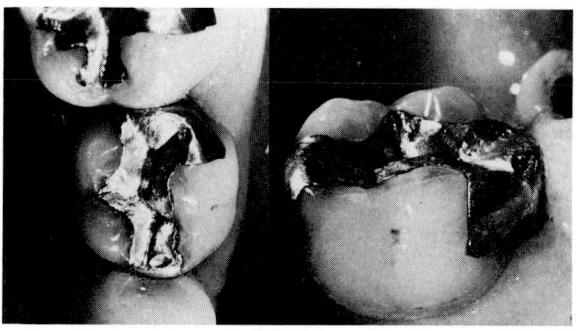

a

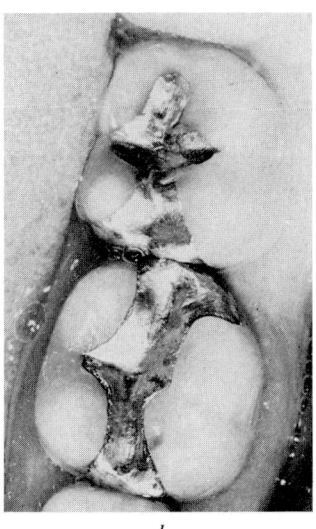

b

Fig. 73.—*a*, 3½-year-old fine cut with overlay of distobuccal cusp |E̅. Note wear facets. *b*, 4-year fine cut on |6̅. 4-year dispersalloy on |7̅ placed same day. Note improved margins with dispersalloy.

Fluoride in Amalgam

At the time of writing the introduction of fluoride into amalgam is an exciting experimental advance. Since Class 2 restorations are constantly in contact with adjacent surfaces, fluoride conceivably could be of value if it is constantly released. However, clinical

139

studies of fluoridated alloys fail to reveal any beneficial effects. It must be realized that the incorporation of fluoride into the alloy should not be detrimental to the physical properties of the material.

Marginal Deterioration

Several causes of amalgam marginal deterioration have been described in Chapter 7. Other causes have been described in this chapter. The causes can be summarized as poor cavity design, faulty manipulation of the alloy and improper selection of the restorative material. (*Fig. 73.*)

Although it takes at least two years to reveal amalgam failures (Mahler et al., 1973), marginal deterioration may occur well before this time, if only at a microscopic level. A defect of 50 microns will encourage the development of secondary caries (Jørgensen and Wakumoto, 1968). Horwitz et al. (1967) evaluated minimal extension Class 2 amalgam restorations in primary molars which were prepared and restored under the rubber dam. Refined television microscopic apparatus evaluated the margins. In the first twelve weeks the gingival margins exhibited rapid breakdown, which was then superseded by a more rapid occlusal breakdown, presumably due to occlusal forces. This study brought into sharp focus the need to finish accurately the restoration to prevent flashes of amalgam which subsequently break down.

REFERENCES

BASKER R. M. and WILSON H. J. (1971) Spherical particle amalgam. *Br. Dent. J.* **130**, 338.

DOYLE W. A. (1967) Esthetic restoration of deciduous incisors: a new Class IV preparation. *J. Am. Dent. Assoc.* **74**, 82.

DOYLE W. A. (1973) Acid etching in pedodontics. *Dent. Clin. North Am.* **17:1**, 93.

EAMES W. B. (1959) Preparation and condensation of amalgam with a low mercury-alloy. *J. Am. Dent. Assoc.* **58**, 78.

GELLER J. S., KLEIN A. I. and McDONALD R. E. (1971) Association between dentinal sclerosis and pulpal floor thickness: television radiographic evaluation. *J. Am. Dent. Assoc.* **83**, 118.

GOING R. E. (1964) Cavity lines and dentin treatment. *J. Am. Dent. Assoc.* **69**, 415.

HARGREAVES J. A. (1969) *Second. Int. Symp. of Dent. for Child.* Proceedings, Sienna, p. 279.

HEALEY H. J. and PHILLIPS R. W. (1949) A clinical study of amalgam failures. *J. Dent. Res.* **28**, 439.

HORWITZ B. A., KLEIN A. I. and McDONALD R. E. (1967) Intra-oral television micromeasurement of cavity margin deterioration. *J. Dent. Res.* **46**, 700.

HUTCHINS D. W. and PARKER W. A. (1972) Indirect pulp capping: Clinical evaluation using polymethyl methacrylate reinforced zinc oxide–eugenol cement. *J. Dent. Child.* **39**, 55.

JINKS G. M. (1963) Fluoride-impregnated cements and their effect on the activity of interproximal caries. *J. Dent. Child.* **30**, 87.

JØRGENSEN K. D. and WAKUMOTO S. (1968) Occlusal amalgam fillings: marginal defects and secondary caries. *Odont. T.* **76**, 43.

KAYE M. A. (1968) Aetiology of mortality of incisor pulps. *Br. Dent. J.* **125**, 59.

KERKHOVE B. C., HERMAN S. C., KLEIN A. I. and McDONALD R. E. (1967) A clinical and television densitometric evaluation of the indirect pulp capping technique. *J. Dent. Child.* **34**, 192.

KORAN A. and ASGAR K. (1967) A comparison of dental amalgams made from a spherical alloy and from a comminuted alloy. *J. Am. Dent. Assoc.* **75**, 912.

McDONALD R. E. (1974) *Dentistry for the Child and Adolescent*, 2nd ed. St. Louis, C. V. Mosby, p. 201.

MACK E. S. (1970) A restorative pedodontic practice without amalgam. *J. Dent. Child.* **37**, 428.

MACK E. S. (1973) Personal communication.

MAHLER D. B., TERKLA L. G. and VAN EYSDEN J. (1973) Marginal fracture of amalgam restorations. *J. Dent. Res.* **52**, 823.

MATHEWSON R. J., RETZLAFF A. E. and PORTER D. R. (1974) Marginal failure of amalgam in deciduous teeth: a two-year report. *J. Am. Dent. Assoc.* **88**, 134.

OSBORNE J. W., PHILLIPS R. W., GALE E. N. and BINON P. P. (1976) Three year clinical comparison of three amalgam alloy types emphasizing an appraisal of the evaluation methods used. *J. Am. Dent. Assoc.* **93**, 784.

PHILLIPS R. W. (1973) Selection of amalgam alloys: Particle form, new formulas. *J. Dent. Child.* **40**, 106.

PHILLIPS R. W. (1974) In: McDonald R. E. *Dentistry for the Child and Adolescent*, 2nd ed. St. Louis, C. V. Mosby, pp. 210–222.

PHILLIPS R. W., AVERY D. R., MEHRA R., SWARTZ M. L. and McCUNE R. J. (1971) One-year observations on a composite resin for Class II restorations. *J. Prosthet. Dent.* **26**, 68.

PHILLIPS R. W., AVERY D. R., MEHRA R., SWARTZ M. L. and McCUNE R. J. (1973) Observations on a composite resin for Class II restorations: three-year report. *J. Prosthet. Dent.* **30**, 891.

RIBBONS J. W. and PEARSON G. J. (1973) A composite filling material. *Br. Dent. J.* **134**, 389.

RIBBONS J. W., PEARSON G. J. and SIMMONS L. H. (1971) Manipulative techniques using a composite filling material. *Br. Dent. J.* **131**, 157.

TONN E. and RYGE G. (1978) Comparison of composite and amalgam in primary molar Class 2 preparations. American Academy of Pedodontics meeting, San Diego, June 1978.

TRAUBMAN, LIONEL (1967) *A Critical Clinical and Television Radiographic Evaluation of Indirect Pulp Capping.* Typed Thesis, Indiana University.

141

WEAVER R. G., JOHNSON B. E., CVAR J. F. and McCUNE R. J. (1970)
I.A.D.R. Programme and Abstracts, Abst., 267.
WEAVER R. G., JOHNSON B. E., CVAR J. F. and McCUNE R. J. (1972)
Clinical evaluation of intermediate restorative materials. *J. Dent.
Child.* **39**, 189.

RECOMMENDED READING

FINN S. B. and RIPA L. W. (1973) In: Finn S. B. *Clinical Pedodontics*,
4th ed. Philadelphia, W. B. Saunders, pp. 168–200.
MATHEWSON R. J., RETZLAFF A. E. and PORTER D. R. (1974) Marginal
failure of amalgam in deciduous teeth: a two-year report. *J. Am.
Dent. Assoc.* **88**, 134.
PHILLIPS R. W. (1974) In: McDonald R. E. *Dentistry for the Child
and Adolescent*, 2nd ed. St. Louis, C. V. Mosby, pp. 210–222.
WEAVER R. G., JOHNSON B. E., CVAR J. F. and McCUNE R. J. (1972)
Clinical evaluation of intermediate restorative materials. *J. Dent.
Child.* **39**, 189.

CHAPTER 13

THE STAINLESS-STEEL CROWN

THE stainless-steel crown is a moderately recent advance in paediatric dentistry which has helped solve the problem of the extensively carious tooth. Because of the alarming rate of failure for extensive Class 2 amalgam restorations in primary molars, particularly the mandibular first primary molar, the paediatric dentist has used the stainless-steel crown as a routine treatment in selected cases. The stainless-steel crown is prefabricated in a variety of sizes for each tooth. Tooth preparation precedes the fitting, contouring and cementation of the crown, all of which is done at one appointment. Unlike the situation with the gold or porcelain crown, the impression is unnecessary and the finished tooth preparation may have undercut areas, which enhance the retention of the crown whose margins are placed gingival to the undercuts.

INDICATIONS

The stainless-steel crown is indicated in a variety of circumstances. To the general practitioner, the thought of placing steel crowns in all of these instances (to be described) may be horrifying. His inexperience and his resulting slow clinical speed with the technique probably are deterrents. However, before passing off the stainless-steel crown as an unnecessary luxury treatment performed only by specialists, he should evaluate the results of his extensive alloy restorations. There are likely to be several large Class 2 alloy restorations which will require replacement before tooth exfoliation; one has to question whether replacement would be necessary if a steel crown had been placed initially. The stainless-steel crown is indicated in the following circumstances:

1. *Extensive Decay in Primary Teeth*
The interpretation of extensive decay is subjective and therefore specific examples must be given. When removal of the lesion leaves insufficient sound tooth structure to retain a restoration, a crown is indicated. The modified Class 2 cavity (Chapter 7) involves replacement of a single weakened or undermined cusp with alloy; it is unwise to replace more than one cusp. Thus a crown is indicated whenever one or more cusps are destroyed or weakened by caries. This commonly occurs in the first primary molar when the distal interproximal lesion is untreated. The decay involves the whole of

the broad flat contact area, weakening both the distolingual and distobuccal cusps. Attempts at a Class 2 cavity preparation would result in a proximal box whose buccal and lingual walls would flare markedly towards the embrasure; this would encourage failure of the amalgam at these margins (Chapter 7). In the primary incisors Class 4 lesions occurring mesially and distally, along with a Class 5 lesion on the same tooth, would be an indication for a crown, either stainless-steel, polycarbonate or resin (*see also* Chapter 9).

A factor to consider in the preoperative evaluation is the dental age of the patient, which is judged by the root development of the underlying tooth. When a primary tooth can be expected to exfoliate within two years of restoration, heroic attempts can be made with amalgam. However, parent, child, and operator may all be frustrated by the failure of extensive amalgam restorations in primary teeth, and everyone would have benefited from the initial placement of the steel crown. The experienced clinician is able to place a stainless-steel crown faster than a four-surface amalgam alloy restoration, and so the disadvantage of additional time is overcome.

2. *Following Pulp Therapy*

In both primary and permanent teeth pulp therapy leaves the treated tooth more brittle. Subsequent fracture of tooth structure has led to the accepted doctrine of cuspal coverage after endodontics in permanent teeth. This doctrine should also apply to primary teeth. Should the fracture occur below the epithelial attachment, subsequent repair of the tooth may be impossible. It is therefore recommended that postoperative failure be prevented by placing a stainless-steel crown in the first place. A tooth that is a candidate for pulp therapy probably will also be a candidate for a crown for reasons described in the previous section.

3. *As a Preventive Restoration*

It has been implied in the preceding sections that the stainless-steel crown is a preventive restoration because it helps avoid amalgam failure or tooth fracture. It can be used also to prevent caries from developing in other areas of the tooth, while an interproximal amalgam restoration cannot protect the buccal and lingual surfaces. Evidence of a developing Class 5 lesion is a sign of a lapse in dietary and oral hygiene habits (Chapter 10). When this occurs in the pre-school age child who also has a Class 2 lesion in the same tooth, the stainless-steel crown should be seriously considered, particularly for the first primary molar. This recommendation is prompted by the failure rate of disto-occlusal amalgam restorations in mandibular first primary molars (Castaldi, 1957) and the length of time required of the alloy. It also ensures final treatment and prevents the need for difficult Class 5 restorations. This application should be fully used in the handicapped child whose lack of oral hygiene may encourage further decay.

The anatomy of the first primary molar accounts for the difficulty in placing durable mesial-occlusal-distal restorations. The marked convergence of buccal and lingual walls towards the occlusal surface close to the mesial contact explains the difficulty in preparing the mesial box. It is extremely difficult to leave the mesiobuccal wall well supported. Also, Castaldi (1957) and MacRae et al. (1962) reported that the distobuccal margin of mandibular first primary molars was most commonly deficient in the analysis of Class 2 primary molar alloys. Therefore many practitioners no longer place MOD restorations in the first primary molars of pre-school children; rather they place a stainless-steel crown.

A further advantage of the stainless-steel crown is that dental plaque is more readily seen than on enamel. This, when pointed out to the child and parent, can stimulate them to improve the oral hygiene.

4. For Teeth with Developmental Defects

Linear hypoplastic defects can undermine the occlusal surface of first primary molars if the systemic upset occurs at or around birth (Jaffe et al., 1973). Similarly, amelogenesis and dentinogenesis imperfecta can alter tooth morphology and predispose the dentition to excessive wear and loss of vertical dimension. Hypoplastic and hypocalcified defects on teeth may be more susceptible to caries because the anatomy encourages plaque retention, although this does not always occur. Often the location and extent of the hypoplastic defect do not lend themselves to amalgam restorations. In all these instances the stainless-steel crown can be considered. The steel crown on the first permanent molar is frequently used as a semi-permanent restoration to last through the teenage years before placement of a gold crown or porcelain bonded to gold crown. Pulp morphology and the length of clinical crown may preclude the use of gold crowns in the child under twelve years of age.

Caution is required in placing steel crowns on hypoplastic teeth. Since the treatment may well involve the crowning of teeth in all four quadrants (often all posterior teeth) there is a very real danger of altering the vertical dimension by impinging on the freeway space. For this reason, it is recommended that the practitioner fit the crowns in quadrants, proceeding to tooth preparation in the next quadrant only when the previous crowns are cemented. In this way there is less likelihood of opening the bite. On the other hand, it is acceptable to open the bite slightly (less than 2 mm) if extensive abrasion has already resulted in loss of vertical dimension; however, leaving the crown excessively high will result in tenderness of the treated tooth and possibly in an adverse pulp response.

The other complication with placement of steel crowns on hypoplastic teeth is the short clinical crown that is available. This occurs commonly in the first permanent molar which presents with a hypoplastic defect. In such instances it may be necessary to overextend the crown margins subgingivally to increase retention and to allow for anticipated eruption and gingival recession of that tooth unit.

5. *As an Abutment for a Space Maintainer or Denture*

The stainless-steel crown can be used as an abutment for a fixed space maintainer in two instances. When the abutment tooth presents an indication in its own right for a steel crown, the space maintainer can be incorporated as a crown and loop; alternatively, a band is fitted over the crown and the space maintainer attached to the band.

When the abutment tooth presents none of the other indications, but also does not lend itself to banding or to clasping, a stainless-steel crown can be considered. An example is the first primary molar whose buccal and lingual walls converge occlusally, thereby presenting little or no undercut. Should the second primary molar need to be lost before the first permanent molar erupts, a band and loop appliance can be fabricated with an intragingival extension into the second primary molar socket to prevent mesial migration of the first permanent molar and guide it into occlusion (Hicks, 1973). Since the first primary molar can seldom be satisfactorily banded, it can be crowned and the appliance constructed over the crown, which is contoured with undercuts that will aid the retention of the band.

TOOTH PREPARATION

1. *Anterior*

The aims of tooth reduction are to provide sufficient space for the steel crown, remove the caries, and leave sufficient tooth for retention of the crown. Mesial and distal slices are required to clear the interproximal contacts. The gingival margin should have no ledge or shoulder; rather the chamfer should merge with uncut apically-placed tooth structure at the free gingival margin. Incisal reduction is required to prevent unnecessary elongation of the tooth. Tooth reduction should not destroy undercuts for mechanical retention; thus labial and lingual undercuts are left whenever possible. Lingual reduction is necessary when the overbite is complete such that the mandibular incisors are in contact with the lingual surfaces of the maxillary incisors. One to two millimetres should be removed uniformly with a diamond stone. When an incomplete overbite or open bite exists, and there are indications that it will not close, the lingual surface need not be reduced; the undercut towards the gingival margin is used for retention. For this same reason the only tooth reduction that should occur on the labial surface is that which will remove caries. A No. 2L plain cut* tapered fissure bur is compatible with the minimal preparation required. A pulp-protecting base is placed in the deepest areas of the preparation. Crown selection and contouring are done in the same way as for posterior crowns.

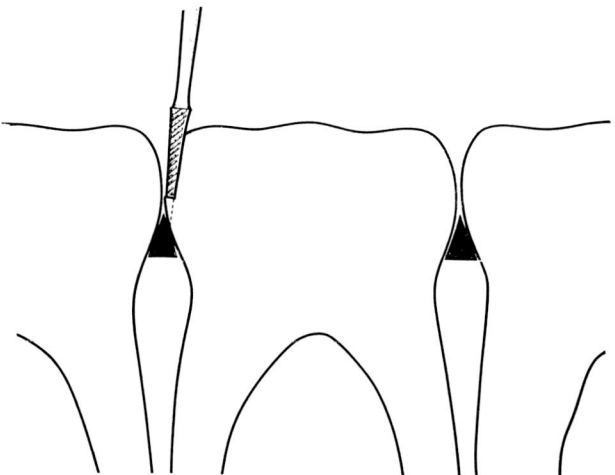

Fig. 74.—A tapered fissure bur is used to cut the interproximal slice. Note the interproximal wedge.

The anterior steel crown can be closed or open-faced, the latter being more aesthetic. In this latter instance, the crown should be fitted up to the point of cementation before the labial surface of the crown is removed. The small dimensions of the anterior steel crown make them most difficult to manage. They must be handled with care to prevent unwanted distortion both whilst contouring and during preparation of the labial window. The labial window is best prepared with a high speed bur out of the mouth, leaving at least 2 mm of labial collar at the gingival margin. The open-faced crown is placed on the tooth and the labial margins burnished with an amalgam condenser against all available sound tooth structure. The crown is removed, polished and cemented. Resin can be used to fill any remaining labial defect; extensive caries will warrant a full resin veneer to produce a result similar to that of a basket crown.

---

* No. 2L plain cut fissure bur = No. 170L American.

2. *Posterior* (*Figs. 74–81*)

The aims of tooth reduction are the same as those described for anterior crowns.

Proximal Slices: Mesial and distal reduction take the form of a ledge or shoulder-free vertical slice which clears the contact area buccally, lingually, and gingivally. Distal reduction is required even when there is no erupted tooth distally, such as occurs in the preschool child's second primary molar. Failure to follow this recommendation will result in an oversized crown being fitted, which may impede the eruption of the first permanent molar.

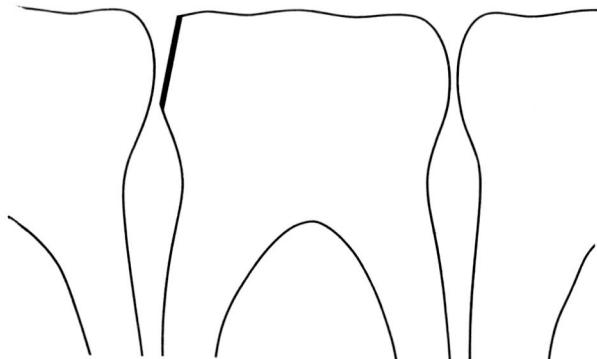

Fig. 75.—Ledge or shoulder free supragingival interproximal slice.

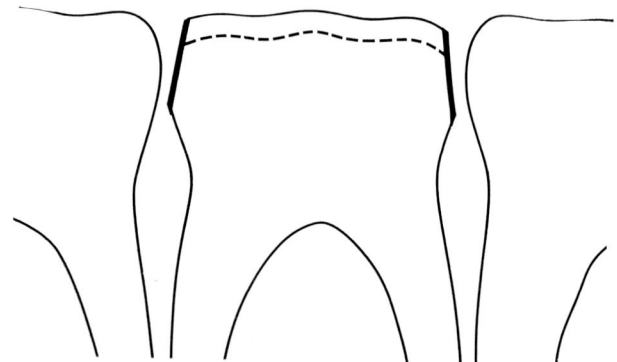

Fig. 76.—Occlusal reduction of 1–2·5 mm follows the occlusal anatomy.

The tapered No. 2L plain cut tapered fissure bur is preferred to a diamond disc for preparation of the slice because of the unwarranted dangers of soft-tissue trauma that can be induced by discs. However, operator preference may encourage the use of discs—if so, they should always be safesided, used with a guard and then only when the preparation is made under the rubber dam. An interproximal wedge facilitates the interproximal reduction by slightly springing the teeth apart and helping prevent damage to the adjacent tooth. The tapered fissure bur is moved in a buccolingual direction starting at the occlusal surface one to two millimetres

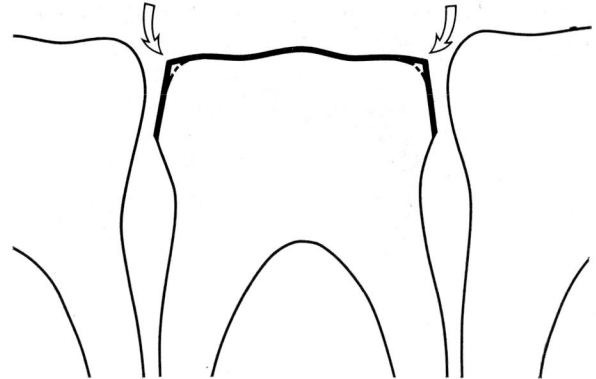

Fig. 77.—Sharp line angles are rounded.

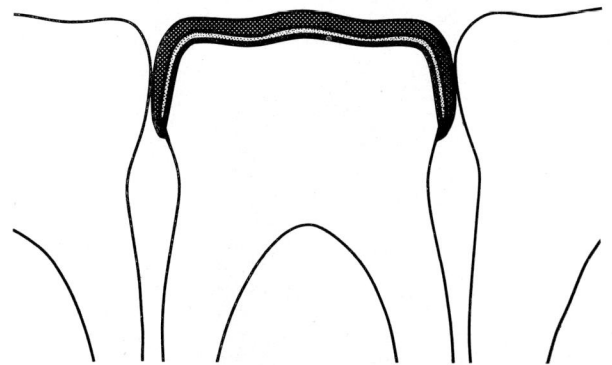

Fig. 78.—Completed preparation and cemented crown—buccal view. Note the rounding of sharp line angles occlusally.

away from the adjacent tooth. As the bur is taken gingivally a ledge will be formed; this will disappear as the slice clears the contact area gingivally. Eventually the bur will touch the wedge; when this is then removed an almost perfect interproximal slice will be seen. As the tooth repositions after removal of the wedge, minimal further reduction will be required to finish the slice.

Occlusal reduction: This should follow the anatomy of the tooth to a depth of 1·5–2·0 mm, which allows sufficient space for the

metal crown. Mink and Bennett (1968) recommended initial placement of 1-mm deep grooves in the occlusal surface to assist in
establishing the correct amount of reduction; undoubtedly this is
the most accurate approach but it is time-consuming. The cusp
height of adjacent teeth gives the operator a good baseline from
which to judge the amount of occlusal reduction; similarly, the
lingual and buccal developmental pits and grooves in maxillary and
mandibular molars are useful reference points.

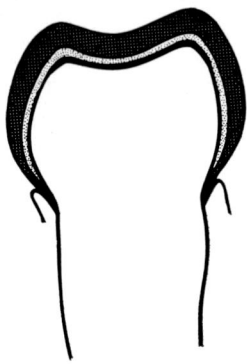

Fig. 79.—Completed preparation and cemented crown—inter·
proximal view. The buccal and lingual surfaces are not reduced:
the crown is retained by the cervical undercut of enamel. The
margins fit in the gingival crevice.

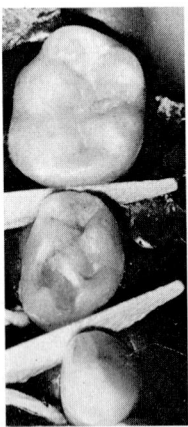

Fig. 80.—Preoperative view of a mandibular primary molar ready
for crown preparation. Note interproximal wedges.

Finishing: Any remaining caries should be removed with a slow
running round bur. The preparation is completed by rounding off
all sharp line angles (*Fig. 77*). These will prevent proper seating of
the stainless-steel crown whose internal contour is free from sharp

angles. Buccal and lingual reduction is not uniformly required to remove undercuts. Retention of the crown is obtained by encompassing the normally gingival bulbosity of primary molars and leaving the crown margins apical to this in the gingival sulcus; thus it is undesirable to remove these undercuts (*Figs. 78, 79*). One exception is the first primary molar, since its marked mesiobuccal bulge of enamel always requires reduction; the enamel is so prominent in this area that it is impossible to contour the crown adequately if the tooth is not reduced.

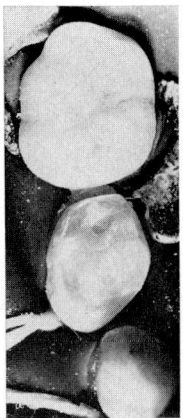

Fig. 81.—Completed stainless-steel crown preparation.

CROWN SELECTION

Several makes of stainless-steel crowns* are available, and the practitioner will make his choice on the basis of experience. A correctly selected crown, prior to trimming and contouring, should cover all the tooth preparation and provide resistance to removal (*Fig. 82*). Some crowns can be purchased either festooned (partially trimmed) or non-festooned (untrimmed); the latter require more reduction to prevent the margins from impinging on the gingivae, but are useful when the preparation extends subgingivally. Handling properties of the various crowns differ markedly; some work harden very quickly while others are almost too readily distorted by contouring pliers. The festooned Unitek or Ion stainless-steel crown* is superior to the other crowns mentioned because it most accurately reproduces the tooth morphology and requires the least

---

* Unitek Corporation, Monrovia, California, U.S.A. Available from Orthomax Ltd., Queens House, Queens Road, Bradford, Yorks.; Rocky Mountain Metal Products Co., Denver, Colorado; Ormco Corporation, Covina, California. Ion Crown, 3M Co., St. Paul, Minnesota, U.S.A.

trimming and contouring, thereby reducing clinical time. This crown will be suitable for the majority of primary and young permanent teeth.

Primary molars with deep interproximal caries extending subgingivally may warrant a non-festooned crown (Rocky Mountain) to encompass the margins of the preparation. However, in an alternative approach, any required pulp treatment can be performed at a preliminary appointment, the tooth being temporarily restored with

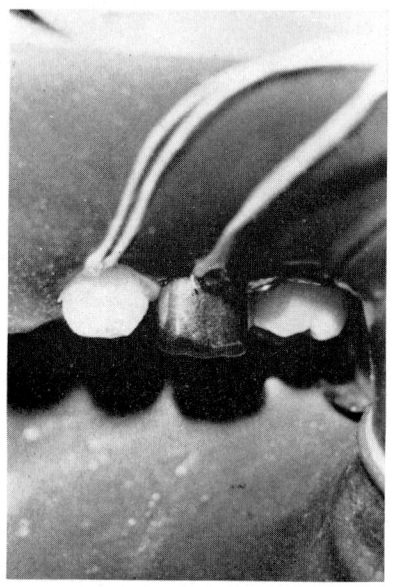

Fig. 82.—A Unitek festooned crown is selected which will cover the preparation and provide some resistance to removal.

amalgam alloy. If that is done, it is unnecessary to remove all the alloy during the subsequent crown preparation; the crown margins can be left on the alloy. This latter approach reduces the need to use non-festooned crowns, which usually require more trimming and contouring than their festooned counterpart.

The preoperative mesiodistal width of the tooth to be crowned can be measured with callipers and this width matched with an appropriate steel crown. A crown that provides considerable resistance to removal or that requires pressure to place initially is probably too small since no allowance is made for subsequent contouring. At the other extreme, it will be impossible to contour satisfactorily a grossly oversized crown. Preoperative assessment should also consider the presence or absence of primate spaces, when first primary molars are being crowned. Impingement upon the primate space by an oversized crown may prevent early mesial migration of the mandibular first permanent molar from a cusp-to-cusp occlusion into an Angle Class 1 relationship (Baume, 1950). Similarly, overcontoured and oversized steel crowns on second primary molars can prevent the normal eruption of the first permanent molars.

CROWN TRIMMING AND CONTOURING

The purposes of crown trimming and contouring are, respectively, to leave the crown margins in the gingival sulcus and to reproduce the tooth's morphology. All preformed crowns will require both trimming and contouring. The amount of gingival reduction can be accurately assessed by scratching on the crown a mark at the level of the free marginal gingivae and reducing the crown with small curved crown and bridge scissors* (*Fig. 83*). This should be done

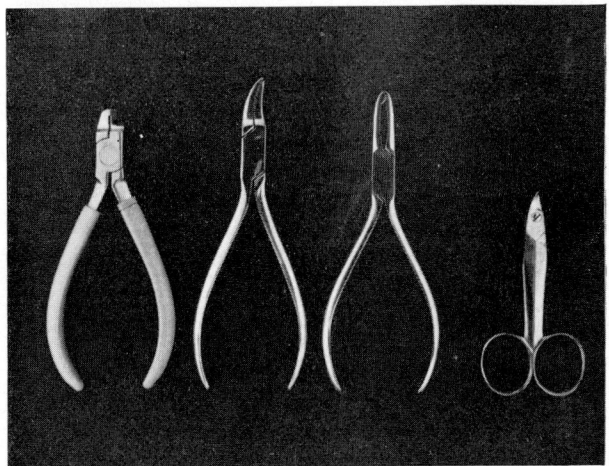

Fig. 83.—Crown trimming scissors and contouring pliers. *From right to left:* scissors, 114, 137, 800–412.

away from the child's face to minimize the danger of slivers of metal lodging in vital organs such as the eye. Crown contouring subsequently will reduce the effective occlusogingival crown height, and so the crown should be left slightly long at this stage. Final gingival trimming is done after crown contouring and is most accurately accomplished with a stone wheel. The whole preparation should be covered by the crown, whose margins fit in the free gingival sulcus. There should be no blanching of the gingivae, which indicates overextension. However, when caries requires a subgingival preparation, it is both desirable and necessary to extend the margins apically.

---

* Unitek Crown and Bridge Scissors.

Initial crown contouring is performed with the 114 plier in the middle one-third of the crown to produce a belling effect. This will give the crown a more even curvature than one which is contoured only in the gingival one-third (*Fig. 84*). During contouring and trimming procedures, the crown is trial fitted and the margins and adaptation are checked both visually and with an explorer. Adaptation of the gingival one-third of the crown is done with the 137 plier. Any marked gingival crimping of the crown can also be accomplished with a Unitek 800–412 plier. Since it is impossible to

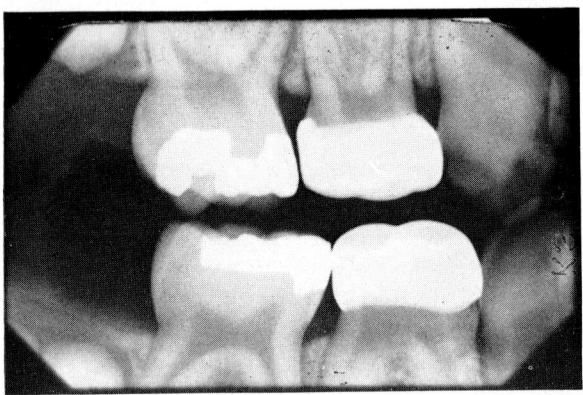

Fig. 84.—Bite-wing radiograph demonstrates properly contoured mandibular crown. Note the even curvature, positive contact and absence of overhang. The maxillary crown is undercontoured and exhibits an open contact distally. This crown has only been contoured in the gingival one-third and not in the middle third.

burnish the margins of the crown in the mouth, all contouring and trimming procedures must be performed out of the mouth. The finally trimmed and contoured crown should be evenly and smoothly shaped with no marked changes in contour (*Figs. 78, 79, 84–87*).

The buccal and lingual margins are more readily evaluated than the interproximal fit. The ability of the crown to fray waxed dental floss indicates an unsatisfactory inaccuracy in interproximal adaptation. The floss also checks the presence or absence of a sound contact (alterations in contact areas will be discussed later). A diagnostic bite-wing radiograph prior to cementation provides excellent evaluation of the interproximal fit; this is recommended for those gaining experience with the stainless-steel crown technique.

During trial fitting and cementation, the crown should be placed from the lingual and rolled towards the buccal whenever possible. In this way, the maximum undercut on the buccal surface is more readily encompassed. As the crown is being rolled from lingual to buccal, the interproximal adaptation can be assessed by looking at

154

right angles to the preparation and comparing the depth of the preparation and the depth and contour of the crown. When the crown margins pass over the cervical bulbosity on the buccal surface, a definite snap or click should be heard; this assures the operator of the crown's retention. The occlusion should be checked to see that

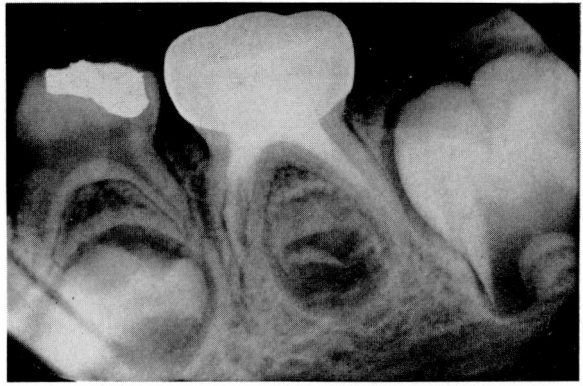

Fig. 85.—Mandibular periapical radiograph of a 3-year-old demonstrating well adapted and contoured stainless-steel crown. The tooth has been treated by partial pulpectomy procedures.

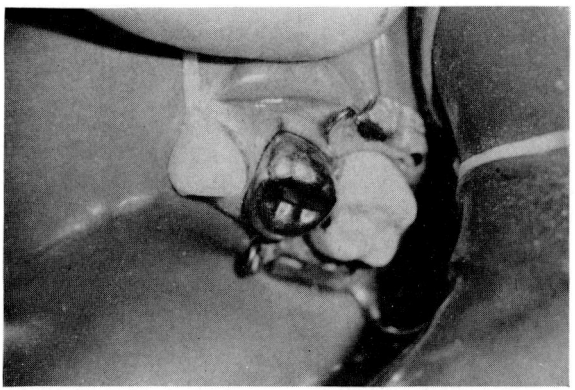

Fig. 86.—Trial fitting of the crown can be performed with the rubber dam in place: the margins are visible when the floss ligature is removed and the interproximal rubber is cut.

the crown is not interfering. Insufficient occlusal tooth reduction or sharp line angles result in inability to seat the crown. The width of a metal crown does not permit reduction without danger of perforation; therefore occlusal adjustment must occur by further tooth preparation, allowing a more gingival positioning of the crown.

155

POLISHING AND CEMENTATION

Prior to cementation the crown should be polished with a rubber wheel to remove all scratches. A final lustre is achieved with a rouge impregnated cloth. The crown margin should be blunt since a knife-edge finish merely produces sharp slivers of stainless steel which act as areas for plaque retention. A broad stone wheel should be run *slowly* across the margins towards the centre of the crown; this improves the adaptation of the crown by drawing the metal closer to the tooth without reducing crown height (Roche, 1970).

Pulp-protecting bases should be placed over the deep areas of the preparation, followed by a cavity varnish prior to cementation when the tooth is vital. This is unnecessary when pulp therapy has been performed. The cementing medium is either zinc-oxyphosphate or a fluoride-impregnated cement (*see* Chapter 12). A consistency similar to that used for cementing gold inlays is recommended, although a thicker mix can be used when only one crown is being cemented. Stainless-steel crowns should be cemented only on clean dry teeth; cotton roll isolation (Chapter 5) is recommended. Floss can be passed interproximally before the cement has set to assist in the later removal of set subgingival interproximal cement. The crown should be left undisturbed during setting by allowing the child to apply pressure through a cotton roll. Cement excess in the gingival sulcus should be removed thoroughly with an explorer prior to final polishing of the crown with pumice and a rubber cup.

THE USE OF CROWNS IN QUADRANT DENTISTRY

The child who presents with extensive decay may require pulp therapy and stainless-steel crowns in adjacent primary molars. A note of the crown size should be made on the patient's records; since tooth size is fairly constant for each individual, this will be of value when selecting appropriate crowns for teeth in other quadrants. As noted in Chapter 1, treatment planning should minimize the number of appointments and readministration of local anaesthesia; therefore it may be desirable to place steel crowns on adjacent primary molars which are also candidates for pulp therapy. This can be performed in one visit, very little additional time being required if the pulps are vital. Confidence in preoperative assessment of pulp status (Chapter 16) may encourage the operator to perform his crown preparation before embarking on pulp therapy, thereby allowing him to contour the crown while formocresol is in the pulp chamber if pulpotomy is performed (*Fig. 87*) (*and see also* Chapter 17). This approach is efficient since the high-speed cutting instruments and water coolant are used only once. However, an error in diagnosing pulp status may necessitate a two-visit pulp procedure, which is indeed unfortunate once the crown preparation has been completed! The alternative operative sequence is to perform the pulp therapy first and later reduce the tooth for crowning. This is less efficient since it requires a second use of high-speed cutting instruments; also the water coolant will dilute any medicament placed in the pulp chamber and the bur may catch the cotton pellet. The former method is recommended only for those who are confident of their preoperative diagnosis and operative speed with both crowns and pulp therapy; it is not recommended for the dental student.

Crown preparation for adjacent primary molars must provide sufficient interproximal clearance to allow for the bulk of two stainless-steel crowns. Completing one preparation before beginning the second usually prevents insufficient interproximal reduction. Although each crown will be trial fitted individually, both crowns must be tried on together prior to cementation. Occasionally one of the crowns has a path of insertion which is hindered if the other crown is already seated; in these cases the insertion sequence must be reversed.

Adjacent stainless-steel crowns are considerably more difficult when there has been longstanding interproximal caries that requires subgingival slices to encompass the depth of caries; furthermore tooth loss from caries leaves little interproximal clearance for both crowns. It is impossible to regain lost space from crowning alone; rather, the crowns have to be adapted to the altered space. During crown selection it may be necessary to reduce the mesiodistal width of the crown by squeezing it with a 110 plier, which will flatten the interproximal contour and provide more bulk of metal buccally and lingually (McEvoy, 1977). Alternatively, the crown can be cut, the margins lapped over, spot welded and soldered to reduce its size (*see* section on Crown Modifications).

The stainless-steel crown is also placed adjacent to Class 2 amalgam restorations; in this type of quadrant dentistry the sequence of operative procedures is most important. A typical example of one-visit quadrant dentistry is the mesio-occlusal alloy on the second primary molar, the stainless-steel crown on the first primary molar, and the distal restoration on the primary canine (*Fig. 87*). If the alloys are completed first, there is danger of amalgam fracture and inadequate contact areas when the crown is trial fitted and cemented. If all cavity and crown preparations are made first and the crown is then cemented, the excess cement from the crown will flow into the cavity preparations and need to be removed. Also, it is easier to overcontour the crown so that its dimensions impinge on the space for the alloy. Furthermore, the Class 2 cavity preparation may require further modification after the adjacent crown has been cemented, in order to make the interproximal margins self-cleansing. Therefore the crown should be prepared and cemented prior to any adjacent cavity preparations. In this way all the above disadvantages are avoided.

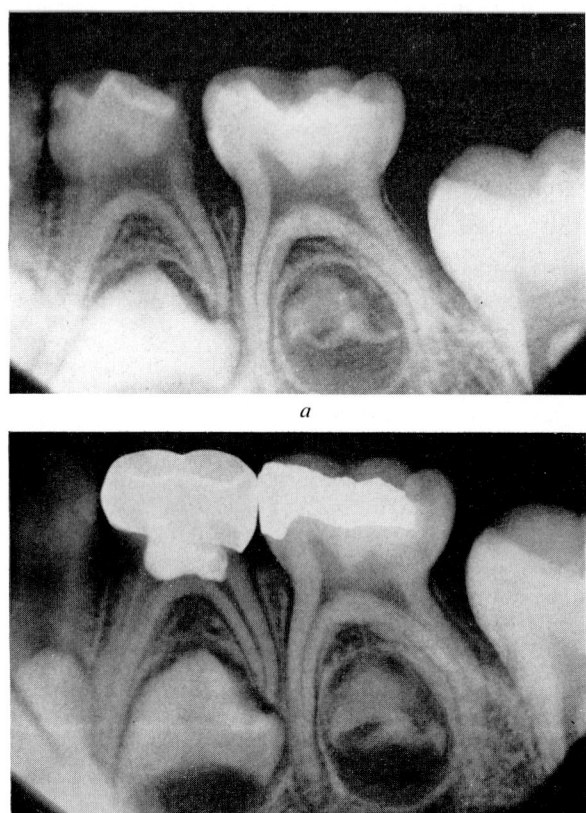

Fig. 87.—*a*, Preoperative mandibular periapical radiograph of a 4½-year-old. *b*, Postoperative mandibular radiograph shows the treated quadrant. The canine has been restored with a composite, the first molar by pulpotomy and crown and the second molar with amalgam. Note the good reproduction of contour.

STAINLESS-STEEL CROWN MODIFICATIONS

Mink and Hill (1971) reported several ways of modifying the stainless-steel crown. These can be summarized as follows:

a. The undersized tooth or the oversized crown: This commonly occurs when space loss has occurred as a result of long-standing interproximal caries. The crown is cut vertically along the buccal wall. The free crown margins are approximated and spot welded to reduce the crown's dimensions. After contouring, the cut and re-located area is soldered and polished.

b. The oversized tooth or the undersized crown: A vertical cut is made on the buccal surface of the crown. The margins are pulled apart and an additional piece of stainless-steel band material is spot welded to the buccal surface, increasing the dimensions of the crown. After contouring, solder is applied to fill any microscopic deficiency in seal. The crown is polished and cemented.

c. Deep subgingival caries: If this occurs interproximally, the un-festooned Rocky Mountain crown will normally be deep enough to encompass the preparation. Failing to stock such crowns or making an error in crown trimming can be compensated for by lengthening the crown with a spot welded and soldered piece of band material, as described in the previous section.

d. The open contact: Inability to establish a closed contact area (except for the primate space) will result in food packing, increased plaque retention, and subsequently gingivitis. Selection of a larger crown may solve this problem. Alternatively, exaggerated inter-proximal contour can be obtained with a 112 (ball and socket) plier to establish a closed contact. Localized addition of solder can also build out the interproximal contour.

COMPLICATIONS

The stainless-steel crown is by no means a panacea for the treatment of extensive caries or a means of avoiding amalgam failure. Handled improperly, these crowns can do as much damage as a poorly finished amalgam alloy. Some of the common complications that arise are mentioned, together with appropriate treatments:

a. Interproximal ledge: Incorrect angulation of the tapered fissure bur can produce a ledge instead of a shoulder-free interproximal slice. Further tooth reduction to remove this ledge should be attempted cautiously, because of the possibility of a traumatic exposure. Failure to remove the ledge will result in inability to seat the crown whose margins will bind on the ledge (*Fig. 88*).

When the adjacent tooth is partially erupted and the contact area is poorly established, the interproximal slice is difficult to prepare. Extensive subgingival tooth reduction is required to clear the contact area; difficulty in access increases the likelihood of establishing a ledge or damaging the erupting tooth, which would be unfortunate if it were the first permanent molar. In such instances it may be wise to delay crowning until the contact areas are properly established, which may occur in as little as three months.

b. Crown tilt: Destruction of a complete lingual or buccal wall by caries or overzealous use of cutting instruments may result in the finished crown tilting towards the deficient side. Lack of tooth support encourages this tilting which is commonly seen on the lingual aspect of mandibular primary molars. Placement of an amalgam alloy restoration prior to crowning provides support to prevent crown tilt, the alloy acting as a core. The clinical significance of crown tilting is minimal unless it occurs on young permanent molars where unfavourable supra-eruption of the opponent tooth may occur.

c. Poor margins: The marginal integrity of the crown is reduced when it is imperfectly adapted. Recurrent caries seldom occurs around open margins. However, as the marginal discrepancy increases, so does the chance of plaque retention and subsequent

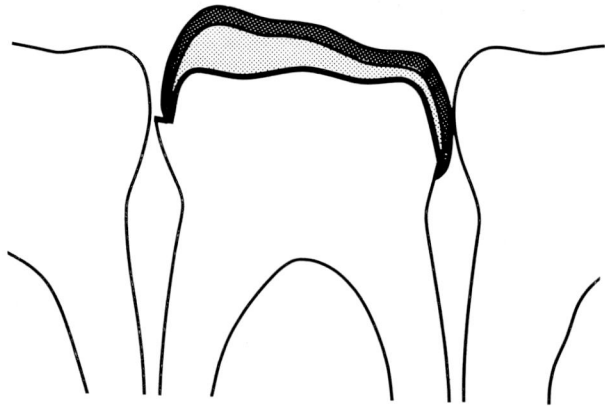

Fig. 88.—Inability to seat the crown results from a ledge on the preparation. This must be removed taking care not to expose the pulp.

gingivitis (Henderson, 1973) (*Fig. 89*). It is speculated that any chronic inflammation of the supporting tissues which is caused by open or overextended margins may result in premature exfoliation of that tooth; however, this speculation awaits clinical verification.

d. Inhalation or ingestion of the crown: This complication fortunately is rare. This is due to the practitioner's careful handling of the small and sometimes slippery crown in a young patient. However, sudden unpredictable movement may result in inhalation or ingestion of the crown. Should this occur, an attempt at removal can be made by holding the child upside down as soon as possible; if this is unsuccessful medical referral for an immediate chest X-ray is mandatory. If the crown is in the bronchi or lung, medical consultation and referral will probably result in an attempt to remove it by bronchoscopy. The presence of a cough reflex in the conscious child fortunately reduces the chances of inhalation, ingestion of the crown being more likely. Ingestion is of less consequence, but none the less must be diagnosed by the absence of the crown on a chest radiograph. The stainless-steel crown will usually pass uneventfully through the alimentary tract within 5–10 days. The parent should assume the unpleasant task of locating the crown.

Anguish and stress to child, parent and clinician are reduced by taking all possible precautions to prevent crown ingestion or inhalation. Therefore, crown preparation, trimming, and trial fitting should be performed with the rubber dam in place (*see Fig. 86*). When a crown is being fitted adjacent to the clamped tooth, the interproximal rubber can be cut and ligature removed so that the gingival margins are visible. Experience with crowns will encourage the

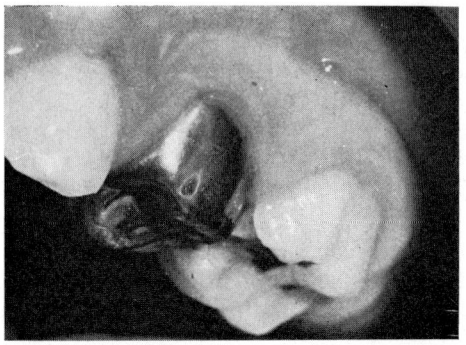

Fig. 89.—Good gingival response to well adapted stainless-steel crown.

operator to cement on the crown with the rubber dam in place; while the cement is setting, the cut rubber dam is removed and the occlusion checked. This technique cannot be used when two adjacent crowns are cemented or a crown is placed on the clamped tooth.

REFERENCES

Baume L. J. (1950) Physiological tooth migration and its significance for the development of occlusion. *J. Dent. Res.* **29**, 123, 331 and 440.

Castaldi C. R. (1957) Analysis of some operative procedures currently being used in paedodontics. *J. Can. Dent. Assoc.* **23**, 377.

Henderson H. Z. (1973) Evaluation of the preformed stainless-steel crown. *J. Dent. Child.* **40**, 353.

Hicks P. E. (1973) Treatment planning for the distal shoe space maintainer. *Dent. Clin. North Am.* **17**: 1, 135.

JAFFE E. C., STIMMLER L. and OSBORNE J. A. (1973) Enamel defects associated with neonatal symptomatic hypocalcaemia. *Proc. Br. Paedodontic Soc.* **3,** 25.

McEVOY S. A. (1977) Approximating stainless steel crowns in space-loss quadrants. *J. Dent. Child.* **44,** 105.

MacRAE P. D., ZACHERL W. and CASTALDI C. R. (1962) Study of defects in Class II dental amalgam restorations in deciduous molars. *J. Can. Dent. Assoc.* **28,** 491.

MINK J. R. and BENNETT I. C. (1968) The stainless-steel crown. *J. Dent. Child.* **35,** 186.

MINK J. R. and HILL C. J. (1971) Modification of the stainless-steel crown for primary teeth. *J. Dent. Child.* **38,** 61.

ROCHE J. R. (1970) In: *Current Therapy in Dentistry*, Vol. 4. St. Louis, C. V. Mosby Co., p. 540.

RECOMMENDED READING

MINK J. R. and BENNETT I. C. (1968) The stainless-steel crown. *J. Dent. Child.* **35,** 186.

MYERS D. R. (1976) The restoration of primary molars with stainless steel crowns. *J. Dent. Child.* **43,** 406.

TSAMTSOURIS A. and WHITE G. E. (1976) The use of preformed crowns for the primary dentition: Part II—The stainless steel crown. *J. Pedodont.* **1,** 10.

CHAPTER 14

PREVENTIVE ASPECTS OF PAEDIATRIC OPERATIVE DENTISTRY

PREVENTIVE aspects of operative dentistry fall into the following categories:

Preservation of tooth structure.

Protection of interproximal surfaces.

Protection of the occlusal surface.

Before these individual units are discussed, it should be stated that a high standard of operative dentistry is one of the best preventive measures that a patient can receive. Well placed and properly contoured restorations whose margins are in self-cleansing areas should provide longer service than those placed less meticulously.

Operative dentistry should be an adjunct to the practitioner's philosophy of preventive care for the child patient. Preventive measures, specifically applicable to the individual patient, must be instituted at the earliest possible time to alter the aetiological factors in caries formation.

PRESERVATION OF TOOTH STRUCTURE

This section will include many examples already described earlier in the text; however, it serves to bring together some important concepts in paediatric operative dentistry.

One aim in paediatric operative dentistry should be to place a restoration which will last as long as the tooth is in the mouth. This may not be possible in either primary or permanent teeth since new lesions may develop on a different surface of the tooth and marginal deterioration of a restoration may result in subsequent replacement. However, every time a restoration is replaced there is a danger of increasing cavity size and weakening cusps or incisal edges.

For example, the mandibular first permanent molar often requires an occlusal restoration within two years of its eruption. This same tooth may subsequently require a mesio-occlusal Class 2 cavity when the second primary molar is present before the second premolar erupts. This restoration may then need to be replaced when the premolar erupts, if the interproximal margins are no longer self-cleansing. When the second permanent molar erupts, the mesio-occlusal restoration may have to be removed for the second time to include any distal lesion. And how many MOD restorations in teenagers are of the classic textbook dimensions?

This exaggerated example demonstrates that one tooth, in this case a first permanent molar, may be subjected to as many as four operative procedures in as little as seven years, between ages 7 and 14. Cavity preparation in primary and young permanent teeth should therefore be conservative of sound tooth structure. Although all cavity margins must be extended into self-cleansing areas and decay must be removed, the preparations should have minimal intercuspal dimensions. As noted in Chapter 6, the intercuspal width of a Class 1 cavity determines the isthmus width of any Class 2 restoration subsequently placed in that tooth. Such minimal cavity preparations leave interproximal margins which are better supported and less likely to fail.

One specific modification to this concept must be made for the mesio-occlusal cavity in a first permanent molar, adjacent to the second primary molar. The interproximal margins of the Class 2 cavity must be made self-cleansing with respect to both the adjacent second primary molar and the anticipated contact with the second

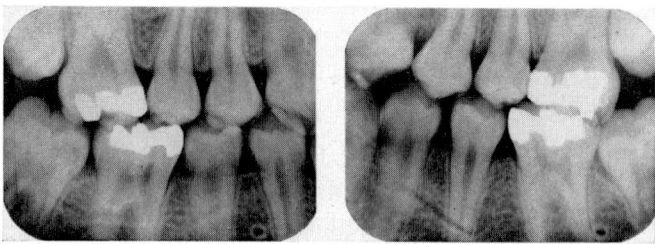

Fig. 90.—Correctly placed mesio-occlusal restorations in first permanent molars. Note the depth of the proximal box.

premolar. Usually the contact area between first permanent and second primary molar is more occlusally located than the one between permanent molar and second premolar. Therefore the gingival seat of the interproximal box should be placed deliberately subgingival in anticipation of the premolar's eruption. Failure to do this means that the floor of the box will not be self-cleansing with respect to the second premolar (*Fig. 90*). The buccal and lingual walls of the interproximal box should be self-cleansing with respect to the primary molar. Because of the subgingival preparation, additional care must be exercised in placing the matrix band and finishing the restoration.

These examples underline the fact that the dimension of time as it relates to paediatric operative dentistry is most important. The need for restorations in adults, and the types of restorations which are placed, may be directly related to the dentistry that the patient received when he was a child. It cannot be overemphasized that early diagnosis of the lesion enables the practitioner to perform minimal cavity preparations.

PROTECTION OF INTERPROXIMAL SURFACES
(adjacent to Class 2 restorations)

The proximal surface adjacent to a Class 2 cavity is put at risk during operative dentistry. Cardwell (1974) found that in more than 90 per cent of cases, dental students traumatically etched this surface when preparing a Class 2 cavity on the adjacent tooth; statistics are not available for dental practitioners. This traumatic damage is of minimal significance in the primary dentition since adjacent primary molars usually require simultaneous restoration of Class 2 lesions, (i.e. disto-occlusal on the first primary molar and mesio-occlusal on the second primary molar). The situation is different when a distal lesion in a second primary molar is being restored and the first permanent molar has erupted. Because of the thicker enamel in permanent teeth, immediate restoration of radio-lucent interproximal areas confined to enamel cannot be justified. It should be realized that the aetiological factors which are responsible for the distal lesion in the second primary molar will invariably cause some demineralization on the adjacent mesial surface of the first permanent molar. This demineralization may not be apparent radiographically but can be observed directly when the distal proximal box of the second primary molar has been prepared (McDonald, 1974).

Two methods can be used to protect interproximal surfaces adjacent to Class 2 cavities. First, precautions must be taken to prevent unnecessary mechanical damage and second, fluoride (in some form) should be applied to the proximal surface.

Prevention of Mechanical Damage

Unnecessary mechanical damage to proximal surfaces adjacent to Class 2 cavities is prevented by a combination of interproximal wedging, matrix protection, correct cavity preparation sequence, and patient control. Interproximal wedges, in addition to retracting the rubber dam and interdental papillae, spring the teeth slightly apart to facilitate cavity preparation. A metal matrix band can be placed before the interproximal box is prepared to protect the adjacent surface. The occlusal lock should be prepared before the proximal box as described in Chapters 4 and 7. The gingival, buccal and lingual extensions of the proximal box should be made before the contact is broken, using hand instruments for this reduces the danger of mechanical damage to the adjacent surface. Unfortunately, the inclination of enamel rods in primary molars necessitates further rotary instrumentation to finish the gingival floor of the box. Sudden movement of the child after the practitioner has used the greatest of care can result in trauma to the adjacent surface and the floor of the proximal box.

Fluoride
Topical

McDonald (1974) compared the ability of directly applied 8 per cent stannous fluoride and silver nitrate to prevent the progression of superficial lesions on the mesial surface of first permanent molars. The solutions were applied to the exposed mesial surface following cavity preparation of distal lesions in second primary molars with the rubber dam in place. Although stannous fluoride was more

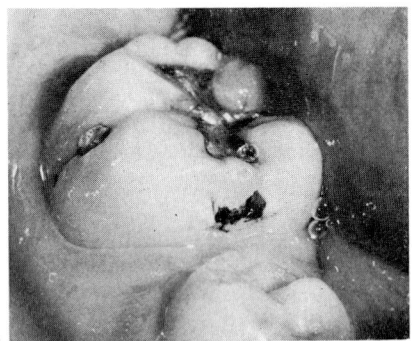

Fig. 91.—Stannous fluoride staining on the mesial surface of the first permanent molar. An incipient lesion has been arrested.

effective than silver nitrate at 1 year, it seemed to lose its effect after this time since both solutions were equally effective in preventing the progression of the lesion at the 2-year evaluation period. It is interesting that in approximately 75 per cent of the untreated (control) teeth, the lesion progressed from an enamel radiolucency to radiographic involvement of the dentine in 2 years. By comparison, a single application of 8 per cent stannous fluoride (or silver nitrate) prevented the progression of the lesion in 43 per cent of teeth after two years (*Fig. 91*).

A similar study comparing direct application of acidulated phosphate fluoride, stannous fluoride, and silver nitrate to the exposed mesial surface of recently erupted first permanent molars was reported by Hyde (1973). All solutions were effective after 1 year although the acidulated phosphate fluoride solution was superior to the others at the 2-year evaluation period. This tends to confirm that stannous fluoride loses its effectiveness after a year and also that silver nitrate is least effective. The protection afforded by

166

fluoride, though beneficial, may be insufficient over the long term since the opportunity to apply it directly occurs only once, namely when the adjacent Class 2 cavity is prepared.

However, this should not discourage the routine application of topical fluoride to quadrants isolated during operative dentistry; certainly any exposed surface will benefit from its application. In addition, 10 per cent stannous fluoride is of benefit in indirect pulp treatment (Nordstrom et al., 1974). It is difficult to assess whether fluoride applied to isolated cavity preparations will reduce recurrent caries. The many variables in cavity preparation and amalgam manipulation make such a study very difficult to structure, although it has been attempted (Alexander, 1968). It seems more likely that recurrent caries is due to marginal failure resulting from faulty operative dentistry rather than lack of fluoride. However, the extent to which fluoride alters the rate of recurrent decay, or even prevents it, remains unknown.

Fluoride-impregnated Cements

Since the second primary molar and first permanent molar may be in contact for as many as five to six years (between ages 6 and 12), other means of protecting the mesial surface of the permanent tooth must be considered. The difficulty of placing a Class 2 restoration in a partially erupted first permanent molar makes this preventive approach even more desirable. Placement of a material which continually releases fluoride would be of benefit. It has been recognized for several years that surfaces adjacent to silicate restorations seldom decay. This is explained by the fluoride flux in the silicate powder which is continually released from the set restoration. The acidic pH of silicate, together with exothermia from setting reaction may, however, produce an unfavourable pulpal response in teeth with inadequate pulp-protecting bases. However the concept is valuable.

1. *Tunnel Preparation*

Jinks (1963) recognized the problem of preventing mesial caries in the first permanent molar in the mixed dentition. He realized that the mesial surface had to receive a constant supply of fluoride, rather than a single application, to be afforded maximum protection. He prepared a tunnel from the occlusal surface to the distal contact area in the second primary molar. This was filled with a fluoride-impregnated cement so that the material was adjacent to the mesial surface of the first permanent molar; the occlusal part of the cavity was restored with amalgam (*Fig. 92*). Long-term results (between 1956 and 1962) demonstrated that approximal caries was prevented in 96 per cent of treated teeth when compared to untreated teeth in opposing quadrants (*Fig. 93*). This procedure unfortunately has two disadvantages: (1) There is a danger of traumatically exposing the pulp while preparing the tunnel under very limited visibility; and (2) The distal marginal ridge is undermined by the preparation and may subsequently fracture.

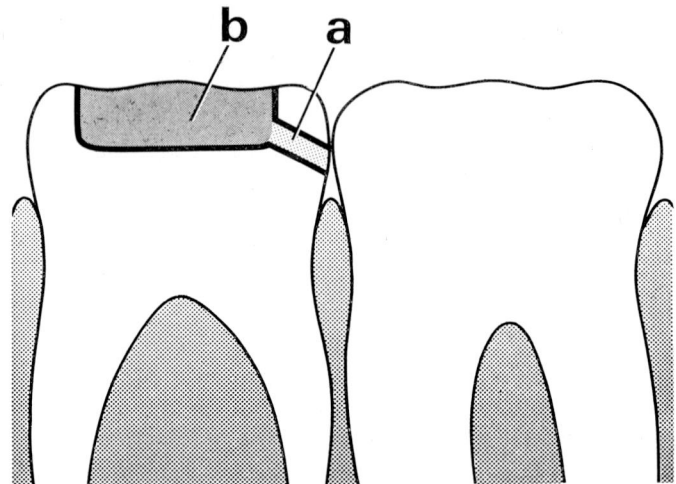

Fig. 92.—Tunnel preparation using fluoride impregnated cement (a) and an occlusal restoration in amalgam (b). *Modified from Jinks, G. M. (1963)*, J. Dent. Child. **30**, 87.

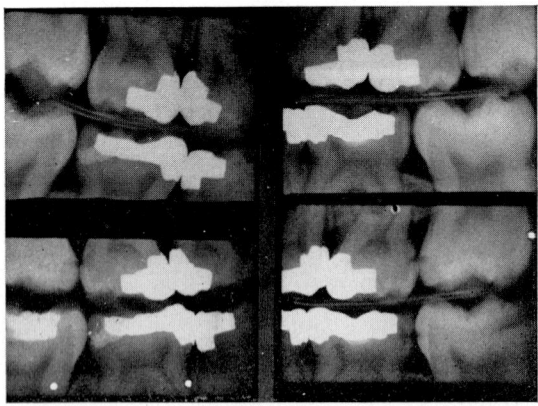

Fig. 93.—Successive bite-wing radiographs demonstrate the ability of fluoride impregnated cement to prevent a mesial cavity in the recently erupted first permanent molars. *By courtesy of Dr. G. M. Jinks and* J. Dent. Child. (1963) **30**, 87.

2. *Laminated Restoration*

This ingenious concept has been further developed by Jinks (1973) to avoid the disadvantages of the tunnel preparation. The concept of maintaining fluoride-impregnated cement adjacent to the mesial surface of the first permanent molar is still used. A distal Class 2 amalgam preparation is made in the second primary molar. The proximal box is filled with fluoride-impregnated cement to the level of the pulpal floor of the occlusal lock. The cement should be mixed to a stiff consistency. A soft mercury-rich mix of amalgam is condensed directly on the partially set cement. Excess mercury is removed from the amalgam before condensation is completed.

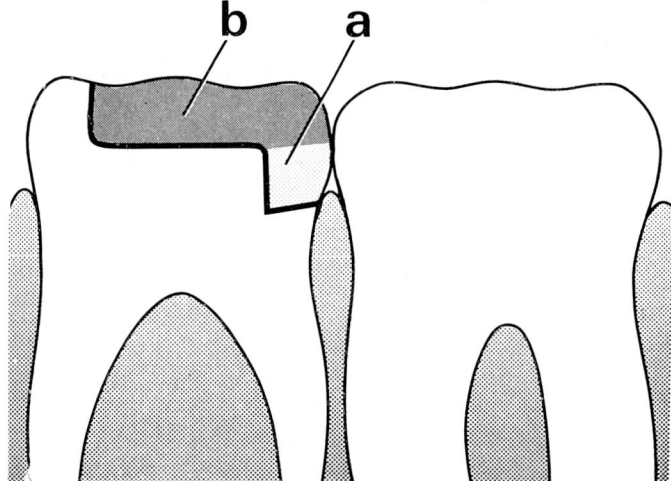

Fig. 94.—Laminated restoration using fluoride impregnated cement (a) in the proximal box of a second primary molar restored by amalgam (b) adjacent to a first permanent molar.

Finishing of the restoration is the same as for any Class 2 amalgam. Jinks (1973) calls this a laminated restoration (*Figs. 94, 95*).

One advantage of this technique is that the occlusal surface of the first permanent molar may require restoration at the same time; in this way two restorations can be performed at one visit with maximum utilization of anaesthesia. Furthermore, if the primary molars have already received Class 2 alloys, providing an occlusal restoration in the first permanent molar and a preventive laminated restoration in the second primary molar will usually eliminate the need of any operative dentistry in that quadrant until the second permanent molars erupt. Of course, this assumes that other routine preventive measures are used. If that treatment sequence is performed in all four quadrants at age 8, the child may go caries-free until age 12 or 13. Of course, this is extremely encouraging to both child and parent.

However, the technique is not without disadvantages. Isthmus fracture can be avoided by grinding the opposing tooth and not carving the marginal ridge area excessively deep. The possibility of adverse pulp response to the fluoride impregnated cement exists although Jinks (1963) reported only 2 clinically observable adverse responses out of 394 tunnel restorations. The main disadvantage is the gradual dissolution of the cement. The earlier the restoration is

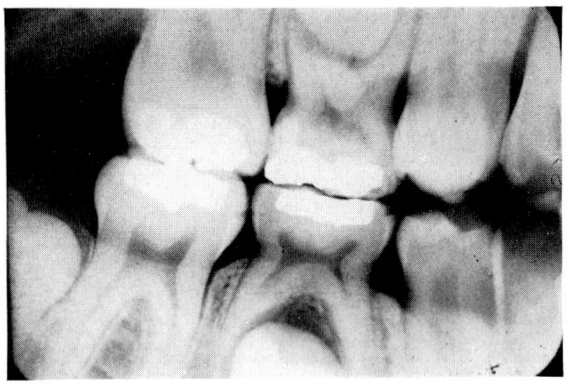

Fig. 95.—Bite-wing radiograph demonstrates the ability of the laminated restoration to prevent mesial caries in the maxillary first permanent molar, when compared to the untreated mandibular area.

placed, the longer the fluoride protection, but also the greater are the chances of washing out of the cement. There is a danger that mesial migration of the first permanent molar may occur, resulting in loss of arch length. However, any mesial migration is unlikely to exceed the leeway space.* Because of potential loss of arch length,* the laminated Class 2 restoration cannot be recommended in the permanent dentition. Also, the procedure is not applicable adjacent to primary molars because primary molar interproximal enamel radiolucencies are indicative of dentinal involvement of the lesion (Dwyer et al., 1973).

A variation of this concept can be used when a stainless-steel crown is placed. A hole is cut in the proximal surface of the crown adjacent to the surface which is to be protected after crown contouring has been completed. The hole is made with a small fissure

---

* *See* Glossary.

bur and should be about 2 mm in breadth buccolingually and 1 mm in height incisogingivally. The crown is then cemented using fluoride impregnated cement.

PROTECTION OF OCCLUSAL SURFACES
General Considerations

The depth and inclination of the occlusal fissures predispose these surfaces to plaque retention and subsequently to caries. The fissure may be impossible to cleanse properly since the diameter of a tooth-brush bristle may exceed the diameter of the fissure orifice. This means that toothbrushing at best will remove superficial dental plaque and at worst will force debris into the depths of the fissure. Since these fissures often extend to the amelodentinal junction, it is not surprising that carious involvement of the dentine can occur soon after eruption. This is verified by Walsh and Smart's observation (Walsh and Smart, 1948) that 50 per cent of mandibular first permanent molars had occlusal lesions by the age of 9 years. This rapid dentinal involvement of the lesion poses a severe problem to the preventive-oriented clinician. If one believes that the carious lesion cannot arrest once the dentine is involved (indirect pulp treatment excepted—*see* Chapter 17), then it is imperative to apply preventive measures as soon as possible after eruption. At this time such measures are usually hindered by a young and sometimes apprehensive child, as well as by an incompletely erupted tooth which cannot be effectively isolated.

Another complicating factor is the lack of agreement on what an occlusal cavity is and what constitutes a stained or sticky fissure that could be observed rather than restored (*see* Chapter 6).

Researchers frequently use the following code in classifying occlusal fissures:

    0—unstained, no catch of explorer.
    1—stained fissure, no catch of explorer.
    2—stained or unstained fissure, some explorer catch but no penetration or sticking.

Groups 0 and 1 are considered to be non-carious, while group 2 is considered a questionable lesion. This writer feels that if there is any catch of the explorer the fissure should be considered carious and treated with a Class 1 restoration. Other criteria such as de-calcification, grey discoloration resulting from enamel undermining, or bite-wing radiolucency assist in the diagnosis (*see also* Chapter 6).

The presence of caries (either occlusal or interproximal) in the tooth is a contra-indication to the use of preventive measures for protecting the occlusal surface. In the case of an interproximal radiolucency, the occlusal fissure would have to be removed to form the occlusal lock. Also, there is questionable value in sealing a permanent tooth which has an interproximal lesion confined to enamel, if previous decay experience indicates that such a lesion will progress to dentine involvement. Only those surfaces and those teeth which are definitely free of decay should be considered for preventive measures.

The methods of protecting the occlusal surfaces from decay are:
1. Prophylactic odontotomy.
2. Reshaping the fissures.
3. Fluoride.
4. Sealants.

Since these preventive measures are best applied as close as possible to the eruption of the tooth, they should be available at ages 6 and 7 and 12 and 13 to coincide with the eruption of first permanent molars, premolars, and second permanent molars, respectively. Since primary molars do not have as severe a prevalence of occlusal caries as permanent molars, these preventive measures should be applied only to permanent teeth.

Prophylactic Odontotomy

Hyatt (1923) recommended eliminating all susceptible fissures by cutting a shallow, minimal width Class 1 cavity in enamel. Since the cavity floor is left in enamel, local anaesthesia is not required, but the outline form must include all deep fissures. The cavity is then filled with amalgam. This procedure has the following disadvantages: cutting instruments must be used; the tooth is always committed to a restoration; and there is a risk of sealing caries if the preoperative diagnosis is inaccurate or if the fissure extends to the amelodentinal junction. For these reasons and because of the encouraging results with fissure sealants, prophylactic odontotomy cannot be recommended.

Reshaping of the Fissures

It has been recommended that the fissures be reshaped by reducing the steep cuspal inclines so that the occlusal surface is more readily cleansed by the child (Bodecker, 1929). This has many of the disadvantages of prophylactic odontotomy; also, the benefits of such reshaping are very limited in that the caries reduction is not proportionate to the time and effort invested. On these grounds the technique cannot be recommended on a universal basis.

Fluoride

Fluoride, either systemic or topical, is most effective in preventing caries on smooth surfaces; the least benefit is to the occlusal surface. Systemic fluoride may be responsible for producing teeth with less steep occlusal fissures (Lovius and Goose, 1969). However, epidemiological studies indicate that any modification of occlusal anatomy caused by systemic fluoride does not result in a significant occlusal caries reduction.

Some benefit will occur if the enamel in the depths of the fissure is exposed to fluoride topically. Marthaler (1969) found a 36 per cent reduction in DMFT in children who chewed fluoride tablets; it is speculated that the crushed tablets can force fluoride into the embrasures and into the depths of the occlusal fissures to obtain a topical effect from this systemically taken fluoride.

The avenue of saturating the fissures with topical fluoride has been further investigated, but the minimal reduction in occlusal caries is disappointing. It is speculated that neither stannous nor acidulated fluoride is able to impregnate the enamel at the depths of the fissures. This disappointing finding has prompted the evaluation of fluorides in concentrated polyurethane coatings or fissure-protecting lacquers. Three materials have been developed.

*Epoxylite 9070** is a long-lasting topical fluoride coating, although it was originally marketed as an occlusal sealant. The basis of the material is 10 per cent sodium monofluorophosphate in a polyurethane coating, which is applied following prophylaxis and a 60-second application of 50 per cent citric acid. No significant reduction in occlusal caries was reported by Rock (1972) after a one year trial in 11–13-year-old English children.

Elmex Protector† advertised as a combined sealant and topical fluoride, contains amine fluoride in a self-polymerizing varnish. Its retention must be questioned since no prior acid conditioning is used; it is ineffective in reducing occlusal caries (Rock, 1974).

Duraphat‡ yields 2·26 per cent fluoride and is a varnish which is applied to the tooth surface. This high fluoride concentration (in comparison to APF solutions which contain 1·23 per cent available fluoride) supposedly affords more protection. Another advantage claimed for Duraphat is an ability to adhere to moist teeth. Initial reports indicate 30 per cent caries reduction over a 15-month period (Heuser and Schmidt, 1968). A 36·7 per cent reduction was noted after 36 months with a three-treatment-a-year regime (Mainwald et al., 1978).

Sealants

Development of Sealants: The present-day fissure sealants are an exciting advance in preventive dentistry since they attempt to prevent caries in those areas where fluoride, either systemic or topical,

---

* Lee Pharmaceuticals, South El Monte, California.
† Vivadent Company, Liechtenstein.
‡ I.C.N., 1956 Bourdon St., Montreal, Quebec.

is least effective. However, attempts to protect the occlusal surface are not new. In addition to the methods previously described, various materials have been advocated for placing in the pits and fissures. These materials include copper cement, silver nitrate and zinc chloride with potassium ferricyanide; none is well retained without cavity preparation and their ability to prevent caries has proved even less encouraging.

An ideal sealant should adhere to all sound tooth surface around a fissure. Such a seal would theoretically provide the key to prevention of bacterial invasion and subsequent caries formation. The problem of retention and adaptation is magnified by the irregular anatomy of the occlusal surface, both at a macroscopic and microscopic level. Acid conditioning of the enamel surface before the sealant is applied improves the resin's retention. This acid conditioning is almost universally used in all present day sealants to enhance retention and to improve the marginal seal.

The most recently developed sealants are:
1. The cyanoacrylates (no longer clinically available).
2. The polyurethanes (discussed under fluorides).
3. The reaction product of Bisphenol A and glycidyl methacrylate (*see* p. 178).

Before these materials are discussed, the important matter of acid conditioning prior to sealant application will be reviewed.

Enamel Conditioning with Acid Solutions

Buonocore (1955) demonstrated the improved retention of simple acrylic resin to enamel that had been conditioned by acid. Since that time, acid conditioning or etching of enamel has been used in the retention of pit and fissure sealants, the attachment of orthodontic brackets directly to teeth, the restoration of fractured incisors, splinting of mobile teeth and the increase in enamel fluoride uptake. Various types and concentrations of acid and durations of application have been studied; as a result, a 60-second application of 50 per cent phosphoric acid was commonly used. Usually a buffered solution is preferred—50 per cent phosphoric acid and 7 per cent dissolved zinc oxide (Buonocore et al., 1968). Silverstone (1974) found that an unbuffered solution of 37 per cent phosphoric acid produced the most favourable conditions for bonding.

Acid etching has two distinct actions on human enamel. Firstly, it removes superficial plaque, debris, and a very shallow layer of enamel, including chemically inert enamel crystallites. Secondly, it renders the enamel surface more porous. A honey-combed latticework is produced within the remaining superficial enamel, where enamel tags are left projecting in different planes and at different angles (*Figs. 96–99*). There is differential demineralization of

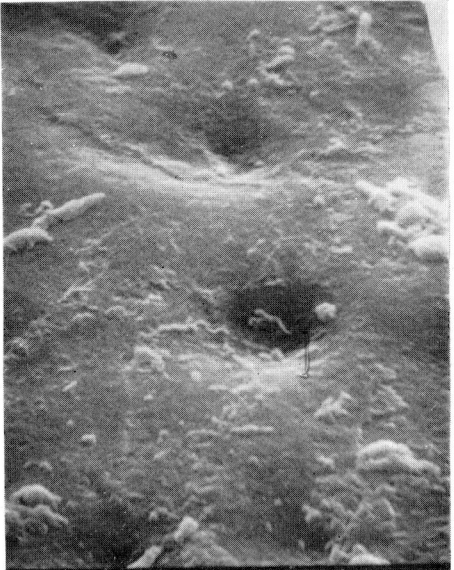

(*Figs. 96–99 by courtesy of Dr. H. Lee, South El Monte, California.*)

Fig. 96.—Photomicrograph of normal enamel: permanent tooth (× 2400).

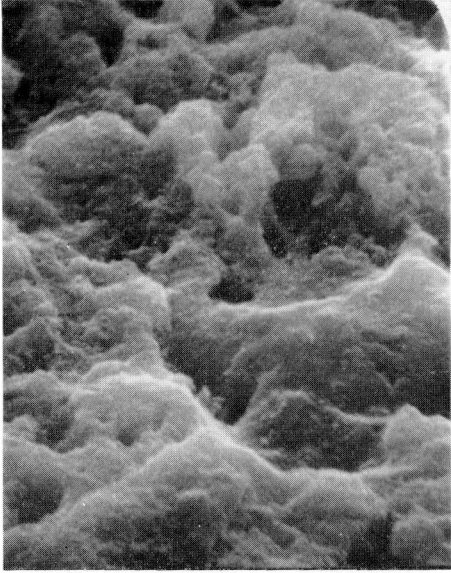

Fig. 97.—Photomicrograph of permanent enamel etched by 50 per cent phosphoric acid for 60 seconds (× 2400). Note the honeycomb effect.

175

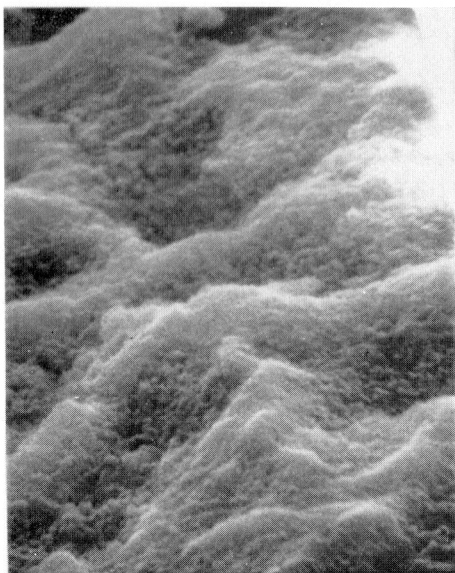

Fig. 98.—Photomicrograph of primary enamel etched by 50 per cent phosphoric acid for 60 seconds (× 2400). Note that the etching is considerably different from that in *Fig. 97.*

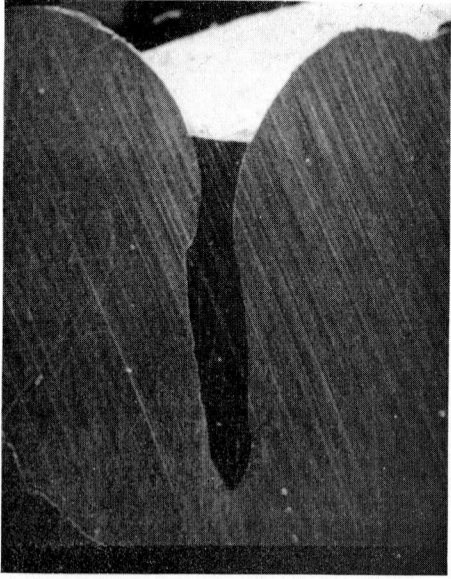

Fig. 99.—Cross-sectional view of a fissure sealed with Epoxylite 9075. Note incomplete extension into the fissure: the retention is mainly from the inclined planes of the fissure.

176

the prisms because the primary attack occurs on the cores of enamel rods to produce the microspaces. However, this depends on the incident angulation of the enamel rods to the tooth surface. On an average, the etching is about 25 microns deep in permanent teeth.

Primary teeth react differently to acid etching. After etching for 60 seconds with 50 per cent phosphoric acid, the microspaces in primary teeth are smaller and finer, which reduces the retention of resins to primary teeth (*Fig. 98*). It was thought that the outer prismless layer of enamel (Ripa, 1966) prevented the penetration of resins in the surface of etched primary enamel (Hinding and Sveen, 1974; Sheykholeslam and Buonocore, 1972). There is not universal agreement that prismless enamel occurs in all surfaces of all primary teeth (Mortimer, 1970; Silverstone, 1970). To obtain a comparable pattern of etching as found in permanent teeth Silverstone and Dogon (1976) found it necessary to etch for 120 seconds.

Retention of the sealant is by mechanical locking into the microspaces produced in the outer enamel surface by etching. This occurs on the inclined planes and not at the depth of the fissures (*Fig. 99*). Differential dissolution of the enamel of teeth treated with fissure sealants reveals tags of resin penetrating into the enamel; this confirms the mechanical locking that produces retention. The depth of the resin tags is related to the strength of the bond. Three factors influence the sealant's retention to the etched enamel of the pits and fissures: those which influence etching, debris in the fissure, and viscosity and handling of sealant.

Factors which influence etching

When the etched surface is contaminated with saliva or moisture from the breath before the sealant is applied, the result is reduced bond strength for the sealant. The contamination prevents adaptation of the sealant, and causes remineralization of etched enamel. This is a strong indication for the routine use of the rubber dam during application. However, Buonocore (1971) reports good retention of the sealant with cotton roll rather than rubber dam isolation. Also, using rubber dam for sealant application requires additional time; and when the procedure is not being done in conjunction with operative work, cost effectiveness is reduced. Oil contamination of the etched surface can occur from a faulty air syringe; this also reduces the strength of the sealant's bond. It is therefore advisable to clear the air hose into a cotton roll to observe whether any oil droplets stain the white cotton before drying the etched surface.

Exposing the enamel to fluoride can significantly alter the strength of the bond. Teeth that have been exposed to either systemic or topical fluoride, or both, are more resistant to acid etching. Therefore, the teeth should not be cleaned with a fluoride prophylaxis paste before the sealant is applied, nor should topical fluoride be used. Fluoride applied to an etched surface reduces the size of the microspaces and so reduces bond strength of the sealant. Thus, although it might seem a good idea to seal fluoride into the fissures, such an attempt would result in reduced retention of the sealant. However, it is acceptable and even advisable to apply fluoride topically after sealant application. Any etched enamel that is not covered by sealant will quickly incorporate this fluoride and remain well protected.

Debris within the fissure

Prior to acid etching, the pits and fissures must be thoroughly cleaned with a non-fluoridated paste. All debris and remnants of polishing paste must be completely removed from the pits and fissures beforehand by an explorer and by thorough irrigation. Some manufacturers recommend a cavity cleanser for this step. This cleansing is most important along the inclined planes of the fissures which provide the main retention of the sealant.

Viscosity and Handling of the Sealant

The strength of the bond depends on the sealant's ability to flow both into the microspaces produced by acid etching and into the depths of pits and fissures. The more viscous materials will not flow and their retention is consequently reduced. Improper mixing or application will make the material porous, and if this occurs adjacent to the etched surface, the seal will be imperfect.

The Reaction Products of Bisphenol A and Glycidyl Methacrylate

These materials are very similar to composite resins, although they are usually less viscous and permit flow into the depths of pits and fissures. Their viscosity is reduced by the incorporation of the alphatic diacrylate type. Resin systems (whether they be of the sealant or the composite resin type) are polymerized either by the action of ultraviolet light or benzoin methyl ether (e.g. Nuva-Seal*) or by chemical activation with benzyl peroxide as the catalyst (e.g. Delton†). Both use an activator or catalyst system which accelerates the intra-oral setting time while maintaining adequate shelf life and working time. Sealants are applied after initial prophylaxis and enamel pre-treatment with a 60-second application of 50 per cent buffered phosphoric acid. However, most commercially available etchants consist of 37 per cent unbuffered phosphoric

---

* L.D. Caulk Company, Milford, Delaware.
† Johnson and Johnson, East Winsor, New Jersey.

acid. The acid can be applied by a fine camel hair paint brush or by a small cotton pellet maintaining a moist surface for the required time. The tooth is washed with water for 15 seconds and air dried,

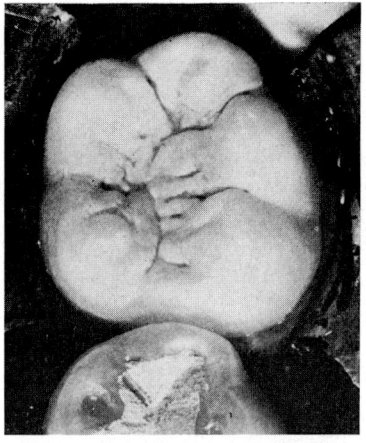

Fig. 100.—Preoperative view of isolated tooth suitable for a fissure sealant. Note absence of caries.

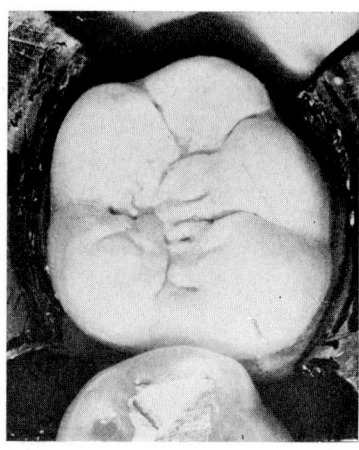

Fig. 101.—Following acid etching with 50 per cent phosphoric acid for 60 seconds, the occlusal surface appears chalky.

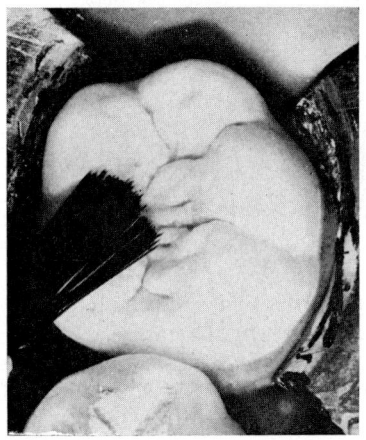

Fig. 102.—The sealant is applied with a camel hair brush.

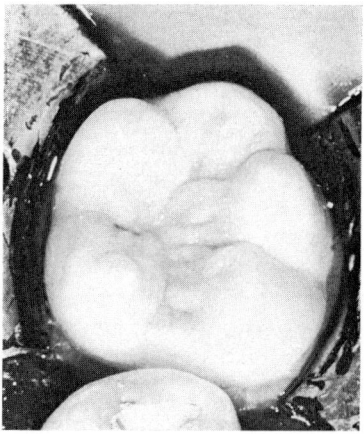

Fig. 103.—Completed fissure sealant.

and the treated enamel should then appear chalky, dull, and opaque with loss of natural lustre. Acid must be re-applied if this appearance is not observed. Rubbing the surface dry with a cotton pellet is not recommended since this will smooth over the etched surface

179

and close the microspaces to resin penetration. Rubber dam isolation is preferred by this author since it provides the most efficient working environment and prevents remineralization of etched enamel by saliva. The materials should be mixed and applied according to manufacturer's instructions; however, some points of clinical significance should be discussed separately here, since materials differ in their manner of polymerization.

Ultraviolet Polymerized Sealants (Figs. 100–104)

They are polymerized by exposure to long wave ultraviolet light at 360 Angström units in wavelength; the light-sensitive catalyst is benzoin methyl ether which is added prior to application. This light-sensitive material will not set until exposed to the U-V light gun (Nuva-Lite), which allows the clinician adequate working time.

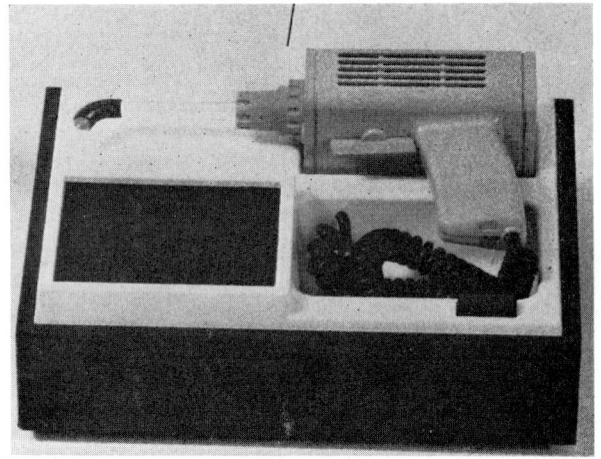

Fig. 104.—U-V gun.

It is painted into the fissures with a camel-haired brush prior to polymerization. The gun is held 2 mm from the occlusal surface for 30 seconds to obtain polymerization. Once the catalyst has been added, the light-sensitive material, stored in a dark bottle, will remain stable for only 24 hours. Accordingly, the clinician would be well advised to schedule patients requiring sealants at one treatment session to minimize waste. The U-V light gun must reach full output before it is ready for use; it has a 5-minute warm-up time. The gun should be left on in between patients, since it can be turned on only when the lamp is cool. If it is turned off when warm, the clinician will have to wait until it cools and then a further 5 minutes until full output is reached.

Chemically Polymerized Sealants

They use a benzoyl peroxide catalyst which is mixed with the resin. Because polymerization occurs immediately the catalyst is added, the operator is faced with reduced working time. An advantage of this is that there is less time in which saliva contamination of etched enamel can occur; also time is not taken up with applying the sealant and then reaching for the U-V light source. Therefore, the chemically polymerized sealant must be very accurately positioned, unlike U-V light polymerized materials which do not harden until the light source is placed.

Provided that gross excess of resin has not been used, there should be no occlusal interference. Selective grinding with a green stone will relieve any prematurities. The polymerized sealant should appear very smooth and shiny. Any air bubbles can be removed by grinding or by filling in the void with additional sealant. The margins should be indiscernible to an explorer. At this time the two sealants given approval by the American Dental Association Council on Dental Materials are Nuva-Seal and Delton.

Selection of Teeth

Maximum benefit is obtained when the sealant is applied as close as possible to eruption time. There is little value in sealing a tooth which has been erupted for three years in a child whose caries incidence is low. The depth and inclination of the fissures must also be considered since they will determine the likelihood of developing caries. The child's previous decay experience will also help the clinician predict whether a tooth is at risk and if so would benefit from a sealant.

Selection of teeth on the basis of freedom from caries has already been described (*see* p. 171). These rigid criteria for application of sealants are in contradiction to the results of deliberately sealed deep carious lesions using Nuva-Seal (Handelman et al., 1973). A comparison of sealed and untreated non-sealed lesions revealed a marked reduction in cultivatable bacteria in the sealed lesions 6 months postoperatively. This speaks highly of the sealant's marginal integrity over the first 6 months, since it can be presumed that the bacteria within the lesion could no longer remain viable in the absence of nutrients and saliva which were denied by the effectiveness of the seal. However, this study should not encourage the clinician to seal active lesions. The temptation to do this is greater when the child presents a behaviour problem; but application of the sealant may be more difficult in such a child and the clinical result imperfect. Should that sealant fail and decay progress in that tooth, the clinician is faced with the problem of treating a large lesion, frequently in the critically important first permanent molar, in a difficult child.

Postoperative Evaluation

Since most materials are clear, they are very difficult to see and this makes postoperative evaluation difficult. Bite-wing radiographs must be obtained at each 6-month recall visit; and besides observing interproximal surfaces the clinician must look for radiolucencies beneath the depths of occlusal fissures. Any alteration in radiographic appearance compared to the baseline preoperative radiograph should prompt removal of the sealant and restorative treatment. In the absence of any such radiolucency, re-application of the sealant is indicated if the margins are deficient and no lesion is apparent clinically.

Sealant Effectiveness

The ability of various fissure sealants (mainly Epoxylite 9075 and Nuva-Seal) to be retained in the occlusal fissures and to prevent caries in those fissures has been clinically evaluated (Buonocore, 1971; Rock, 1974). These studies are significant since study periods of at least two years were used; these allowed detailed evaluation of the need for sealant reapplication, of sealant leakage, and of subsequent caries formation both occlusally and interproximally.

In young permanent teeth complete retention of Nuva-Seal can be expected in 80 per cent of fissures; 15 per cent demonstrated partial retention after two years (Rock, 1974). By comparison, Epoxylite 9075 was only fully retained in 51 per cent of permanent teeth, 15 per cent showing partial retention. Buonocore (1971) reported 50 per cent retention of Nuva-Seal to primary teeth and 87 per cent to permanent teeth after two years. Caries reduction, due to the sealant was in the order of 99 per cent for permanent teeth and 87 per cent for primary teeth (Buonocore, 1971). Hinding (1974) and Rock (1974) found that extended protection against caries is provided to occlusal surfaces which have lost sealant. Retention of resin tags within the superficial enamel may be responsible for this. The use of Nuva-Seal in an exclusively paedodontic practice was studied over a 5-year term by Doyle and Brose (1978). They concluded that 57 per cent of primary teeth that were sealed were eventually restored; failure was attributed to the high abrasion seen on primary teeth. By comparison only 29 per cent of permanent tooth sealants were replaced by restorations. The highest failure rate occurred in second molars; this is consistent with Rock's finding (1974) that the distal pit of maxillary molars has the highest failure of sealant retention. Retention of the sealant was not influenced by oral hygiene or by refined carbohydrate increase.

No one preventive measure is totally effective—sealants are no exceptions. Their real effectiveness in paediatric dentistry should not be overestimated at a time when many dentists are eager to jump on a preventive dentistry bandwagon that perhaps benefits the manufacturer more than the patient.

REFERENCES

ALEXANDER, W. E. (1968) M.S.D. Thesis: *Effect of a Stable 30% Stannous Fluoride Solution on Recurrent Caries Around Amalgam Restorations.* Indiana University.

BOLECKER C. F. (1929) The eradication of enamel fissures. *Dent. Items Int.* **51**, 859.

BUONOCORE M. G. (1955) A simple method of increasing the adhesion of acrylic filling materials to enamel surfaces. *J. Dent. Res.* **34**, 849.

BUONOCORE M. G. (1971) Caries prevention in pits and fissures sealed with an adhesive resin polymerized by ultraviolet light: a ten-year study of a single adhesive application. *J. Am. Dent. Assoc.* **82**, 1090.

BUONOCORE M. G., MATSUI A. and GWINNETT A. J. (1968) Penetration of resin dental materials into enamel surfaces with reference to bonding. *Arch. Oral Biol.* **13**, 61.

CARDWELL J. A. (1974) Personal communication, results available from a study reported by J. A. Cardwell and B. J. Roberts (1972). *J. Dent. Res.* **51**, 1269.

DOYLE W. A. and BROSE J. A. (1978) A five-year study of the longevity of fissure sealants. *J. Dent. Child.* **44**, 127.

DWYER D. M., BERMAN D. S. and SILVERSTONE L. M. (1973) A study of approximal carious lesions in primary molars. *J. Int. Assoc. Dent. Child.* **4**, 41.

HANDELMAN S. L., BUONOCORE M. G. and SCHOUTE P. C. (1973) Progress report on the effect of a fissure sealant on bacteria in dental caries. *J. Am. Dent. Assoc.* **87**, 1189.

HEUSER H. and SCHMIDT H. F. M. (1968) Zahnkariesprophylaxe durch tiefenimprägnierung des zahnschmelzes mit fluor-lack. *Stoma* **21**, 91.

HINDING J. (1974) Extended cariostasis following loss of pit and fissure sealant from human teeth. *J. Dent. Child.* **41**, 201.

HINDING J. H. and SVEEN O. B. (1974) A scanning electron microscope study of the effects of acid conditioning on occlusal enamel of human permanent and deciduous teeth. *Arch. Oral. Biol.* **19**, 573.

HYATT T. P. (1923) Prophylactic odontotomy. *Dental Cosmos* **65**, 234.

HYDE E. J. (1973) Caries-inhibiting action of three different topically-applied agents on incipient lesions in newly erupted teeth: results after 24 months. *J. Can. Dent. Assoc.* **39**, 189.

JINKS G. M. (1963) Fluoride-impregnated cements and their effect on the activity of interproximal caries. *J. Dent. Child.* **30**, 87.

JINKS G. M. (1973) Personal communication.

LOVIUS B. B. J. and GOOSE D. H. (1969) The effect of fluoridation of water on tooth morphology. *Br. Dent. J.* **127**, 322.

McDonald R. E. (1974) *Dentistry for the Child and Adolescent*, 2nd ed. St. Louis, C. V. Mosby, p. 132.

Mainwald H. J., Kunzel W. and Weatherell J. (1978) The use of a fluoride varnish in caries prevention. *J. Int. Assoc. Dent. Child.* **9,** 31.

Marthaler T. M. (1969) Caries-inhibiting effect of fluoride tablets. *Helv. Odont. Acta* **13,** 1.

Mortimer K. V. (1970) The relationship of deciduous enamel structure to dental disease. *Caries Res.* **4,** 206.

Nordstrom D. O., Wei S. H. and Johnson R. (1974) Use of stannous fluoride for indirect pulp capping. *J. Am. Dent. Assoc.* **88,** 997.

Ripa L. W. (1966) The histology of the early carious lesion in primary teeth with special reference to a 'prismless' outer layer of primary enamel. *J. Dent. Res.* **45,** 5.

Rock W. P. (1972) Fissure sealants. *Br. Dent. J.* **133,** 146.

Rock W. P. (1974) Fissure sealants: further results of clinical trials. *Br. Dent. J.* **136,** 317.

Sheykholeslam Z. and Buonocore M. G. (1972) Bonding of resins to phosphoric acid-etched enamel surfaces of permanent and deciduous teeth. *J. Dent. Res.* **51,** 1572.

Silverstone L. M. (1970) The histopathology of early approximal caries in the enamel of primary teeth. *J. Dent. Child.* **37,** 17.

Silverstone L. M. (1974) Fissure sealants: laboratory studies. *Caries Res.* **8,** 26.

Silverstone L. M. and Dogon I. L. (1976) The effect of phosphoric acid on human deciduous enamel surfaces *in vitro*. *J. Int. Assoc. Dent. Child.* **7,** 11.

Walsh J. P. and Smart R. S. (1948) Relative susceptibility of tooth surfaces to dental caries and other comparative studies. *N.Z. Dent. J.* **44,** 17.

RECOMMENDED READING

Gwinnett A. J. (1971) Caries prevention through sealing of pits and fissures. *J. Can. Dent. Assoc.* **37,** 458.

Hyde E. J. (1973) Caries-inhibiting action of three different topically-applied agents on incipient lesions in newly erupted teeth: Results after 24 months. *J. Can. Dent. Assoc.* **39,** 189.

Rock W. P. (1974) Fissure sealants: further results of clinical trials. *Br. Dent. J.* **136,** 317.

CHAPTER 15

PRINCIPLES OF PULP THERAPY

THIS chapter and the two following will deal with pulp treatment of primary and young permanent teeth. Principles of pulp therapy will be discussed in the present chapter; Chapters 16 and 17 will deal with diagnosis of pulp pathology and treatment techniques, respectively. As background information to these chapters, the various treatment procedures are outlined briefly in the following chapter and they will be discussed in detail in Chapter 17.

Indirect Pulp Treatment

The technique is to remove all decay, except that which, in the clinician's experience, would expose the pulp if it were removed. A pulp-protecting base, such as zinc oxide or calcium hydroxide, is placed over the deep aspects of the cavity, whose margins are well supported and finished. An intermediate or permanent restoration is placed depending on whether a two- or one-visit procedure is being used. Elimination of the majority of the bacteria from the lesion and the substrate by an efficient seal of the restoration will hopefully diminish the rate of progression of the lesion. Since the pulp is no longer insulted by the carious lesion it is also hoped that it will respond physiologically to this protective layer by depositing secondary dentine, rather than pathologically, were the lesion left untreated. For this treatment to be successful, the pulp must be vital and free of inflammation; at least, if any inflammation is present, it must be reversible so that the secondary dentine can act as a barrier to further insult.

Direct Pulp Capping

Direct pulp capping is the placement of material over an exposed vital pulp. It is hoped that the pulp will respond by remaining free from pathosis and preferably will lay down secondary dentine. For this to be successful the pulp adjacent to the exposure site must be vital and capable of repair. If the inflammation extends throughout the pulp chamber, the chances of success obviously diminish. Therefore the technique is most applicable to small carious or traumatic vital exposures.

Pulpotomy

Pulpotomy is the removal of *vital* pulp from the coronal chamber. This is followed by placing some medicament over the radicular pulp stumps which either stimulate repair in, fix, or mummify the remaining vital radicular pulp. When the pulp is vital and local anaesthetic is used the treatment can be performed in one visit; this pulpotomy technique is referred to as vital amputation. Mortal amputation refers to: 'a method of root treatment in which the pulp is first devitalized. Then after removal of the coronal parts, the amputated radicular parts are covered with an antiseptic drug. This permeates the remaining devitalized tissues and preserves them without undue irritation of the viable tissues beyond the demarcation line which is now forming.' (Castagnola and Orlay, 1951.) Effectively this method was a two- or-more visit mummification procedure commonly used in Europe—it was used prior to the introduction of formocresol and prior to the recognition of a need for local anaesthesia in paediatric dentistry.

Pulpectomy

Pulpectomy is the removal of *vital* tissue from the coronal pulp chamber and root canals. Following mechanical and chemical preparation of the root canals they are filled. As with pulpotomy, through common usage, pulpectomy refers to débridement and subsequent filling of the root canals irrespective of preoperative vitality. Pulpectomy can either be partial or complete depending on the extent of instrumentation of the root canals. The thin, tortuous and branching path of the primary molar pulp filaments (Hibbard and Ireland, 1957) preclude the possibility of complete removal of all radicular pulp. Therefore, theoretically any pulpectomy in a primary molar is partial. Through common usage, complete pulpectomy refers to those instances when successful biomechanical preparation and obliteration result in an effective apical seal. Partial pulpectomy is removal of pulp and debris and subsequent filling of the canals short of the apex. The pulpectomy for primary and permanent teeth can be performed in one or many visits. Pulpectomy techniques are applicable to those teeth with inflamed vital radicular pulps or to non-vital teeth.

Successful pulp therapy for primary teeth is one of the most valuable services a child patient can receive, since there is no better space maintainer than the retained primary tooth. The practitioner must be aware of the dangers of retaining untreated carious primary molars. A carious primary molar which is left untreated merely invites chronic infection which may at any time become an acute alveolar abscess. The underlying permanent tooth is put at unnecessary risk during its development by the surrounding inflammation; the possibilities of hypoplasia and hypocalcification are increased. In addition, the tooth and surrounding periodontium are

186

a focus of chronic inflammation, which is of serious consequence in children with congenital and acquired heart conditions because of the risk of developing subacute bacterial endocarditis. Space loss can also occur as a result of untreated interproximal caries.

The orthodontic implications of premature loss of primary teeth have been outlined in Chapter 1.

ASSESSMENT

Thorough preoperative assessment is essential to determine whether pulp therapy or extraction is indicated. If conservation is indicated, the assessment will indicate which type of pulp therapy (e.g. pulpotomy) is applicable. The following should be considered:

1. Medical conditions.
2. Space management decisions and parental attitudes toward dental health.
3. Assessment of the individual tooth.

1. *Medical Conditions*

A thorough medical history may reveal a systemic problem or disease which will influence treatment. For example, every effort should be made to conserve teeth in haemophiliacs to prevent the hospitalization that would be required if extractions were to become necessary. Another systemic abnormality which influences pulp treatment and operative dentistry is congenital and acquired heart disease. Failure to eliminate any infected pulp or periapical tissue poses a serious health hazard in these children by increasing their chances of developing subacute bacterial endocarditis. Also, the trauma of operative dentistry results in a transient bacteraemia from the gingivae which places the cardiac patient at further risk. From 75 to 90 per cent of bacterial endocarditis cases are caused by the alpha haemolytic streptococcus of the viridans group, an organism commonly found in the gingival sulcus (Sorenson, 1973).

There will never be unanimity on the advisability of endodontic therapy in patients with congenital or acquired heart conditions. Each child, each mouth, and each individual tooth must be evaluated. For example, a child may present with three out of four carious primary molars in one arch already committed to removal. Attempts to save the fourth tooth may be unwarranted if its loss can be incorporated into any early orthodontic or space management plan involving the loss of the other three teeth.

The ideal pulp treatment for cardiac patients is indirect pulp treatment, since this avoids exposure. Direct pulp therapy should be avoided whenever possible in cardiac patients. The treatment of non-vital primary teeth does not carry a high enough success rate to justify its use in cardiac patients; these teeth should be extracted. Whenever pulp treatment is performed, the clinician must be convinced that the chances of success are high and postoperative results must be carefully monitored. If there is any suspicion that the pulp treatment might fail, the tooth should be extracted.

Although it is generally accepted that patients with cardiac anomalies must receive a course of antibiotics prior to dental treatment, opinions differ on the exact dosage, its timing, and the route and duration of administration. The objective of an antibiotic régime is to obtain a high blood level at the time of any dental procedure which will result in a transient bacteraemia above the physiological limit. The antibiotic must be continued postoperatively to prevent sensitization and development of resistant strains.

The most effective and certain means of ensuring a high blood level is by intramuscular injection one hour preoperatively. This is followed by an oral course of antibiotics for a minimum of 3 days postoperatively. Penicillin is the antibiotic of choice unless allergy exists, in which case erythromycin should be used. Tetracycline should not be used, since it is only bacteriostatic and not bactericidal; also there is unnecessary danger of intrinsic staining in developing permanent teeth.

Intramuscular injection is best given in the upper and lateral quadrant of the buttock to avoid damage to the sciatic nerve. Unfortunately, it is not the most painless procedure and therefore does little to enhance cooperation in the young child. Because of the viscosity of erythromycin, its intramuscular injection is even more painful than that of penicillin. Some practitioners may wish to refer the patient to a physician for this intramuscular injection; if this is done, the appointment times must be accurately co-ordinated to ensure maximum blood level of antibiotic at the time of operative dentistry. Because of these problems, an oral route of administration is commonly used in preference to the intramuscular.

The newest American Heart Association guidelines for the prevention of bacterial endocarditis have been accepted by the American Dental Association (1977). The recommended doses for children are penicillin G (30,000 units/kg I.M) plus procaine penicillin G (600,000 units/kg I.M) followed by penicillin V 250 mg every 6 hours for eight doses. As an alternative regimen which does not require I.M. injection, they recommended penicillin V (2 grams) one hour prior to dental surgery followed by 500 mg every 6 hours for eight doses. For penicillin allergy erythromycin (1 gram) is given $1\frac{1}{2}$–2 hours before the dental visit followed by 500 mg every 6 hours for eight doses. Doses should be halved for the child under six. Infants require similar consideration.

It is both courteous and advisable to consult with the child's physician, paediatrician, and cardiologist when contemplating treatment for any child with a congenital or acquired heart anomaly. Collaboration can only result in improved care for the child.

An interval of 4–6 weeks between appointments is usually sufficient to prevent sensitization to the antibiotic. It is also possible to alternate penicillin and erythromycin as the antibiotics for each visit. Every effort should be made to reduce the number of visits and obtain maximum usage from the antibiotic by performing quadrant dentistry at least, and complete arch dentistry whenever possible. In some instances, consideration must be given to performing the work under general anaesthesia. If so, a hospital is the only place adequately equipped to deal with any emergency that might arise during anaesthesia.

2. *Space Management Decisions and Parental Attitudes to Dental Health*

Before each tooth is individually evaluated as to its suitability for pulp therapy, an overall assessment of the mouth must be made. The practitioner must ask himself why the child has so many untreated carious teeth, all of which may be possible candidates for pulp therapy. It may be that the parent has been unable, despite every effort, to locate a dentist who is prepared to treat the child. Perhaps the child has been examined on various occasions by a visiting school dentist but the parent has ignored the recommendation for dental care, finally being driven to seek an appointment by the child's pain. The latter parent, unlike the former, will probably not be receptive to extensive appointments for pulp therapy and conservative dentistry. The practitioner must attempt to evaluate each parent's attitude towards dental health. If it is negative, he should attempt to improve it by motivation and education. However, it may be fruitless to attempt extensive work because of parental apathy manifested by poor appointment-keeping and poor response to preventive recommendations. In these cases, the treatment plan may have to be more radical and include extractions.

Since the effects of space loss are most extreme prior to the completed eruption of the first permanent molar, every effort should be made to conserve the primary molars in a child under 7 years old. However, when a child presents with primary molars that are candidates for extraction the effects of premature loss on the developing occlusion must be considered (*see* Chapter 1). Orthodontic evaluation can be made only with adequate radiographs to permit observation of the developing succedaneous teeth. Well taken intraoral periapical radiographs will permit the most accurate evaluation

189

of the tooth's suitability for pulp therapy, as well as the presence or absence of the developing permanent dentition, the dental age of the child, the possibility of ectopically erupting teeth, the eruption sequence, and the presence of crowding. The alternative radiographic survey is extra-oral and can take the form of bi-molar, lateral jaw and panoral films, such as the panorex or orthopantomograph. These techniques take less time and are generally easier to perform on an anxious child than an intra-oral survey. Also, gonadal radiation dosage is reduced with extra-oral films. The bi-molar and lateral oblique films require no additional X-ray equipment. Extra-oral films, particularly the bi-molar and lateral oblique film, can also demonstrate the presence or absence of 'stacking' in the permanent molar region which is indicative of potential crowding. However, the practitioner must realize that the detail of the pulp and periodontal tissues is of superior quality in intra-oral films.

When extractions are unavoidable, compensating and balancing extractions of other primary molars must also be considered. Compensating extractions are those performed in the opposing arch but on the same side of the mouth. The objective is to obtain equal mesial movement of the first permanent molars on that side and good cuspal interdigitation of the permanent dentition. Balancing extractions are those performed within the same arch but on the opposite side. The objective is to maintain symmetry in space loss within the affected arch; the subsequent localization of crowding may later necessitate bilateral loss of permanent teeth. The location of other carious primary molars, the extent of tooth destruction and the tooth's suitability for pulp therapy must be taken into account when considering the use of compensating and balancing extractions. These extractions may also be indicated in children whose parents are negative towards dental health. It should be remembered though, that wholesale compensating and balancing extractions do little to improve the parents' attitude; rather, they are likely to become more convinced that primary teeth are not worthy of restoration. Unfortunately, manpower resources sometimes leave no alternative.

The use of space-maintainers should also be considered when primary molar extraction is necessary. They have the same ability to maintain symmetry in an arch as do balancing extractions. While there will never be uniform agreement on the value of space-maintainers, they do have a definite place in paediatric dentistry. The problems they pose can be minimized by correct planning, construction and supervision of the appliance, Those who are experienced with their use tend to advocate them while those who are skilled in correcting the malocclusions that develop from early loss of primary molars tend to deprecate them (Holloway et al., 1969). It is hoped that the final decision on their use is made with the best

190

interests of the child at heart and not the ability or whims of the dentist.

3. *Assessment of the Individual Tooth*

Three considerations must be kept in mind: (1) Can the tooth be restored if pulp therapy can be performed? (2) Does the dental age of the child warrant retention of the particular tooth? (3) Is the pulp status amenable to pulp therapy? (This third question will be discussed in Chapter 16).

The stainless-steel crown has increased the number of primary teeth that can be restored after pulp therapy. A minimum of supragingival tooth structure may be all that is necessary to retain a stainless-steel crown. However, caries extending on to the root surface may be untreatable. Similarly, extension of caries to the furcation defies all attempts at conservation and necessitates extraction.

The dental age, judged by root development, also influences the decision to perform pulp therapy or extract the tooth. When the roots of primary molars have been more than half resorbed by the erupting succedaneous teeth, extraction should be seriously considered. However, the effects of an unfavourable eruption sequence on the occlusion of the first permanent molar must be critically analysed.

REFERENCES

AMERICAN HEART ASSOCIATION (1977) Prevention of bacterial endecarditis: A committee report of the American Heart Association. *J. Am. Dent. Assoc.* **95,** 600.

CASTAGNOLA L. and ORLAY H. G. (1951) Mortal amputation of the pulp. *Br. Dent. J.* **90,** 280.

HIBBARD E. D. and IRELAND R. L. (1957) Morphology of the root canals of the primary molar teeth. *J. Dent. Child.* **24,** 250.

HOLLOWAY P. J., SWALLOW J. N. and SLACK G. L. (1969) *Child Dental Health.* Bristol, John Wright, p. 97. (2nd ed. (1975) by Holloway P. J. and Swallow J. N., p. 110).

SORENSON H. W. (1973) The pedodontic patient with heart disease. *Dent. Clin. North Am.* **17:1,** 173.

RECOMMENDED READING

JOLLY M. and DRUCKER D. B. (1971) Prevention of bacterial endocarditis. *Br. Dent. J.* **131,** 539.

CHAPTER 16

DIAGNOSIS OF PULP PATHOLOGY

GENERAL CONSIDERATIONS

No single type of pulp therapy will be uniformly applicable or successful. The success of the treatment used depends mainly upon an accurate preoperative assessment of pulp status. Once this has been established, a treatment procedure can be selected which will eliminate the pathology believed to be present. For example, a non-vital primary tooth with premature root resorption should be extracted. Attempts to pulp-cap that non-vital primary molar will fail because any drainage that may have occurred previously through an open lesion will be prevented. On the other hand, complete root-canal therapy may be unnecessary on a primary molar which has a minute traumatic exposure. In these last two examples, the treatment performed in no way relates to the pulp status.

The clinician is faced daily with emergency patients who require a prompt, accurate diagnosis of pulpal pain so that a palliative service can be rendered. Unfortunately, the most accurate diagnosis of pulp status is by microscopic evaluation of the extracted tooth. Since this is obviously impractical, the clinician must use a variety of diagnostic aids, including an accurate history, to determine the true extent of the microscopic pathosis of the pulp. Various diagnostic aids have been evaluated by correlating clinical data with the histological diagnoses in primary and permanent teeth. These individual aids will be discussed and related to the preoperative decision regarding suitability for treatment and to the postoperative evaluation of success.

DIAGNOSTIC FEATURES

Pain

An accurate history must be obtained of the type of pain experienced, including its duration, frequency, location and spread, as well as aggravating and relieving factors. Since pain is subjective, the clinician must be aware of the varying responses given by the child and parent. A fearful child may have been kept awake the previous night with a toothache only to report that he has no pain when faced with the immediate dental experience. On the other hand, a parent who has neglected seeking dental care for the child may describe agonizing pain of three weeks' duration in the hope that comprehensive care will be performed immediately for the child. Indeed, it

192

is often difficult to elicit an accurate history from the parent, who is effectively the third party and who is eventually responsible for, and feeling guilty about, the child's oral condition.

The absence of toothache does not preclude a histological pulpitis, either in primary (Prophet and Miller, 1955; McDonald, 1956; Hobson, 1970) or permanent teeth (Hasler and Mitchell, 1970). For example, children are seen who have non-vital primary molars with fistulae, although their parents will truthfully deny any history of toothache. The active life of the child, together with his short attention span, may mean that minor discomfort passes without comment in his whirlwind of activities. However, the clinician should be sensitive to the extreme pain that some patients report. Its severity can probably be attributed to increased pressure within the enclosed hard tissue parameters of the tooth and supporting structures.

A positive history of toothache suggests definite pulp pathology. However, it is difficult to correlate the type of pain with the degree of pathosis. Sensitivity to thermal stimuli indicates that the pulp is vital. The immediate response to hot or cold which disappears on removal of the stimulus (momentary pain) indicates that the pathosis is limited to the coronal pulp; in such cases pulpotomy would be appropriate treatment. Momentary pain in response to thermal stimuli may also be due to the exposure of dentine from a leaking restoration or an open lesion; sealing the exposed dentine may relieve this type of pain. Persistent pain from thermal stimuli would indicate widespread inflammation of the pulp, extending into the radicular filaments to contra-indicate single visit pulpotomy techniques (Koch and Nyborg, 1970).

Spontaneous pain in primary teeth has been linked with extensive inflammation extending throughout the radicular filaments (Prophet and Miller, 1955; McDonald, 1956), and microscopic internal resorption in the root canals (Guthrie et al., 1965). Spontaneous pain refers to that pain which is not elicited by any direct stimulus, such as thermal changes; it occurs well away from meal times and frequently at night. Single-visit pulpotomy techniques are contra-indicated in such teeth, since inflamed tissue within the root canals would not be removed or mummified.

Pain on chewing or biting will be discussed later.

Swelling

Swelling may present intra-orally, localized to the infected tooth, or extra-orally in the form of cellulitis (*Figs. 105, 106*). It is caused by the inflammatory exudate associated with a non-vital tooth. Since swelling may not exist at the time of examination the clinician must thoroughly question both child and parent to uncover any history of swelling. The relationship of muscle attachments, particularly the buccinator, to the interradicular and periapical areas determines whether the swelling has an intra-oral or extra-oral location.

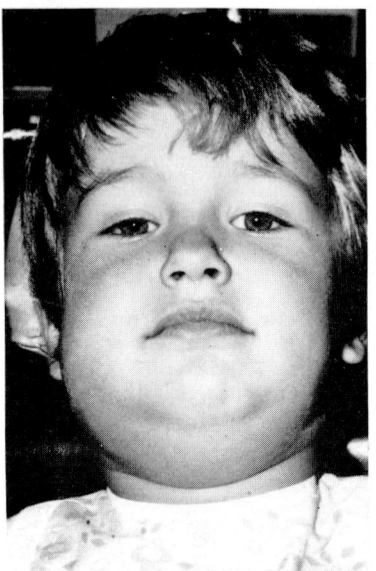

Fig. 105.—Extra-oral swelling (cellulitis). The mandibular right second molar is non-vital.

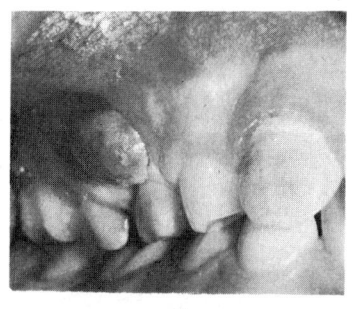
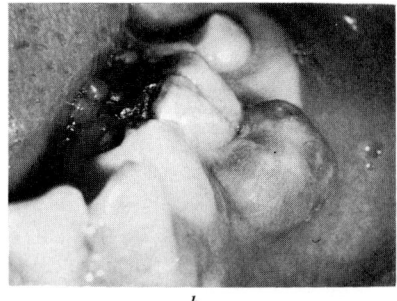

| *a* | *b* |

Fig. 106.—*a*, Fistula adjacent to a non-vital D|. *b*, Swelling draining through gingival margin.

Intra-oral swelling is usually apparent on the buccal aspect, although it may in rare instances present lingually or palatally. There is less buccal than lingual or palatal bone through which the inflammatory products from the periapical or interradicular regions penetrate, taking the path of least resistance. The pressure of the swelling will eventually result in spontaneous drainage if treatment is not rendered. Drainage may occur through an open lesion in the tooth, although the fine apical foramina of primary molars usually preclude this possibility. Most commonly, drainage occurs intra-orally either via the gingival margin or by the establishment of a fistula.* The fistula is a small elevated nodule of tissue which is patent to permit drainage. It is generally seen at or near the junction of the attached gingivae and alveolar mucosa since that site is adjacent to the interradicular region where the inflammatory products are normally located in non-vital primary molars. The tissue adjacent to a fistula is frequently inflamed to give the appearance of a white nodule surrounded by an erythematous base. The fistula's patency may be tested by the ability to milk serous exudate or pus from it. Once a fistula is present, the infection is seldom acute since drainage has already occurred. Therefore radical decisions (which may include surgery) regarding treatment of an asymptomatic tooth with a fistula should be delayed until a treatment plan has been formulated.

Extra-oral swelling presents as a cellulitis, the location of which is dependent on the spread of infection along fascial planes. In the mandibular arch, the submandibular region is commonly involved as a result of non-vital second primary or first permanent molars. In the maxillary arch, the swelling from non-vital primary canines and first primary molars can be so severe as to close the child's eye. Drainage of the extra-oral swelling would eventually occur through the path of least resistance, which may unfortunately be the skin. The pyrexia associated with such swellings, together with the obvious abnormality, usually stimulates parents to seek care before extra-oral drainage occurs.

The pulp of a tooth having either an intra-oral or extra-oral swelling or a fistula will be non-vital. However, it is possible for vital tissue, although inflamed, to be present in one canal while an adjacent canal will be non-vital; the fistula will be adjacent to the non-vital canal. For treatment purposes, the whole pulp must be considered non-vital.

Mobility

Mobility in a primary tooth may result from physiological or pathological causes. Radiographic evaluation of the remaining root of a primary tooth, the crown position, and the amount of root formation of the underlying permanent successor will determine whether any mobility is physiological or pathological. Physiological root resorption of more than one-half the root length contra-indicates pulp therapy and extraction should be considered.

---

* Fistula—*see* Glossary.

Pathological mobility is due to root or bone resorption or both, and it is associated with a non-vital pulp. Bone resorption is identified radiographically by a periapical or interradicular radio-lucency or both; most commonly the radiolucency appears in the furca. The degree of pathological mobility is of no particular value in ascertaining the degree of microscopic pathosis (Guthrie et al., 1965).

Percussion

Pain from pressure on a tooth indicates that the supporting perio-dontal structures are inflamed. Depression of the tooth into this inflamed tissue results in this type of pain. Occasionally the radio-graph will demonstrate that the tooth has been slightly extruded from its socket and is in premature occlusion. As the teeth occlude, the inflamed tissue around the apex is irritated by trauma. As with pathological mobility, pain from percussion indicates that the tooth is most likely non-vital and that the surrounding periodontium is inflamed. It is possible, however, to have an inflamed vital pulp associated with apical periodontitis in permanent teeth (Seltzer et al., 1963).

It is not necessary to perform a percussion test by hitting a tooth with a mirror handle; indeed this may be overly traumatic, especi-ally if the child reports that the tooth is sensitive to pressure. Rather, a definite history will often reveal the diagnosis. A useful clinical test is to apply finger pressure to the tooth and observe the child's response by watching the eyes. Constricted pupils are indicative of pain.

Vitality Tests

Vitality tests, either thermal or electrical, are of little value in primary teeth. While they may sometimes give an indication of pulp vitality, the response does not identify the degree of pathosis present. Fear of the unknown may make the child patient apprehensive of the electric vitalometer; he may then give the response he feels is correct rather than an accurate response. Also normal healthy primary teeth may not respond to vitality tests.

The real value of vitality tests, either thermal or electrical, is in permanent teeth when comparison can be made with normal anti-meres over a time period. The obvious example involves traumatized incisors, when serial testing may reveal that a fractured tooth requires additional current to effect a response compared to its untraumatized antimere. If identical responses have been obtained with the same current at a previous appointment, a *trend* is developing which would indicate that the fractured tooth may become non-vital. However, since no one single diagnostic aid is pathognomonic of

196

the true histological status of the diseased pulp, the clinician should be wary of relying solely on this one particular diagnostic aid.

It is important that the results of vitality tests be compared to those for normal antimere teeth. Even so, the thickness of tooth structure separating the pulp chamber from the vitality tester influences the possible degree of response. Also, recently erupted permanent teeth, particularly lateral incisors, have failed to produce responses to vitality tests up to three years after eruption, even though they were clinically and radiographically normal. Furthermore, the liquid contents of a necrotic tooth's pulp chamber may account for a positive electric vitality test response from some non-vital permanent teeth (Stephan, 1937; Reynolds, 1966).

Radiographs

Recent preoperative radiographs are essential prerequisites to pulp therapy in primary and young permanent teeth. Besides providing information on the child's dental development (*see also* Chapter 15), they may demonstrate pathological entities which contra-indicate some forms of pulp therapy or indicate failed treatment. As noted earlier, the position of the succedaneous permanent tooth will dictate the decision on performing pulp therapy for primary tooth retention. Let it be emphasized again (as in Chapter 15) that intra-oral radiographs of the periapical type provide the best detail of the pulp and the supporting structures. Extra-oral radiographs, though excellent for demonstrating the developing dentition, are inadequate for diagnosis of pathology in the pulp and supporting tissues.

Despite its immense diagnostic value, the radiograph can deceive the clinician into thinking that periapical or interradicular pathosis is absent when in fact it may be histologically present. This is because the microscopic lesion must be of certain dimensions before it is manifested radiographically. Furthermore, superimposition of permanent successors masks the true appearance, particularly in maxillary primary teeth. A bite-wing radiograph should be used to supplement the maxillary periapical primary molar film, since less superimposition of the developing premolars occurs in the critical trifurcation region.

Experimentally produced lesions in exarticulated bones become radiolucent only when the cortical plate is perforated (Adran, 1951; Bender and Seltzer, 1961; Ramadan and Mitchell, 1962). The observation of histologically present but radiographically absent periapical pathosis was also confirmed in permanent teeth by Bender et al. (1966).

The following abnormalities are sometimes observed in conjunction with carious primary teeth:

197

Pulp calcifications occasionally occur in the primary pulp horn area of extensively carious primary molars. They represent the pulp's response to a long-standing lesion by the laying down of very irregular dentine. These calcifications are associated with advanced pulpal degeneration extending into the root canals, contra-indicating single visit pulpotomy techniques (McDonald, 1956).

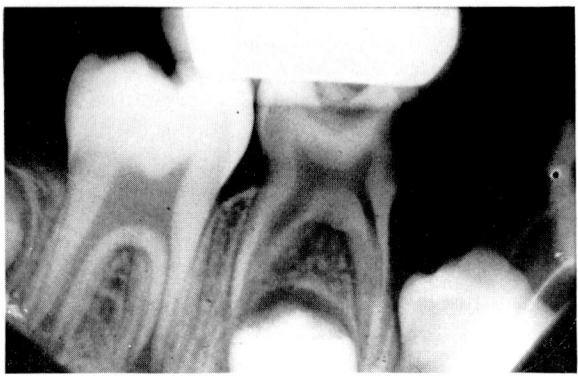

Fig. 107.—Internal resorption in distal root of mandibular second primary molar: this was undiagnosed and a pulpotomy was performed, *see Fig. 108.*

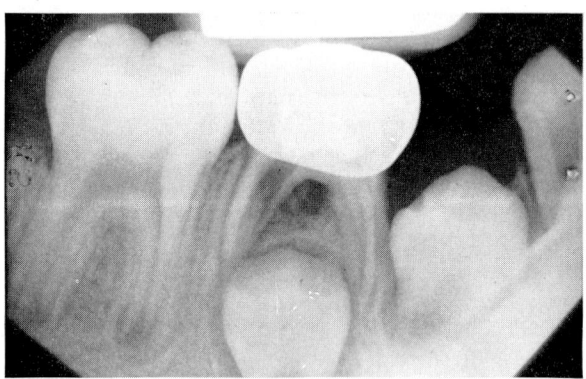

Fig. 108.—Three month postoperative radiograph of *Fig. 107* demonstrates progression of internal resorption despite pulpotomy procedures. The pulp treatment failed.

Internal resorption will be radiographically apparent only when the resorption occurs on the mesial or distal aspects of the root canal; buccal or lingual resorption may pass undetected due to the angulation of the radiograph. Microscopic internal resorption is associated with spontaneous pain at night and inflammation extending

198

throughout both the vital coronal and radicular pulp to contra-indicate single visit pulpotomy procedures. The radiographic post-operative presence of internal resorption after pulp capping or pulpotomy would indicate failure (*Figs. 107, 108*); it is likely that the resorption was present preoperatively but was not radiographically apparent.

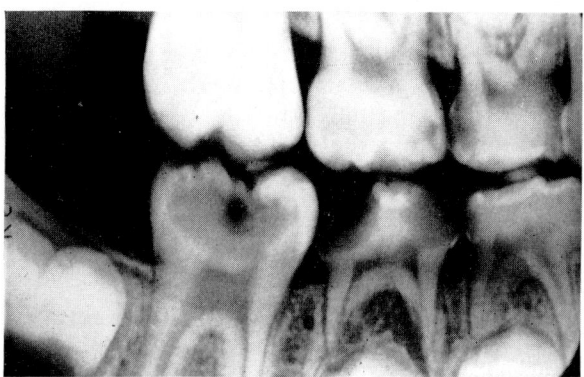

Fig. 109.—Early resorption of the mesial root of the mandibular second primary molar. This tooth was considered for pulpectomy, *see Fig. 110.*

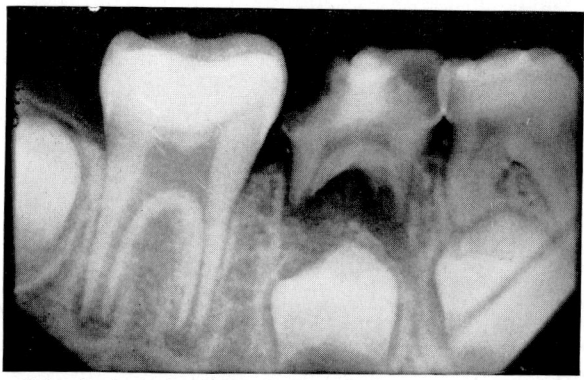

Fig. 110.—Periapical radiograph 4 weeks later, at the time the first permanent molar was treated by indirect pulp treatment demon-strates marked progression of external root resorption of the second primary molar. This tooth had to be extracted. Note the speed at which resorption occurred and therefore the need for recent radiographs.

External root resorption can occur physiologically or pathologically (*see* section on Mobility). The clinician should be familiar with the normal appearance of primary molar roots and their physiological resorptive pattern. It is not uncommon, however, for the distal root of a mandibular first primary molar to be foreshortened to almost one-half the length of the mesial root. This should not be interpreted as pathological if a normal periodontal membrane space is seen, with no radiolucency. Pathological root resorption is invariably associated with periapical radiolucency (*Figs. 109, 110*). It is indicative of a non-vital pulp and extensive inflammation in the supporting tissues; the only viable treatment is pulpectomy or extraction.

Bone resorption will present as a radiolucency if the cortical plate has been penetrated. It indicates that there is inflammation extending beyond the tooth and into the supporting periodontium. The pulp will probably be non-vital although it is also possible that the canals contain vital inflamed pulp. In either circumstance, a pulpectomy procedure would carry the highest chance of success. When bone loss is extensive, extraction is indicated.

Radiolucency in primary molars is usually seen at the furcation and not at the periapex. It is possible that the inflammatory exudate cannot penetrate the fine branching ramifactions of the primary molar root canals. This is not the case in the young permanent molar where it is more common to see periapical than interradicular radiolucency. The high incidence of furcation radiolucency in primary molars has been attributed to the presence of accessory canals in the bifurcation region of human primary molars (Winter, 1962). Also, the pulpal floor in infected primary molars may be more porous and permeable (Moss et al., 1965). The accessory canals and porous pulpal floor, which is thinner in primary than in permanent teeth, may permit the diffusion of inflammatory exudate more readily, which would explain the high incidence of interradicular rather than periapical pathology in necrotic primary teeth.

Depth of the Lesion

The proximity of the lesion to the pulp can be estimated preoperatively by a radiograph. If the lesion is radiographically very close to the pulp, there is a 75 per cent chance of an exposure when all the caries is removed (DiMaggio and Hawes, 1963). A broken down marginal ridge is indicative of probable pulp exposure in Class 2 lesions in primary molars (Stoner, 1967) (*Fig. 111*). The clinician should therefore plan on some form of pulp therapy when the clinical and radiographic appearances indicate a deep lesion. Correct preoperative assessment will permit accurate scheduling of appointment times and reduced stress during the clinical technique.

The clinician should also be aware of the possibility of an undetected avascular microscopic pulp exposure. Whenever the pulpal floor of the cavity is so thin that the pulp outline is shown by pink coloration, there may well be a microscopic pulp exposure. This phenomenon should encourage the clinician either to err on the conservative side by performing indirect pulp treatment or to be radical and proceed to pulpotomy, rather than risk pulp capping these teeth. The more conservative method of stopping short of exposure is recommended, since successful treatment will maintain the pulp's vitality.

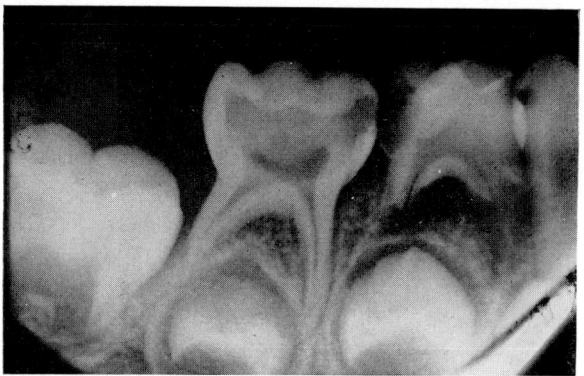

Fig. 111.—Periapical radiograph of a 3-year-old. Note that when the marginal ridge is broken down the lesion is in close proximity to the pulp. Note also the premature root resorption.

THE EXPOSURE SITE

Both the size of the exposure site and the nature of exudate expressed from it are useful diagnostic aids (McDonald, 1956; Koch and Nyborg, 1970). Exposure sites in excess of 1 sq mm do not lend themselves to direct pulp capping. Indeed, only traumatically induced exposure sites and those whose surrounding dentine is bacteria-free in asymptomatic teeth are suitable for pulp capping. The colour and amount of blood at the exposure site have been shown to be a reliable guide to the extent of pulpal inflammation in primary teeth. Light-red blood whose haemorrhage can be arrested easily is associated with inflammation that is limited to the coronal pulp in primary teeth. Profuse haemorrhage from the exposure site, with deep-red blood, is histologically associated with inflammation extending into the root canals of primary molars. The former instance would be compatible with pulpotomy procedures while the latter would not.

THE AMPUTATED PULP STUMPS

In pulpotomy procedures, the coronal pulp is removed and amputated from the radicular filaments at the entrance to the root canals.

Uncontrollable haemorrhage from these pulp stumps will occur if the blood vessels are dilated, as seen in the inflamed pulp. It is therefore imperative that no astringent or vasoconstrictor be placed over these pulp stumps since observing the ability to arrest this haemorrhage is useful to the clinician in assessing radicular pulp status and the extent of inflammation.

REFERENCES

ADRAN G. M. (1951) Bone destruction not demonstrable by radiography. *Br. J. Radiol.* **24,** 107.

BENDER I. B. and SELTZER S. (1961) Roentgenographic and direct observation of experimental lesions in bone. *J. Am. Dent. Assoc.* **62,** 152, 708.

BENDER I. B., SELTZER S. and SOLTANOFF W. (1966) Endodontic success —A reappraisal of criteria. *Oral Surg.* **22,** 780.

DIMAGGIO J. J. and HAWES R. R. (1963) Continued evaluation of direct and indirect pulp capping. *I.A.D.R. Abst.* **41,** 38.

GUTHRIE T. J., MCDONALD R. E. and MITCHELL D. F. (1965) Dental pulp hemogram. *J. Dent. Res.* **44,** 678.

HASLER J. E. and MITCHELL D. F. (1970) Painless pulpitis. *J. Am. Dent. Assoc.* **81,** 671.

HOBSON P. (1970) Pulp treatment of deciduous teeth. *Br. Dent. J.* **128,** 232.

KOCH G. and NYBORG M. (1970) Correlation between clinical and histological indications for pulpotomy of deciduous teeth. *J. Int. Assoc. Dent. Child.* **1,** 3.

MCDONALD R. E. (1956) Diagnostic aids and vital pulp therapy for deciduous teeth. *J. Am. Dent. Assoc.* **53,** 14.

MOSS S. J., ADDELSTON H. and GOLDSMITH E. D. (1965) Histologic studies of pulpal floor of deciduous molars. *J. Am. Dent. Assoc.* **70,** 372.

PROPHET A. S. and MILLER J. (1955) The effect of caries on the deciduous pulp. *Br. Dent. J.* **99,** 105.

RAMADAN A. E. and MITCHELL D. F. (1962) A roentgenographic study of experimental bone destruction. *Oral Surg.* **15,** 934.

REYNOLDS R. L. (1966) The determination of pulp vitality by means of thermal and electrical stimuli. *Oral Surg.* **22,** 331.

SELTZER S., BENDER I. B. and ZIONITZ M. (1963) The dynamics of pulp inflammation: Correlations between diagnostic data and actual histologic findings in the pulp. *Oral Surg.* **16,** 846.

STEPHAN R. M. (1937) Correlation of clinical tests with microscopic pathology of the dental pulp. *J. Dent. Res.* **16,** 267.

STONER J. E. (1967) Dental caries in deciduous molars. *Br. Dent. J.* **123,** 130.

WINTER G. B. (1962) Abscess formation in connexion with deciduous molar teeth. *Arch. Oral Biol.* **7,** 373.

RECOMMENDED READING

HASLER J. E. and MITCHELL D. F. (1970) Painless pulpitis. *J. Am. Dent. Assoc.* **81,** 671.

KOCH G. and NYBORG H. (1970) Correlation between clinical and histological indications for pulpotomy of deciduous teeth. *J. Int. Assoc. Dent. Child.* **1,** 3.

MCDONALD R. E. (1974) *Dentistry for the Child and Adolescent.* St. Louis, C. V. Mosby, Chapter 8.

CHAPTER 17

PULP THERAPY — TREATMENT TECHNIQUES

THE EMERGENCY PATIENT

THE child with a toothache, who presents as an emergency patient, manifests special problems. Unless time has been allotted in the appointment book for emergencies, the emergency patient will disrupt the daily schedule. This problem is compounded by the fact that both parent and child may be upset from a sleepless night. These factors contribute to the possibility of a negative experience for the child.

The principles of management for the child with a toothache can be listed as follows:
1. Identify the urgency of the problem.
2. Take a history and make a diagnosis.
3. Be aware of both parental and child anxiety.
4. Relieve the pain (without extraction if possible).

1. *Urgency*

The receptionist should screen all incoming telephone calls to determine the urgency of the problem. The dental office should have firmly established guidelines for the receptionist who handles these calls. The following set of guidelines has withstood the test of time: Emergency patients are asked a series of questions with regard to their toothaches. The response to the questions determines whether the emergency is classified as 'same day' or 'next day'.

The following formula has been successfully used in clinical practice:

Crying child
Child awake at night
Swelling
Fractured teeth
} Same day emergency

Intermittent pain of long duration
Fistula
} Next day emergency

2. *Diagnosis*

A diagnosis of the pulpal condition must be made prior to initiating any treatment. A history must be taken followed by a clinical examination and the taking of appropriate radiographs. Many of the above procedures can be accomplished by properly trained auxiliaries if laws permit. In this manner the disruption to the daily schedule is minimal and children receiving routine care do not have their treatment compromised.

3. *Anxiety*

Both parent and child may have had sleepless nights as a result of toothache. Unnecessary waiting can seem an endless time for those with a true emergency problem. During both the initial telephone call and the history taking, the dental staff must be sensitive to the parents' feelings regarding the dental emergency. Apart from the guilt felt by parents because of their child's toothache, the emergency dental appointment may constitute a severe upset to the family routine. Sometimes parents may express their concerns for immediate care in a hostile manner; they are often unable to realize the disruption they cause to the dental office and act as though theirs was the only child who required treatment. This aggressive behaviour must not be misinterpreted by the staff; rather, the staff should have empathy towards the parents' problem associated with the dental emergency.

4. *Relief of Pain*

The main purpose of the emergency visit is the relief of pain. If definitive treatment can be provided in a manner that will not endanger either the child's future cooperative behaviour or the developing occlusion, this is also advantageous. Personal experience reflects an opinion that too frequently the dentist tries to accomplish too much at an emergency visit only to realize several visits later his errors. Because of the child's apprehension associated with an awareness of an existing dental problem (Wright and Alpern, 1971), a minimum of operative dentistry should be attempted.

Relief of pain from non-vital teeth with associated swelling is achieved by establishing drainage and the use of antibiotics, if the temperature is elevated by 2 degrees or more and if lymphadenopathy is present. In some teeth, drainage can be established through the root canals, while in others fluctuant intra-oral swellings may be drained using topical anaesthesia. Because the pulp is non-vital, local anaesthesia is unnecessary. Because injection of local anaesthetic into inflamed tissues is contra-indicated on the grounds that it may spread infection and the solution is neutralized by pus, it may be necessary in severe instances to resort to extraction using general anaesthesia to establish drainage. This may be most appropriate when a cellulitis is associated with a non-vital maxillary tooth.

Relief of pain from vital inflamed teeth can be achieved by a variety of techniques dependent upon the aetiology of the pain. In some instances, such as a lost restoration with no underlying caries, simply closing the exposed dentine to the oral environment will prevent the pain from changes in pH and thermal changes. In teeth with deep carious lesions, the superficial necrotic layers of decay can be removed without local anaesthesia and a temporary restoration placed. In other teeth, the vital inflamed coronal pulp may have to be removed as in a pulpotomy procedure.

In most instances pain relief can be accomplished without extraction; wherever possible this should be done. Extraction identifies to the parent that once a toothache occurs, an extraction is necessary. Psychologically this may not be a desirable association to make for either the child or the parent. Furthermore, consideration has to be given to the need for space management. If the toothache has prompted the child to a first visit, it is quite likely that there may be several carious teeth in addition to the one causing the pain. The extraction of the single offending tooth may be performed without consideration of management of the developing occlusion.

Parents may be very demanding in their desire for definitive treatment. The receptionist may be frequently asked, 'Will the tooth be extracted?' 'Telephone' diagnoses cannot be made, and the receptionist should assure the parent that pain will be relieved. However, extraction should *not* be promised over the telephone. Similarly, if the patient is offered an appointment on the following day, the reason for the delay in scheduling must be tactfully explained.

INDIRECT PULP TREATMENT
(PRIMARY AND PERMANENT TEETH)

This treatment is applicable to vital primary and young permanent teeth with large carious lesions closely approximating the pulp. The aims of treatment are to remove the bulk of the lesion and to protect the pulp so that it can repair itself by laying down secondary dentine. In this way pulp exposure is avoided.

Indications

1. Deep asymptomatic lesions which are radiographically close to but not involving the pulp, in vital primary and/or young permanent teeth.

2. Signs of neglected mouths, including rampant caries, severe breakdown, or nursing bottle syndrome (for definition, *see* Chapter 1).

The first indication follows logically from the material presented in Chapters 15 and 16. The second warrants further discussion.

When the practitioner is faced with mouths which exemplify problems of this type, he may find that several teeth are possible candidates for some form of pulp therapy. The rate of carious attack is a potential source of frustration to child, parent, and practitioner since attempts to tackle the problem tooth by tooth result in permanent treatment to individual teeth while the overall disease process progresses unhindered. Indeed, several teeth, which may have been rescued at the time of initial examination, may be committed to extraction when they finally receive treatment, since the decay has progressed unchecked while other teeth have been treated. Stabilizing the mouth by indirect pulp treatment in these instances results in the following advantages:

1. The decay process in each treated tooth is arrested or at least slowed down, which gives the pulp a chance to repair in the absence of the gross lesion.

2. The bacterial content of the mouth is markedly reduced since the superficial aspects of the lesion contain most of the bacteria; by reducing the bacterial flora, the oral environment is less conducive to active plaque metabolism.

3. With all lesions closed, time is available to present a preventive philosophy and assess the patient's response to this.

4. The mouth is restored to function and the threat of dental pain reduced or removed.

5. Pulp exposure is avoided by successful indirect pulp treatment.

Contra-indications (individual teeth)

1. Spontaneous pain—pain at night.
2. Swelling.
3. Fistula.
4. Tenderness to percussion.
5. Pathological mobility.
6. External root resorption.
7. Internal root resorption.
8. Periapical or interradicular radiolucency.
9. Pulp calcifications.

Technique

The technique can be performed as a two- or single-visit procedure. The two-visit approach is recommended for those who are inexperienced with indirect pulp treatment. Re-entry into the treated tooth at the second visit will allow them to evaluate the success or otherwise of treatment and hence the accuracy of the preoperative assessment. The two-visit approach permits the placement of a

207

large and often time-consuming final restoration with more confidence since the healthy state of underlying pulp is confirmed. This is obviously very important in the case of young permanent teeth with incompletely formed apices. Once confidence and success have been attained, a single-visit approach can be used; however, in the single-visit technique, postoperative evaluation must be more critical.

Local anaesthesia is recommended since all the decay except that which would expose the pulp is to be removed. However, some clinicians doubt the necessity of local anaesthesia for this technique since the superficial layers of gross lesions are necrotic; and the onset of pain elicited by instrumentation indicates vital tissue which is supposedly capable of repair. Unfortunately, it may be difficult in some children to determine what is pain and what is restlessness in response to instrumentation. This certainly justifies the use of local anaesthesia.

Indirect pulp treatment differs markedly from gross caries removal. In the latter treatment, superficial caries is excavated without anaesthesia and a dressing of questionable retention is placed. This treatment is often performed as an emergency procedure, and cavity preparation is not refined to include the use of burs.

After anaesthesia and isolation, the cavity outline form is made. All margins are left adequately supported and all peripheral caries is removed with a large round bur. The amelodentinal junction must be free from all softened material and any stain, even if the latter is firm. All decay, except that which in the operator's experience lies immediately over the pulp, should be removed. The remaining carious material should not be soft, moist or have a leathery texture. Massler (1978) approaches this problem by recommending the removal of only the bacteria-laden superficial necrotic layer of demineralized dentine. He recommends using a basic fuchsine dye which stains this demineralized infected dentine layer a deep red. By contrast, the deeper, vital, relatively bacteria-free dentine is stained light-pink by the dye. Knowledge of pulp morphology and clinical experience allows the practitioner to estimate at which point he will stop. The mesiobuccal pulp horns of second primary and first permanent molars are often superficially placed; the preoperative radiograph may often indicate the location of these pulp horns. No doubt the dental student and those gaining experience with the technique will inadvertently expose some pulps; if this occurs, the primary tooth which is a candidate for indirect pulp treatment will also be a candidate for a formocresol pulpotomy, while the permanent tooth will be suitable for pulp capping.

A protective base must be placed prior to restoration; this restoration can either be intermediate as in the two-visit procedure or permanent as in the single-visit method. Both zinc oxide/eugenol and calcium hydroxide/methyl cellulose sub-bases stimulate secondary dentine formation (Kerkhove et al., 1967). Ten per cent stannous fluoride is also effective for this (Nordstrom et al., 1974), and should be applied to the cavity before the base is placed. Nordstrom et al. (1974) demonstrated that no adverse pulp response is elicited. The clinician must be aware of the possibility of undetected microscopical avascular exposure (Chapter 16) when excavating deep lesions. Since zinc oxide induces an inflammatory reaction in direct pulp capping, a calcium hydroxide/methyl cellulose sub-base is recommended. It is as effective as zinc oxide/eugenol in indirect pulp capping, and it is the material of choice for direct pulp capping. Although most researchers have used pure calcium hydroxide compounds, the commercially available products are also successfully used. They have adequate strength to withstand the condensation pressures of amalgam. In primary teeth there may be inadequate room for amalgam, a cement base, and calcium hydroxide.

The sequence of treatment, including successful results, is shown diagrammatically (*Figs. 112–114*). The removal of bacteria and substrate, together with an effective seal of restoration (either intermediate or permanent), provide the means by which the pulp can recover by laying down secondary dentine. When an intermediate restoration is placed in the two-visit procedure, its retention and marginal seal must be assured. Failure of the restoration prior to the second re-entry visit will result in unnecessary pulpal irritation and an increased risk of ensuing pathosis. Where necessary, the intermediate restoration should be supported with an orthodontic band cemented on to the tooth. The choice of intermediate restorative material lies with the clinician, subject to the recommendations in Chapter 12.

Parental acceptance of the technique is largely determined by the way the practitioner explains it. The additional appointment of the two-visit approach inconveniences the parent; however, the avoidance of direct pulp therapy, particularly in young permanent teeth with incompletely formed apices, is sufficiently attractive to justify the two-visit approach. It is important that the parent realize the significance of the treatment; thus the intermediate restoration can be presented as a 'treatment filling' rather than a 'temporary filling'. The latter term is avoided since it implies that the filling required little effort; this belittles the importance of maintaining pulp vitality. Also, the public has justifiably little confidence in temporary fillings. The term 'treatment filling' implies that an active process is occurring and it leads logically to the need of a second visit to evaluate the treatment.

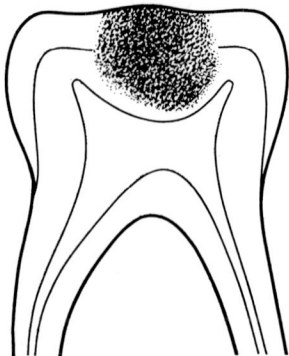

Fig. 112.—Indirect pulp treatment. Preoperative appearance of a deep lesion close to the pulp in an asymptomatic vital tooth.

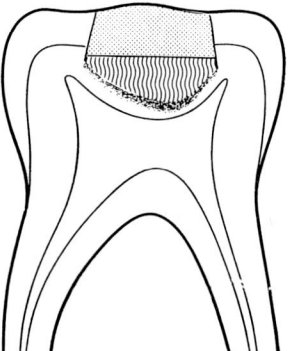

Fig. 113.—All decay is removed except that which may expose the pulp. A calcium hydroxide base is placed followed by a treatment restoration.

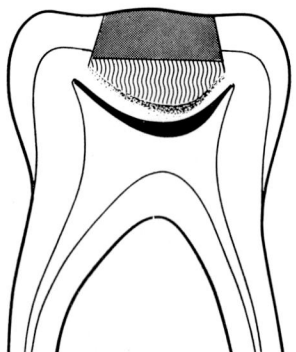

Fig. 114.—Upon re-entry at least 6 weeks later the residual decay is arrested. The base is replaced followed by a final restoration. Note that the pulp has repaired by laying down secondary dentine.

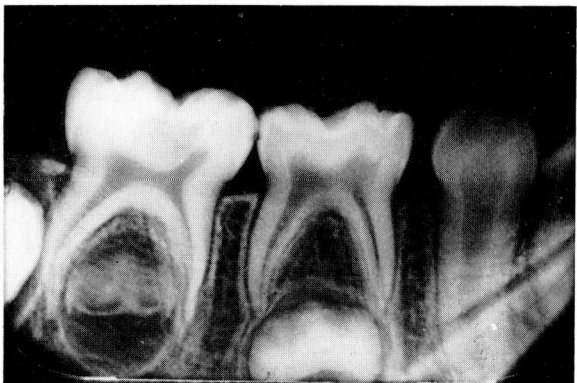

Fig. 115.—Preoperative radiograph demonstrates a deep lesion closely approximating the pulp in a mandibular second primary molar. The child is 3½ years old. Indirect pulp treatment was performed (*see Fig. 116*).

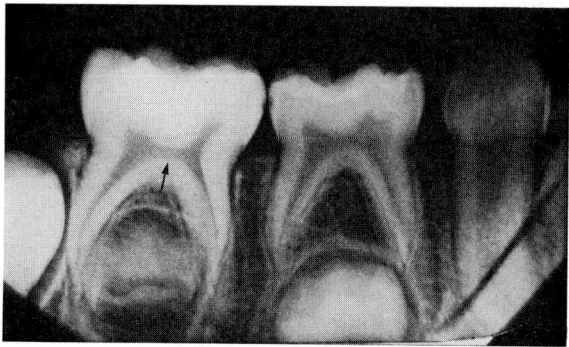

Fig. 116.—Postoperative radiograph taken 3 months after *Fig. 115* demonstrates secondary dentine formation narrowing the pulp chamber; this is evidence of successful treatment.

Postoperative Evaluation

Successful indirect pulp treatment is evaluated by the absence of signs and symptoms, the radiographic evidence of secondary or reparative dentine formation, and the arrest of the lesion judged clinically and by bacterial and micro-hardness evaluation. Before the second re-entry visit the signs and symptoms should be checked, as with preoperative evaluation. In young permanent teeth vitality tests should be performed. Radiographs need not be taken prior to re-entry since their value is mainly of academic interest. However, a radiograph prior to re-entry will *sometimes* demonstrate a radio-opaque area pulpal to the sub-base of the intermediate restoration (*Figs. 115, 116*). This is interpreted as secondary or reparative

211

dentine. However, radio-opacities which remain undetected to the eye can be demonstrated by more refined laboratory techniques (Kerkhove et al., 1967; Geller et al., 1971). Thus the clinician should not rely too heavily on the absence of this radiographic finding.

The tooth should be re-entered after a *minimum* of six weeks. Traubman (1967) demonstrated that the rate of reparative dentine formation was highest during the first month and steadily diminished with time. The thinner the pulpal floor, the faster was the rate of reparative dentine. He also found that reparative dentine continued to form, although at a slower rate, over a time period of up to 9 months to 1 year. Traubman stated that apparent pulp exposures can be avoided by allowing significant amounts of protective secondary dentine to form before complete caries excavation. Provided the intermediate restoration is sound, no harm is done by leaving this restoration for up to 1 year. Because of such factors as inconvenience and lost parental income due to dental appointments, expense of travel, geographic location and financial status, this author recommends delaying re-entry until 4–6 months after initial treatment. Other restorations and preventive care can be performed during this period while it is hoped that more secondary dentine is being formed.

Upon re-entry, the carious material below the sub-base will appear less moist, a darker brown in colour or even grey, and much harder. These clinical findings are indicative of successful treatment. Any remaining soft material should be removed with slow running round burs; it is acceptable to leave firm stained material on the pulpal floor, but not, of course, around the amelodentinal junction. A reduced bacterial content of the residual dentine has been shown after indirect pulp treatment using calcium hydroxide/methyl cellulose (King et al., 1965; Fisher, 1972). However, arrest of bacterial activity can occur under amalgam (King et al., 1965), which indicates that the success of the treatment is attributable not to the medicament used but to the pulp's ability to repair physiologically. Indeed the success of the treatment is directly related to an accurate pulp diagnosis and a technique which denies ingress of substrate to the remaining bacteria.

The increased hardness of this arrested lesion has been demonstrated experimentally (Mjor, 1967). This has been interpreted as remineralization of the carious lesion (Eidelman et al., 1965). Pressure from the slowly running round bur should be avoided when removing any residual caries. If the bur skids off stained material, this should be left. The success of the technique judged clinically, as above, and radiographically, has been reported from 76 per cent (Law and Lewis, 1961) to 92 per cent (Kerkhove et al., 1967), and to 99 per cent (DiMaggio and Hawes, 1963) in primary and young permanent teeth, and 98 per cent in permanent teeth (Jordan and Suzuki, 1971).

For those electing a single-visit approach, the postoperative follow-up is even more critical since success or failure is not verified by re-entry. Therefore, vitality tests (for permanent teeth only) and radiographs should be made at 6 months postoperatively. A positive vitality response and the absence of radiographic pathology, together with absence of all other signs and symptoms are indicative of success.

Failure of the treatment is manifested either by toothache or by pulp exposure at re-entry. Failure of the lesion to arrest and the pulp's inability to repair indicate that the coronal pulp is inflamed to the extent that physiological repair is impossible. In both primary and young permanent teeth pulpectomy procedures or extraction must be considered.

DIRECT PULP CAPPING
(PRIMARY AND PERMANENT TEETH)

These treatments are applicable to teeth with small mechanical or carious exposures when it is believed that there is no pulp pathology adjacent to the exposure site so that the pulp can remain healthy and even repair in response to the pulp capping medicament.

Indications

1. Mechanical exposures less than 1 sq mm surrounded by clean dentine in asymptomatic vital primary teeth.

2. Mechanical or carious exposures less than 1 sq mm in asymptomatic vital young permanent teeth.

Because of the rapid spread of inflammation throughout the primary coronal pulp (Hobson, 1970) it is not surprising that direct pulp capping is less successful in primary teeth (*Figs. 117, 118*). For this reason, it should be used only for clean mechanical exposures, and not for carious exposures in primary teeth. When considering the treatment of a deep carious lesion in a primary tooth, the clinician usually must choose between indirect pulp therapy, direct pulp capping and pulpotomy as each treatment relates to the pre-operative assessment. In fact, the contra-indications for all of these treatments are very similar. Clinical research data indicate that the success of direct pulp capping is considerably less than with indirect pulp treatment or the formocresol pulpotomy in primary teeth. If a primary tooth requires maintenance for several years, the role of direct pulp capping becomes even more questionable.

Direct pulp capping and pulp curettage enjoy a considerably higher success rate in permanent teeth. In the child, it is hypothesized that the increased blood supply from the wide open apical foramina of young permanent teeth increases the pulp's ability to respond favourably to direct pulp capping.

Contra-indications
(*Primary and Permanent teeth*)

(1–9 are contra-indications to indirect pulp treatment.)
1. Spontaneous pain—pain at night.
2. Swelling.
3. Fistula.
4. Tenderness to percussion.

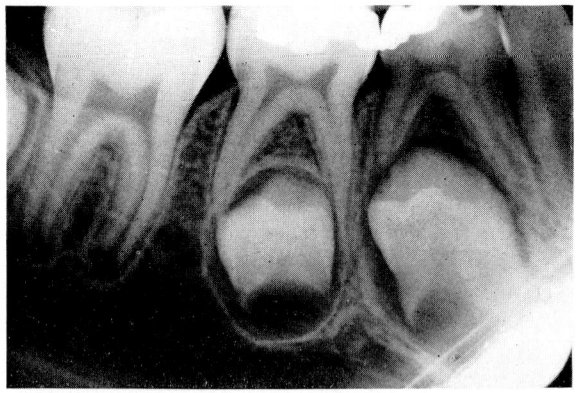

Fig. 117.—Radiograph of a calcium hydroxide pulp cap in a mandibular first primary molar. Six months after the restoration was placed. Apparent success.

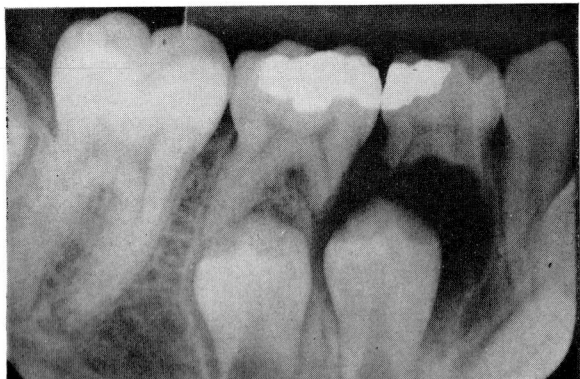

Fig. 118.—Radiograph of the child in *Fig. 117* 18 months after a calcium hydroxide pulp cap. A fistula was present in addition to the radiolucency and premature resorption.

214

5. Pathological mobility.
6. External root resorption.
7. Internal root resorption.
8. Periapical or interradicular radiolucency.
9. Pulp calcifications.
10. Mechanical exposures where an instrument has been pushed inadvertently into the pulp.
11. Profuse haemorrhage from the exposure site.
12. Pus or exudate at the exposure site.

The success of the treatment is dependent upon:

1. Making an accurate preoperative assessment.
2. Preventing unnecessary bacteria from reaching the pulp.
3. Avoiding pressure on the exposed pulp (*see* Technique).

The presence of bacteria has been shown to reduce the chances of successful pulp capping in animals (Kakehashi et al., 1965). For this reason mechanical exposures where a contaminated instrument is pushed inadvertently into the pulp is a contra-indication to pulp capping. The traumatic insult, along with the introduction of bacteria, significantly reduces the chances of success. Similarly, forcing infected carious dentine chips into the pulp reduces success.

Technique

The rubber dam provides the only means of working in a sterile environment. Thus the anticipated success of pulp capping will be increased when the rubber dam is used, although this remains clinically undocumented. However, should an exposure be encountered when working under cotton roll isolation, the operator should continue with treatment and not attempt to place the dam. Bacterial contamination of the exposed pulp would be inevitable during its application even if the exposure were covered with a cotton pellet. Under these circumstances the clinician should seriously consider the use of pulpotomy procedures in primary teeth.

Once an exposure is encountered, further manipulation of the pulp should be avoided. The cavity should be irrigated with saline, chloramine T or water and the haemorrhage arrested with *light* pressure from sterile cotton pellets. While the pulp capping material is being placed pressure, which would force it into the pulp chamber, should be avoided. Calcium hydroxide compounds are recommended for direct pulp capping, although other materials have been recommended (*see* following section). Since further pressure is to be avoided, a cement base should be placed prior to any amalgam restoration whenever possible.

The small dimensions of primary tooth cavity preparations may not provide sufficient space for calcium hydroxide, a cement base, and amalgam, and therefore a hard setting calcium hydroxide (e.g.

Dycal) is preferred. Even then, the clinician should be careful not to apply unnecessary condensation pressure over the exposure site. The marginal seal of the final restoration must adequately prevent ingress of saliva and bacteria to ensure success.

Choice of Direct Pulp Capping Material

1. Calcium Hydroxide

Short-term results (up to 12 months) of pulp capping cariously exposed primary teeth indicate a 75 per cent success, when judged clinically (Hargreaves, 1969; Jepperson, 1971). By comparison, the formocresol pulpotomy is successful in over 90 per cent of cases (Berger, 1965; Redig, 1968).

The pulp beneath a calcium hydroxide pulp cap has a characteristic microscopic appearance. After 24 hours there is a necrotic zone adjacent to the paste whose pH is about 11. At 7 days postoperatively there is much cellular and fibroblastic activity; at 28 days postoperatively a dentine barrier is formed (Glass and Zander, 1949). This dentine barrier may be apparent radiographically as a radio-opaque bridge. However, such a radiographic calcific barrier may be histologically incomplete in the form of a partial bridge (Spedding, 1963).

Failures in pulp capping primary teeth with calcium hydroxide are usually demonstrated by internal resorption radiographically. Hargreaves (1969) attributed the failures to saliva contamination of the exposed pulp prior to placement of the pulp cap. This finding encourages routine use of the rubber dam. However, it is also likely that in these failed cases the undiagnosed preoperative pulpal inflammation precluded the possibility of pulp repair by a dentine bridge.

2. Corticosteroid/Antibiotic Cements

Many clinicians use Ledermix cement for pulp capping. It consists of (1) a powder made up of demethylchlortetracycline hydrochloride and triamcinolone acetonide with zinc oxide and calcium hydroxide; (2) a liquid catalyst made up of eugenol and rectified oil of turpentine.

Hargreaves (1969) found this superior to pure calcium hydroxide in pulp capping primary teeth. It is assumed that the corticosteroid and antibiotic suppress the inflammatory response in the pulp and restore favourable conditions for pulp repair.

PULPOTOMY PROCEDURES (PRIMARY TEETH)

Pulpotomy procedures involve removing vital, partially inflamed coronal pulp tissue, placing a dressing over the amputated pulp

216

stumps, and then placing the final restoration. Various medicaments have been recommended for covering the radicular filaments. The initial recommendation of these materials was empirically based. Since then, assessments of animal and human research by clinical, radiographic, and microscopical means have allowed us to rank the different pulpotomy procedures using different materials. A brief review of the recommended treatments is relevant.

In primary teeth, the pulpotomy procedure can be performed in a single visit when local anaesthesia is used. In this instance, the technique is one of vital amputation. Either calcium hydroxide or, more recently, formocresol is used to cover the amputated radicular pulp stumps (the latter drug is used universally on the North American continent).

In the approach involving two or more visits, the coronal pulp is only partially removed at the first visit; a devitalizing medicament is placed in the pulp chamber in between visits. This multi-visit approach is referred to as mortal amputation and local anaesthesia has not been universally used or even recommended. The mortal amputation, or multi-visit approach is commonly used in Europe where the devitalizing paste recommended was either Gysi's Trio-paste (Hess, 1929), Easlick's paste (Easlick, 1943; Andrew, 1955), or more recently, the devitalizing pastes studied by Hobson (1970).

Single-visit Formocresol Pulpotomy
(*Vital Primary Teeth*)

Indications

Carious or mechanical exposures in vital primary teeth.

Contra-indications

(1–9 are contra-indications to indirect pulp treatment and direct pulp capping.)
  1. Spontaneous pain—pain at night.
  2. Swelling.
  3. Fistula.
  4. Tenderness to percussion.
  5. Pathological mobility.
  6. External root resorption.
  7. Internal root resorption.
  8. Periapicular or interradicular radiolucency.
  9. Pulp calcifications.
  10. Pathological external root resorption.
  11. Pus or serous exudate at the exposure site.
  12. Uncontrollable haemorrhage from the amputated pulp stumps.

217

Technique (Figs. 119–127)

The procedure is carried out in one visit using local anaesthesia and rubber dam isolation. Following cavity outline form, all peripheral caries is removed before the pulp is exposed. This important step prevents unnecessary bacterial contamination once the pulp is exposed and improves visibility of the exposure site. Following pulp exposure and evaluation of it, the roof of the coronal pulp chamber is removed. A fissure bur in the high speed with water coolant is used to locate the pulp horns. Bur cuts are made between these pulp horns so that the roof of the chamber is removed. The coronal pulp can be removed either with a sharp excavator or with a large round bur run at low speed. No attempt should be made to arrest haemorrhage at this stage. The

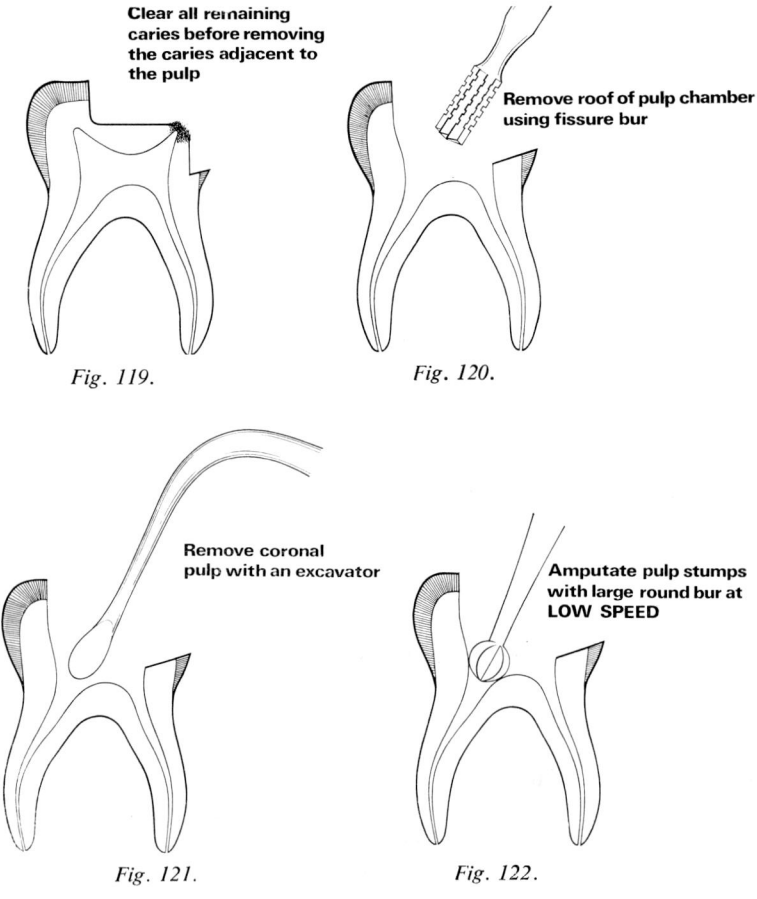

Clear all remaining caries before removing the caries adjacent to the pulp

Fig. 119.

Remove roof of pulp chamber using fissure bur

Fig. 120.

Remove coronal pulp with an excavator

Fig. 121.

Amputate pulp stumps with large round bur at **LOW SPEED**

Fig. 122.

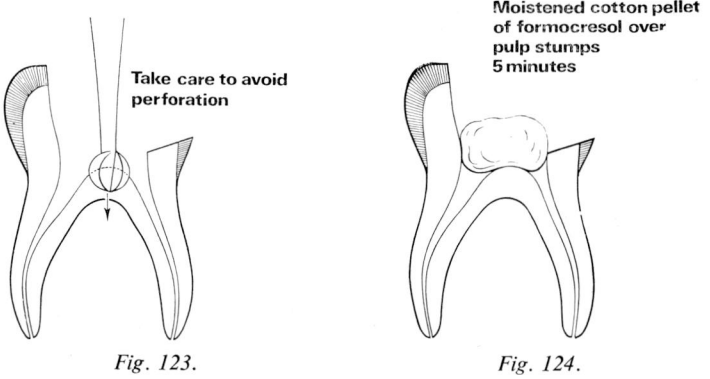

Take care to avoid perforation

Moistened cotton pellet of formocresol over pulp stumps 5 minutes

Fig. 123.   *Fig. 124.*

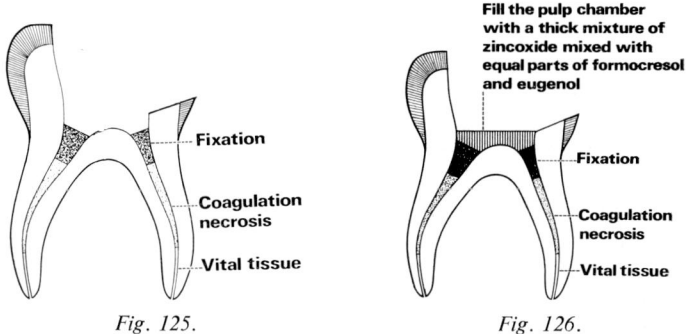

Fixation

Coagulation necrosis

Vital tissue

Fig. 125.

Fill the pulp chamber with a thick mixture of zincoxide mixed with equal parts of formocresol and eugenol

Fixation

Coagulation necrosis

Vital tissue

Fig. 126.

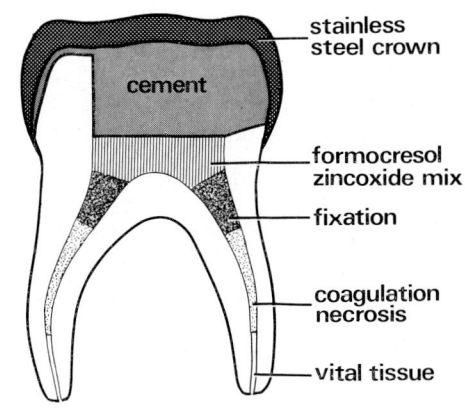

stainless steel crown

cement

formocresol zincoxide mix

fixation

coagulation necrosis

vital tissue

Fig. 127.

Figs. 119–127.—Single-visit formocresol pulpotomy

219

pulp is amputated at the entrance to the root canals. This step is facilitated by knowing the location of the root canals and the depth of the coronal pulp chamber, assisted by the preoperative radiograph. Copious irrigation of the pulp chamber with water will prevent dentine chips from being forced into the radicular pulp, which would occur if air were used. The whole coronal pulp must be removed, paying special attention to pulp filaments left under ledges of dentine. If they are not removed they would continue to haemorrhage and therefore cloud the diagnosis of the radicular pulp stumps. Care must be exercised not to perforate either the thin pulpal or interproximal wall by using excessive force with the round bur (*Fig. 128*). A large round bur (No. 6) run at slow speed with a light touch is recommended; there is less danger of inadvertently forcing it down the canals as its dimensions would exceed those of the canal entrance in most instances. Post-amputation bleeding is controlled by moistening cotton pellets with a non-irritating solution such as saline or water and placing them over the amputated stumps for 3–5 minutes. The status of the radicular pulp stumps is then assessed. It is important that no material is placed over them which would alter the stasis of haemorrhage, such as a local anaesthetic with vasoconstrictor. The tooth may be considered suitable for a single-visit formocresol pulpotomy only if haemorrhage is arrested naturally (*see* Chapter 16). The pulp stumps are sensitive to indelicate handling and the clinician must prevent iatrogenic traumatic haemorrhage when removing the cotton pellet. This problem will be more pronounced in young primary molars with very wide orifices to the root canals. If post-amputation haemorrhage persists, a two-visit pulpotomy or pulpectomy should be performed (*see* following sections).

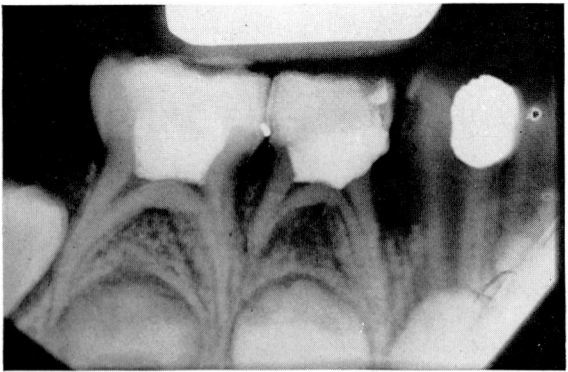

Fig. 128.—Perforation of the mesial wall in the first primary molar: note the interseptal bone loss. The tooth must be extracted

The orifices of the root canals are covered for 5 minutes with cotton pellets moistened with formocresol. The pellets are first saturated with formocresol and later compressed between gauze to remove excess so that they are just moistened with the liquid (*Figs. 129, 130*). Excess formocresol is undesirable since it serves no other purpose than to increase the likelihood of a soft-tissue burn should any leakage occur. Buckley's formocresol is made up of cresol (35 per cent) and formalin (19 per cent) in aqueous glycerine; it can be made up at the local chemist or pharmacy in small 10-ml dark bottles. It has an indefinite shelf life, although the screw cap should always be immediately replaced to prevent evaporation of formaldehyde and also to minimize its pungent odour.

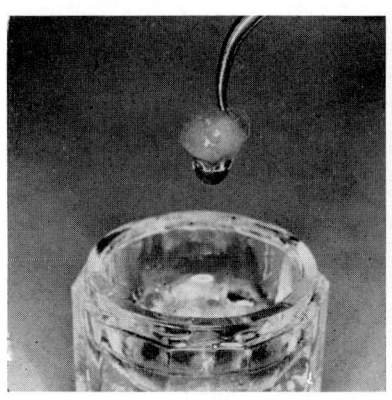 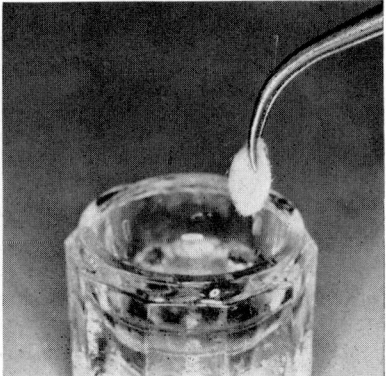

Fig. 129   *Fig. 130*

Fig. 129.—Cotton pellet saturated with formocresol. This should be compressed between gauze to remove excess. Such saturated cotton pellets should *not* be used.

Fig. 130.—Dampened formocresol pellet. This is the correct amount of drug for placing in the chamber. Compare to *Fig. 129.*

When the formocresol pellet is removed, the radicular pulp stumps should appear dark brown or even black as a result of fixation caused by the drug. A creamy mix of zinc oxide powder and one part eugenol, one part formocresol is placed over the pulp stumps and tapped gently into place. Oxypara paste has been used as an alternative to a formocresolized zinc oxide base; the powder consists of zinc oxide, barium sulphate, iodine, and paraformaldehyde, while the liquid consists of phenol, formalin, creosote and thymol. If a crown is not placed at the same visit as the pulpotomy, the restoration that is used must prevent the ingress of bacteria and oral fluids which may further irritate the pulp.

221

Histology

The histological reaction of the radicular pulp to formocresol is represented diagrammatically (*Figs. 125–127*). There is universal agreement that pulp fixation occurs after formocresol application. The histochemical study of Loos and Han (1971) confirms that the drug suppresses metabolism, acting as a cytotoxic agent to account for the fixation. Just below the zinc oxide formocresol mix, in the coronal one-third of the canal, is a narrow band of homogeneous eosinophilic tissue; apical to this is a broader band of pale eosinophilic tissue which fills the bulk of canal. The loss of cellular detail accounts for the microscopical interpretation of coagulation necrosis. The apical one-third of the canal contains vital tissue, but opinions differ as to whether this is vital pulp (Doyle, 1961) or ingrowth of connective tissue (Berger, 1965; Hannah and Rowe, 1971). Because these two tissues are histologically similar and because the mechanical disturbance caused by extraction may account for microscopical misinterpretation, no answer can be given. However, the vitality of this apical tissue may be important in the resorption process.

The above description refers to a single-visit (five-minute) application of the drug. When formocresol application extends beyond 3 days in the two-visit technique, there is an increase in linear vertical calcific degeneration (Emmerson et al., 1959). This may narrow the radicular pulp canal and it is speculated that there is an increased potential problem with resorption. Willard (1976) observed this in human primary molars treated by four-minute formocresol application in a single-visit pulpotomy technique. Of 30 treated teeth, 29 demonstrated calcification of the root canal as early as 6 months postoperatively.

Microscopical study of the supporting tissues of teeth treated by single-visit formocresol pulpotomy indicates that there is no untoward effect of the treatment on the developing permanent tooth (Spedding, 1963; Kennedy, 1971). Obviously such research was done in animals so that microscopical evaluation was possible; caution must be exercised in translating these results directly to humans. A relationship between formocresol pulpotomy in primary teeth and enamel defects on their permanent successors has been demonstrated (Pruhs et al., 1977). These defects take the form of mild enamel opacities which are seldom aesthetically undesirable since they commonly occur on premolars.

Variations in Technique

Time of formocresol application:

It is of historical interest that the formocresol pulpotomy as first advocated by Sweet (1936) was a multi-visit technique. Also, pre-

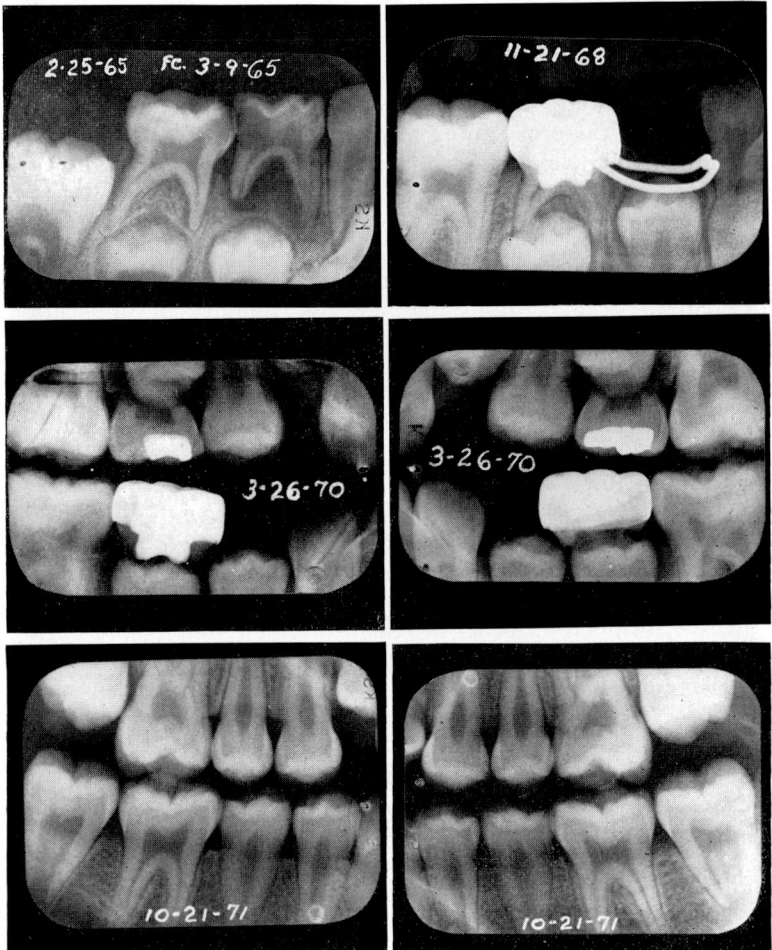

Fig. 131.—Successive radiographs demonstrate successful formocresol pulpotomy (*Top left and right*). Note that the tooth is retained until normal eruption of the premolars has occurred (Bite-
wings *middle* and *lower*). (*By courtesy of Dr. Wayne Moldenhauer,
Dubuque, Iowa, U.S.A.*)

operative criteria were less stringent than those previously mentioned
and included non-vital teeth. The aim of treatment was to sterilize
the pulp chamber by a rotation of drugs (mainly formocresol and
beechwood creosote) before filling it with zinc oxide. The multi-
visit approach was reduced to two visits in vital teeth, a formocresol
pellet being left in the chamber in between appointments. The
treatment was further reduced from two visits to a single-visit,
five-minute application of the drug. Direct comparison of the

two-visit and single-visit formocresol pulpotomy in human primary molars was made by Redig (1968); neither treatment was superior. However, the convenience of the single-visit technique for child and parent, the reduction in the need for further anaesthesia and isolation, and the opportunity to perform quadrant dentistry make the single-visit (five-minute) formocresol pulpotomy superior to a two-visit technique.

Variations in time of formocresol application from days to minutes have been studied (Emmerson et al., 1959; Doyle, 1961; Venham, 1967). Microscopical evaluation indicates that the main action of formocresol occurs within the first five minutes of application (Emmerson et al., 1959). However, since no real attempt is made to monitor the volume of the drug, there seems little sense in accurately timing the five minutes of application. Indeed, Venham (1967) found identical microscopical appearances in the pulps of monkey teeth exposed to five minutes and to 15 seconds of formocresol application; however, Venham always incorporated formocresol in the zinc oxide mix that was placed over the pulp stumps. The author believes that five minutes is the minimum time required, and that anything beyond will not be detrimental. Since the final restoration of choice is the stainless-steel crown, it is clinically convenient to allow the formocresol pellet to remain over the pulp stump during crown contouring and trial fitting. Only rarely does this take less than five minutes.

Dilution of formocresol:

Some researchers are concerned with the cytotoxic damage caused by formocresol and have recommended a 1/5 dilution. Clinical evaluation was made of human primary molars treated by pulpotomy; the amputated stumps were exposed to 1/5 formocresol for five minutes followed by a zinc oxide/eugenol mix to which 1/5 formocresol was added. Results were equivalent to using full strength formocresol (Morawa et al., 1975).

Omission of formocresol from sub-base:

A further variation in clinical technique is the omission of formo-cresol from the zinc oxide mix placed over the radicular pulp stumps, after five minutes direct contact of the wet drug. Micro-scopical evaluation shows that teeth with only a zinc oxide sub-base and those with formocresol/zinc oxide mixes have identical results, provided of course the radicular pulp stumps were covered by formocresol for at least five minutes (Beaver et al., 1966). Thus this omission is of minimal clinical consequence, although this author prefers to include formocresol in the zinc oxide sub-base as added security of pulp fixation.

Other paraformaldehyde compounds:

The concept that 5 per cent paraformaldehyde is the key constituent in primary molar pulpotomy has been studied (Hannah and Rowe, 1971). Using excellent preoperative criteria, they experienced a 98 per cent success over five years using N2 as the material placed over the amputated radicular pulp stumps; this was not preceded by wet contact of the amputated stumps with formocresol although the pulpal haemorrhage was controlled by adrenaline-soaked cotton pellets. These results compare very favourably with the success of the single-visit or two-visit formocresol pulpotomy; they are superior to the two-visit mummifying technique reported by Hobson (1970).

Calcium hydroxide:

Calcium hydroxide has also been recommended for capping the primary radicular pulp stumps. Comparative studies of calcium hydroxide and formocresol in pulpotomy have been performed in animals (Spedding, 1963) and in humans (Doyle, 1961) using microscopical and radiographic means of evaluation; it is significant that these works were performed on non-carious teeth with normal pulps using a sterile technique to obtain the best possible results from each material. In both instances, calcium hydroxide was inferior to formocresol. Clinical evaluation of calcium hydroxide pulpotomy in human primary teeth reveals failures of 51–69 per cent (Via, 1955; Law, 1956). The failures are usually manifested as radiographic internal or external resorption. Comparing these results to those obtained with formocresol and other paraformaldehyde drugs, it can be concluded that there is no place for the calcium hydroxide pulpotomy in *primary* teeth. Of course, this does not apply to permanent teeth.

Two-Visit Devitalizing Pulpotomy Technique
(Vital Primary Teeth)

This is the technique of mortal amputation diagrammatically shown in *Figs. 132, 133.* The procedure was advocated in Europe in the early part of the century, using Professor Gysi's Triopaste as the mummifying agent. As with all pulp therapy at that time, the rationale for treatment was empirical and was not based on any microscopical evaluation. Since then, the two-visit mummification technique has been scientifically studied and developed (Andrew, 1955; Hobson, 1970), although it must be admitted that microscopical evaluation is less well documented than with formocresol.

The medicaments used to devitalize the exposed primary pulp are all similar in that they contain some formalin or paraformaldehyde.

225

This drug has a devitalizing, mummifying and bactericidal action The formula of each agent used in this two-visit technique is given below in chronological order of study.

1. *Gysi's Triopaste* (Hess, 1929)

Tricresol	10 ml
Cresol	20 ml
Glycerin	4 ml
Paraformaldehyde	20 g
Zinc oxide	60 g

2. *Easlick's Paraformaldehyde Paste* (Easlick, 1943; Andrew, 1955)

Paraformaldehyde	1·00 g
Procaine base	0·03 g
Powdered asbestos	0·50 g
Petroleum jelly	125·00 g
Carmine	To colour

3. *Paraform Devitalizing Paste* (modified Easlick's Paste)

Boots Pure Drug Co. Ltd., Code No. E13498 (Hobson, 1970).

Paraformaldehyde	1·00 g
Lignocaine	0·06 g
Propylene glycol	0·50 ml
Carbowax 1500	1·30 g
Carmine	To colour

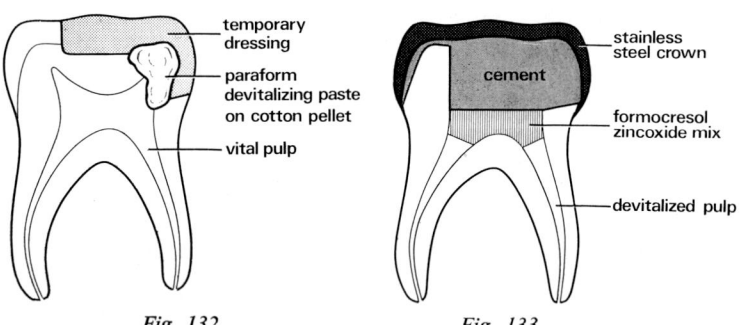

Fig. 132.   *Fig. 133.*

Two-visit devitalizing pulpotomy technique.
Fig. 132.—At the first visit a cotton pellet is used to retain the devitalizing paste over the partially exposed pulp. The dressing is retained by cement. Note the incomplete removal of coronal pulp tissue.

Fig. 133.—Second visit, 7–10 days later. The coronal pulp is removed, the pulp chamber is filled with a formocresol/zinc oxide mix and a final restoration is placed. A stainless-steel crown is preferred.

At present, the only devitalizing paste that has been adequately studied is that recommended by Hobson (1970). Other commercial products (e.g. Caustinerf) are available but cannot be recommended at present because of the lack of scientific data available from the manufacturers. It cannot be emphasized too strongly that devitalizing pastes should be free from any arsenic compounds. The effects of arsenic pastes sealed in the pulp chamber extend outside the root canals into the supporting tissues to cause necrosis; failure of the child to attend the second re-entry visit could have disastrous consequences.

Indications and Contra-indications

The preoperative criteria for suitability are similar to those identified for the single-visit formocresol pulpotomy. However, less emphasis is placed on the type of preoperative pain and on the pulpal haemorrhage at the exposure site. It will be seen that a two-visit mortal amputation pulpotomy procedure is one recommended approach to the treatment of vital primary teeth with inflammation extending into the radicular filaments. Because of the extended effect of the devitalizing paste, these preoperative criteria for suitability are less critical.

Technique

The clinical procedure differs from the single-visit formocresol pulpotomy, first because two visits are required and second because the coronal pulp need not be completely removed at the first visit. Also local anaesthesia and rubber dam placement are not universally recommended (Hobson, 1970). The technique is suggested when the time factor or lack of cooperation from the child make it difficult to complete a single-visit pulpotomy procedure. It may also be indicated when an exposure is encountered at the end of a long visit on a young child, who is becoming restless. It has been recommended for use when the child does not readily accept local anaesthesia (Parkin et al., 1970). However, this author vehemently disagrees with the concept of exposing unanaesthetized pulps in young children; a properly handled local anaesthetic is less traumatic than a painful vital exposure on a tired child. Correct treatment planning should have included the possibility of pulp therapy and therefore a local anaesthetic should have been administered at the outset. Of course, once a local anaesthetic has been given, there is little justification for not performing a single-visit formocresol pulpotomy.

In the mortal amputation pulpotomy (*Figs. 132, 133*), the partially exposed pulp is covered by devitalizing paste held by a cotton pellet. The cavity is filled with a temporary cement and the child is reappointed in 7–10 days. By this time the coronal pulp will be devitalized, although the root-canal tissue will remain vital (Hargreaves, 1959). There should be no signs or symptoms from the tooth at the re-entry visit; the devitalized coronal pulp should be removed and the pulp chamber thoroughly cleansed. Local anaesthesia is not required for this, provided devitalization has been complete. The radicular stumps are covered with a formocresolized zinc oxide/eugenol sub-base, as with the single-visit formocresol pulpotomy. Final restoration with a stainless-steel crown is recommended at the second visit.

Complications

Postoperative pain may result if the devitalizing paste exerts too much pressure on the exposed pulp. The parent should be routinely warned to give the child aspirin as required (dosage—under 5 years, 150 mg; over 5 years, 300 mg).

Occasionally the coronal pulp will be incompletely devitalized after 7–10 days. This can occur if the devitalizing paste is dislodged by the temporary cement, or if the exposure is so small that the paste does not exert its full effect. Under such circumstances, the clinician must choose between administering a local anaesthetic and proceeding with the single-visit formocresol pulpotomy or resealing the devitalizing paste and completing the mortal amputation at a third visit.

PULPOTOMY AND PULPECTOMY FOR PARTIALLY VITAL AND NON-VITAL PRIMARY TEETH

Once the primary pulp has degenerated so that the radicular pulp can no longer be considered healthy, there is controversy concerning the recommended treatment. The treatment techniques used are the pulpotomy involving two or more visits or the pulpectomy procedure. Unfortunately there is insufficient evidence to recommend one technique over the other; neither is universally successful and each has potential complications. It should be remembered that

Fig. 134.—Non-vital mandibular second primary molar with interradicular radiolucency. A cotton pellet of formocresol has been sealed in the pulp chamber as emergency treatment. The tooth was finally treated by a two-visit pulpotomy. A formocresol pulpotomy has been performed on the first primary molar.

Fig. 135.—Six-month postoperative radiograph demonstrates bone healing in the bifurcation region.

Fig. 136.—Eighteen-month postoperative radiograph demonstrates good response of supporting tissues to a two-visit pulpotomy on the non-vital second primary molar. Note the resorption on the distal root of the first primary molar: this tooth must be watched carefully.

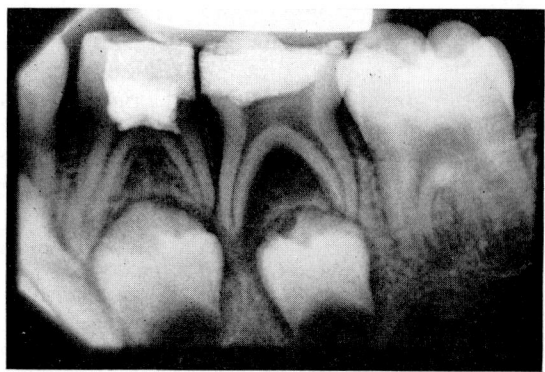

Fig. 134

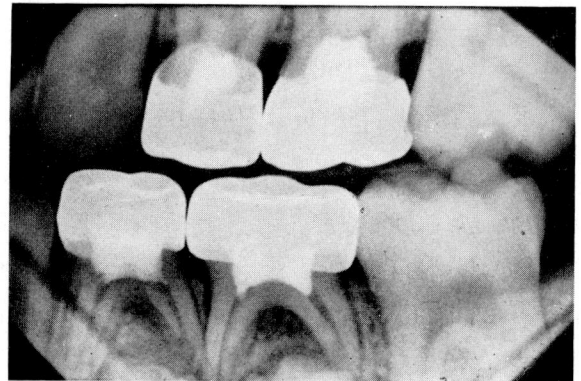

Fig. 135

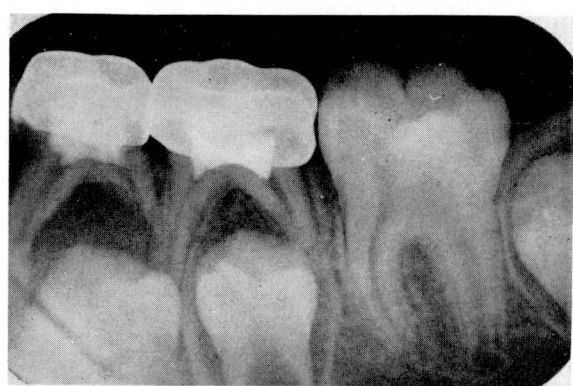

Fig. 136

the terms 'pulpotomy' and 'pulpectomy' refer only to the removal of *vital* pulp tissue from the coronal pulp chamber and radicular canals, respectively. However, through common usage, the terms 'pulpotomy' and 'pulpectomy' refer to techniques in which the coronal pulp chamber and radicular canals are débrided and later filled irrespective of pulp status. For simplification of reading the common terminology, though not strictly accurate, will be used.

The success of treating partially vital primary teeth is considerably less than those with vital uninflamed pulps. The success is in the order of 50–60 per cent in non-vital primary teeth (Wittich, 1956; Nicholls, 1963; Hobson, 1970). Therefore, the clinician should refer to Chapters 1 and 15 and reconsider the orthodontic implications of extractions. However, the retention of a non-vital second primary molar in a pre-school child is one of the most valuable services that can be provided for the child. The retention of this tooth by heroic pulp therapy during the critical period of first permanent molar eruption can have extensive benefits, if symmetry is maintained by the retention of all other primary teeth (*Figs. 134–138*).

TWO (OR MORE)-VISIT PULPOTOMY
(PARTIALLY VITAL AND NON-VITAL
PRIMARY TEETH)

Indications and Contra-indications

The indications for a two (or more)-visit pulpotomy or pulpectomy procedure in primary teeth are:

1. Inability to arrest haemorrhage from the amputated pulp stumps during a single-visit formocresol pulpotomy.

2. Pus at the exposure site or in the coronal pulp chamber.

3. Non-vital coronal and/or radicular pulp.

The following preoperative conditions reduce the chances of success (Lawrence, 1966):

1. Internal root resorption.
2. External pathological root resorption.
3. Gross bone loss at the apex or at the furcation.
4. Pus in the pulp chamber.
5. Pathological mobility.
6. Cellulitis.

Technique

After coronal pulp amputation (*see* Single-visit Formocresol Pulpotomy) a medicament is sealed on a cotton pellet in the coronal pulp chamber with a temporary cement. This medicament can be either formocresol or paraform devitalizing paste when the pulp is vital. The procedure has been described in the preceding section. When the pulp is non-vital, a devitalizing paste is obviously redundant;

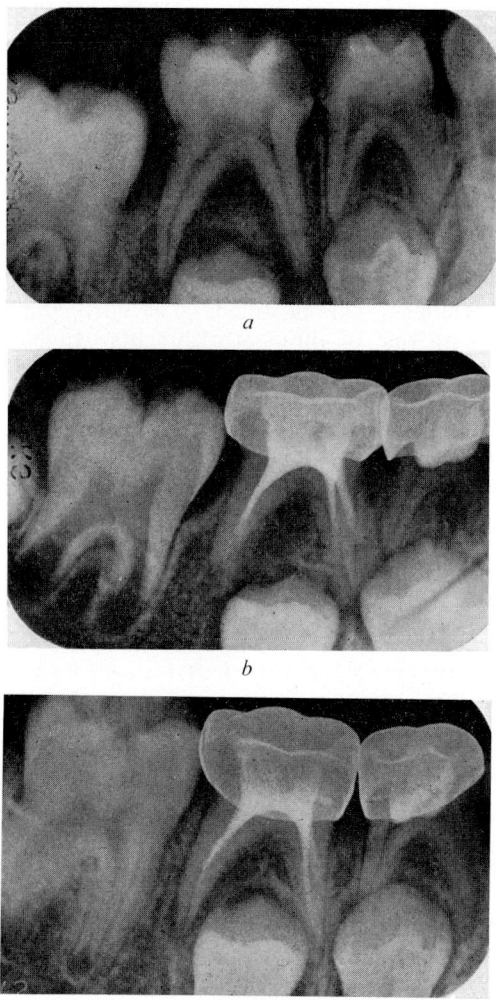

Fig. 137.—Pulpectomy and root-canal filling in non-vital mandibular second primary molar. *a*, Preoperative. Note bone loss and unerupted permanent molar. *b*, 1 year after treatment. Molar erupting. Bone filling in. *c*, 3 years after treatment. Bone healthy. Permanent molar erupted.

rather, some attempt must be made to control the infection both in the coronal pulp chamber and in the root canals. This can be done either with formocresol, camphorated monochlorophenol, KRI liquid, or beechwood creosote. Alternatively, Cresatin, the acetic acid ester of metacresol, is a mild non-irritating antibacterial and

231

antifungal agent. It is an effective pulpal anodyne and thus can be used as an intracoronal medicament in primary teeth. It is assumed that the mechanism of action of these drugs in non-vital teeth is by vapour action as well as wet contact. However, the cotton pellet should not be soaked with any drug; instead it should be moist since excess of the drug may irritate the soft tissues if leakage occurs.

At the second visit, 7–10 days later, a non-vital tooth should no longer be mobile, tender to percussion, or exhibiting a fistula. If any of these signs persist, a further visit is required to control bacterial infection by pharmacological means alone before the coronal pulp chamber can be filled. The coronal pulp chamber can be filled with one of three medicaments. In North America the trend is to use the same formocresolized zinc oxide sub-base as in the single-visit formocresol pulpotomy. In Europe, Hobson (1970) has studied either a zinc oxide/eugenol mix or an anti-septic proprietary brand (Putridomors 22) placed in the coronal pulp chamber. Since this contains the antiseptics thymol, cresol and iodoform in a zinc oxide base, it differs little from the formo-cresolized sub-base in its bactericidal properties. In the two-visit pulpotomy technique, no attempt is made to débride the canals or to force material into them.

PULPECTOMY (PARTIALLY VITAL AND NON-VITAL PRIMARY TEETH)

This can be performed as a single-visit or multi-visit procedure for vital and non-vital primary teeth, respectively. The technique is partial or complete according to the penetration of instrumentation. Pulpectomy differs from pulpotomy in that the infected material within the root canals is both pharmacologically and mechanically treated. This is a more biologically sound approach to the treatment of non-vital primary teeth than a two-visit pulpotomy. Although no proof, in terms of clinical success, exists to support this opinion pulpectomy in primary teeth is successful over short and long term (Gould, 1972; Starkey, 1973).

Single-visit Partial Pulpectomy (Fig. 137)

This is applicable to vital teeth where haemorrhage from the am-putated radicular stumps is uncontrollable. Using local anaesthesia and rubber dam placement, all accessible radicular pulp is removed with broaches. No attempt should be made to instrument beyond the apex. The canals should be filed with the aim of enlarging them to permit condensation of root-canal filling material. A diagnostic wire radiograph is not needed to assess root length, as in endo-dontically treated permanent teeth. Visual comparison of file and root-canal length on the preoperative periapical radiograph will result in sufficient clinical accuracy.

The multiple ramifications of the primary molar radicular pulp make complete débridement impossible. Also, the ribbon shape of the root canals, with a narrow mesiodistal width compared to their buccolingual dimension, discourages gross enlargement of the canals. In permanent teeth the object of mechanical preparation is to provide an even circular apical one-third of the canal which will be obliterated with an accurately fitting master point. In the primary tooth, attempts to mechanically prepare a circular apical one-third may result in lateral perforation of the canal because of its hour-glass shape. Because of the bizarre anatomy of primary molar root canals the use of barbed broaches as in conventional endodontics may be unsuccessful; at the worst there is increased danger of instrument fracture. Rather, a combined biomechanical preparation of the canals is preferred. Instruments used in conjunction with irrigating solutions reduce the possibility of fracture, because of the lubricant action of the solution. A 5 per cent solution of sodium hypochlorite has an excellent solvent action and is dilute enough to cause only mild irritation when contacting periapical tissue (Schilder and Amsterdam, 1970). It can be used in a small (1·5 cc) syringe fitted with a 25 gauge $1\frac{1}{4}$ in (32 mm) needle; provided needle fits loosely in canal there is no danger of forcing debris apically.

Hedstrom files are recommended since they remove hard tissue only on withdrawal, which prevents pushing infected material through the apices. For this reason reamers are not recommended. The limited amount of mouth opening may make access difficult. This can be improved by routinely using a mouth prop and bending the file handles to gain access to the mesial canals of first and second primary molars. The files can also be held by a Porte polisher to facilitate manipulation (Starkey, 1974). The canals should be instrumented to the resistance point; this is evident by tactile sensation and usually corresponds to a curvature in the apical one-third of the root. Each canal should be enlarged three or four instrument sizes greater than the first file capable of working the apex.

After filing, the canals should be irrigated and then dried; saline or chloramine T (Zonite) followed by cotton pellets and paper points can be used. The canals are filled when dry with zinc oxide, a formocresolized zinc oxide, Oxypara paste, or any other resorbable filling paste. A creamy mix of the filling paste can be coated around the walls of the canals with the last used file. A stiffer mix is then pressed into the canal by an amalgam condenser over a cotton pellet at the canal entrance. Another approach is to inject the paste into the canals with a pressure syringe (Spedding, 1973, 1977).

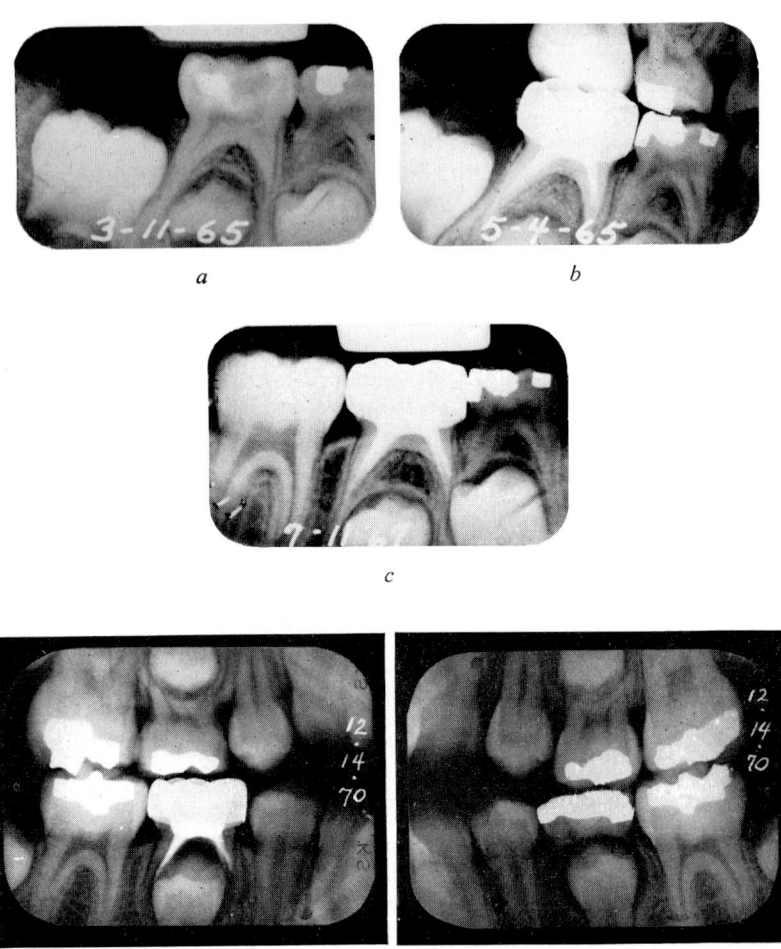

Fig. 138.—Successful pulpectomy and root-canal filling in a mandibular second primary molar. *a*, Preoperative X-ray. *b*, Postoperative X-ray. *c*, 2 years postoperative. *d*, Slightly delayed resorption compared to untreated antimere in *e*. *f*, Treated tooth still present. Compare with bite-wing radiograph in *g*. *g*, Antimere to tooth has exfoliated and succedaneous tooth erupted. *h*, Treated tooth deflected buccally. *i*, Deflected treated tooth. *j*, Erupted bicuspid. *k*, Photographic evidence of freedom from hypoplasia of succedaneous tooth (mirror image). *By courtesy of Dr. Paul Starkey, Indianapolis, Indiana, U.S.A.,* and J. Dent. Child. 1973, **40,** 213).

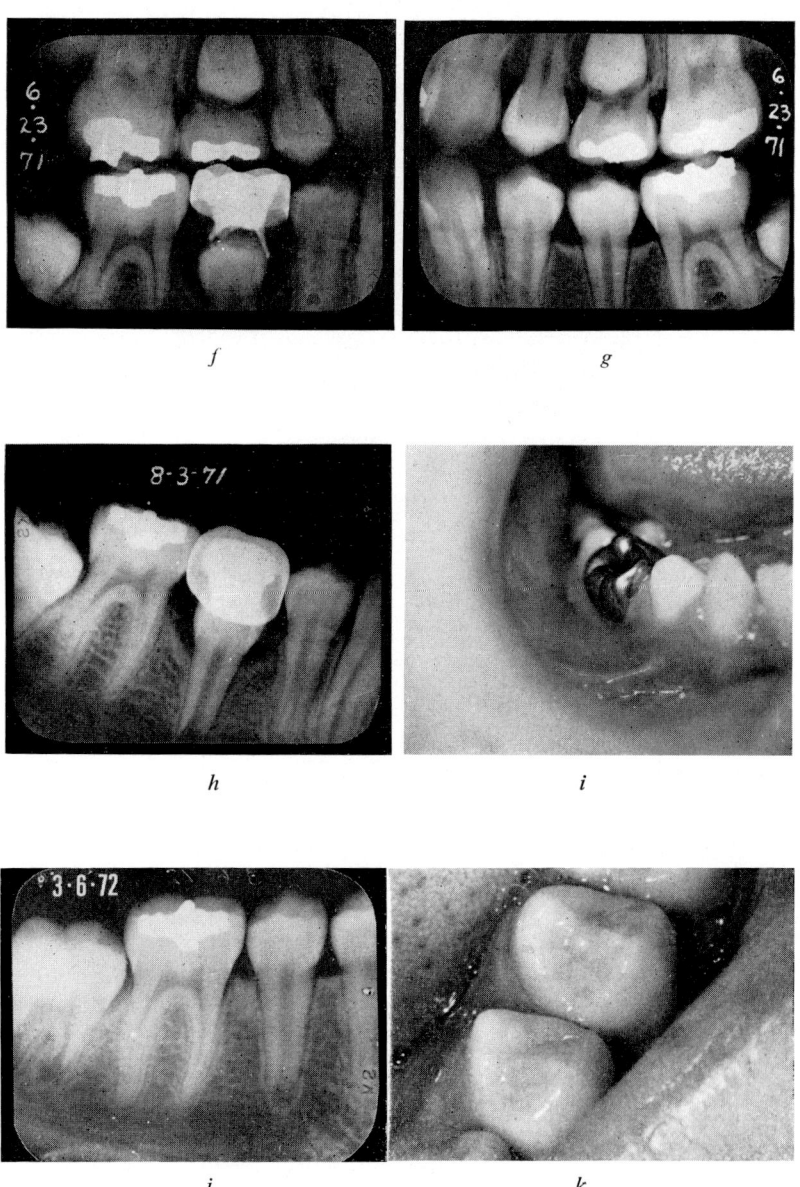

f

g

h

i

j

k

This consists of a syringe barrel, a threaded plunger, a wrench, and threaded needles of gauges 13 to 30. The filling material is mixed to a heavy putty consistency and loaded into the hub of the needle.

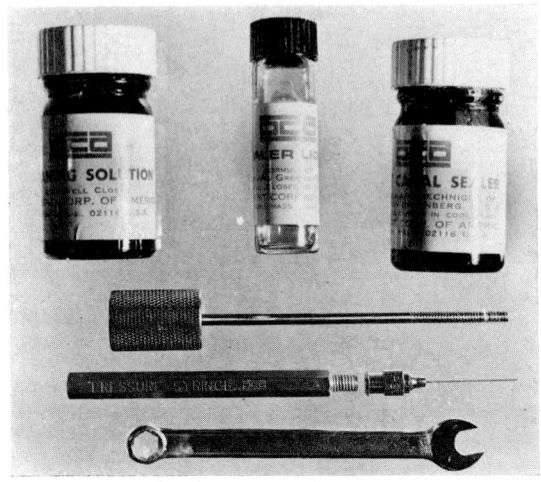

a

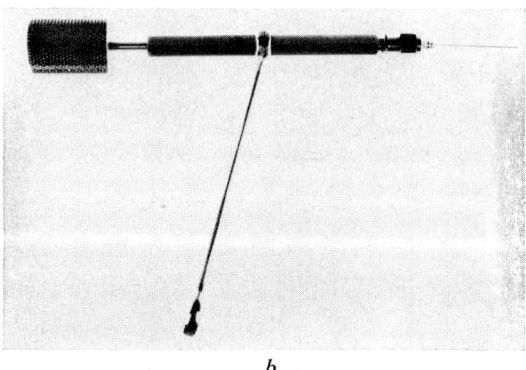

b

Fig. 139.—The pressure syringe. *a*, Parts: barrel, threaded plunger wrench, threaded needles, cleansing solvent, sealer powder and sealer liquid. *b*, Assembled syringe ready to use.

The needle is threaded on to the syringe barrel. The plunger is turned to express the root canal paste. The needle is inserted into the canal with its tip 1 mm short of the working length. The plunger of the syringe is held in one hand while the wrench is held in the other, to stabilize the syringe as force is needed to express the root canal paste. Paste is expressed by turning the knob of the plunger one quarter-turn and gradually withdrawing the tip of the needle. Provided that the apices have not been penetrated, there is little danger of extruding material through the apex into the supporting tissues. The pressure syringe has been shown to be more effective in depositing root-canal paste into fine tortuous canals than the Centulo spiral (Weisz, 1976).

Multi-visit Pulpectomy (*Figs. 138, 140*)

This procedure is used for non-vital primary teeth and has been studied over the short term (Wittich, 1956; Lawrence, 1966; Gould, 1972) and the long term (Starkey, 1973).

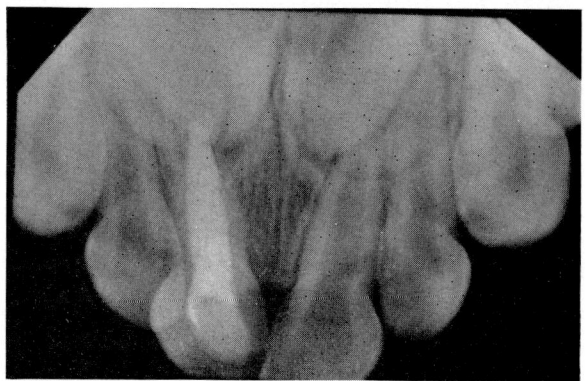

Fig. 140.—One year postoperative radiograph of a pulpectomy in a non-vital maxillary primary central incisor. Treatment was performed when the child was 18 months old to maintain space anteriorly in this crowded mouth.

The clinical technique is similar to the single-visit pulpectomy. Instrumentation of the canals is not recommended at the first visit if the tooth is mobile, if swelling or a fistula is present, or if pus is present in the canals. In the absence of signs and symptoms instrumentation can proceed as described previously; local anaesthesia and rubber dam placement are recommended to ensure the child suffers no pain. This is omitted in cases of swelling and cellulitis. After instrumentation the canals are irrigated as described before.

Between appointments an antibacterial drug is sealed in the pulp chamber, maintained with a temporary cement, as described in the two-visit pulpotomy technique. In rare instances the degree of pre-operative cellulitis will dictate that drainage will have to be established. A smooth broach should be used to perforate the apices and the tooth left open to drain for no more than one day. Leaving the tooth open for longer than 24 hours usually results in food packing into the canal. Local measures include warm saline rinses and parental instruction to prevent food packing in the open cavity. Systemic antibiotic therapy is also indicated. The parent should be advised against applying heat externally since this may result in extra-oral drainage of the infection. In these acutely abscessed teeth, the coronal pulp chamber can be filled with a beechwood creosote-soaked cotton pellet after 24 hours' drainage. In these instances, the clinician must realize that swelling may recur after the tooth is closed, and he should arrange to see the patient, if necessary, during the weekend or in the evening. However, despite pre-operative cellulitis and the need for drainage, pulpectomy in primary molars can be successful and ensure the maintenance of the second primary molar prior to and during the active eruption of the permanent first molar (Cartwright and Bevans, 1970).

Appointments are 7–10 days apart. The number of appointments and the timing and extent of instrumentation will be determined by the signs and symptoms at each visit. The canals should not be filled until they are dry and all other signs and symptoms have been eliminated (Lawrence, 1966). The root-canal filling paste is chosen and inserted as in the single-visit pulpectomy.

FOLLOW-UP—PRIMARY TEETH WITH PULPOTOMY AND PULPECTOMY

Final Restoration

For the reasons given in Chapter 13, the ideal restoration for an endodontically-treated primary tooth is a stainless-steel crown. However, there are instances when it may be acceptable to delay the crown or leave the tooth with an amalgam restoration. For example, extensive occlusal decay in first primary molars due to nursing bottle mouth syndrome may require a pulpotomy; the short cooperation time of the infant may encourage the crowning to be delayed unless general anaesthesia is being used. Also the inadvertent or unplanned traumatic or carious exposure in a small cavity in a second primary molar will encourage maintenance with amalgam after formocresol pulpotomy, especially if additional time had not been scheduled to place a crown.

Assessment of Success

Rarely does pain occur after pulpotomy and pulpectomy in primary teeth. This may lull the clinician into thinking that his treatments are 100 per cent successful. Those who fail to take postoperative radiographs may also claim a low percentage of failures of primary molar pulp treatments (see Figs. 117, 118, Chapter 16).

Postoperative follow-up at 6-month intervals should include an evaluation of signs and symptoms; periapical radiographs should be

238

taken between 12 and 18 months postoperatively. Pathological mobility, the presence of a fistula, and in rare instances pain (usually to percussion) are clinical evidence of failure. Radiographic evidence of failure is judged by the appearance of or increased size of a radiolucency, and by external or internal root resorption. Any bone loss is likely to occur at the furcation region, and not at the apices (*see* Chapter 16). The radiographic observation of bone repair is evidence of success, together with absence of signs and symptoms. Those teeth which show neither an increase nor a decrease in pre-operative radiolucency must be considered successful in the absence of signs and symptoms. However, they must be closely evaluated to observe any changes in size of radiolucency.

Accurate postoperative follow-up requires meticulous maintenance of the patient's records. For example, it is impossible to evaluate a postoperative radiolucency without a preoperative radiograph to serve as a baseline. Preoperative signs and symptoms, such as the type and duration of pain, mobility, and presence of a fistula should be recorded, as well as the medicaments used. With accurate treatment records comes pride in one's work and a superior service for the child.

Vital primary teeth treated by pulpotomy which exhibit fistulae, internal resorption or bone loss should be treated by extraction or by pulpectomy. Most of these teeth have already received a consider-able investment of time. Their value in maintaining the integrity of developing occlusion must be reassessed and appropriate treatment performed.

It is a clinical impression that the succedaneous permanent tooth also erupts prematurely (*Fig. 141*).

Eruption of the Permanent Successor

Sweet (1963) has reported that 6·3 per cent of vital primary molars treated by formocresol pulpotomy were prematurely lost. Hobson (1970) also reported premature exfoliation of primary teeth treated by two-visit mummification pulpotomy when compared to caries-free antimeres. More rapid external root resorption because of failure to control infection and the inflammatory process, accounts for this premature loss. In non-vital teeth treated by pulpotomy and pulpectomy, premature root resorption is more marked.

Any root-filling material placed either in the coronal pulp chamber or in the root canals must be resorbable. Zinc oxide based materials fulfil this requirement. However, the material is not the same tex-ture or hardness as normal tooth or vital pulp. Thus when the erupting permanent successor meets root-filling material, there is increased possibility of deflexion. One major disadvantage of pul-pectomy compared to pulpotomy in primary teeth is the increased likelihood of resorption problems. However, it has been documented that pulpectomy in a primary molar can be followed by proper eruption of the permanent successor (Starkey, 1973). Most problems associated with resorption arise when the erupting tooth has resorbed the pulpal floor of the primary molar and is contacting the material in the coronal pulp chamber. This is the time when the

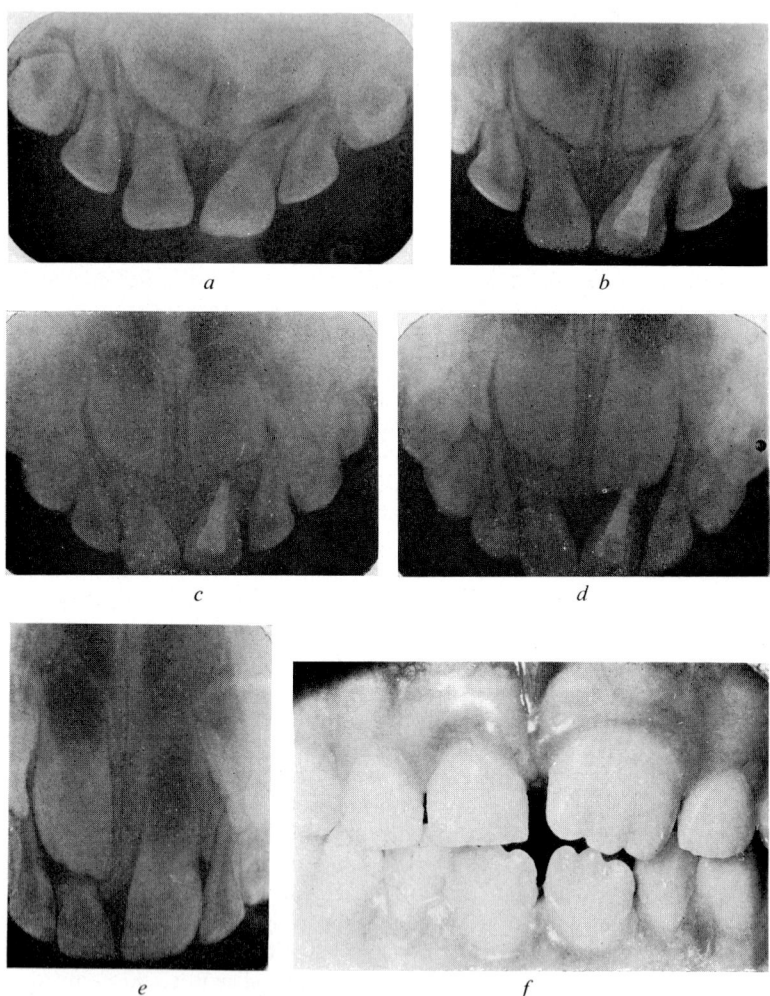

Fig. 141.—*a*, Preoperative. *b*, Pulpectomy and root-canal filling at 21 months. *c*, at 3 years. *d*, At 4½ years. *e*, At 6½ years. Note premature exfoliation of treated tooth and premature eruption of permanent successor. *f*, Absence of enamel defect on erupted permanent incisor.

clinician least suspects trouble. Ankylosis of the primary tooth and deflexion of the permanent successor can occur at this critical stage. The improper eruption of permanent successors can negate the many previous years of successful pulp therapy.

PULP THERAPY IN YOUNG PERMANENT TEETH
General Considerations

When young permanent teeth have large carious lesions which are radiographically close to the pulp or involving it, the clinician should evaluate the patient orthodontically. The aesthetic desirability of maintaining anterior permanent teeth should be obvious. Yet heroic, time-consuming and costly pulp treatment to maintain first permanent molars may not be justified when crowding exists. In crowded or potentially crowded mouths, thought should be given to extracting grossly carious first permanent molars, followed where and when necessary by active orthodontic treatment. It is imperative that the child have the benefit of orthodontic consultation before such a drastic step is taken. Orthodontic treatment planning in relation to the first permanent molar has been excellently outlined (Crabb and Rock, 1971) and the reader is referred to this article for clinical application.

There are instances when pulpally involved young permanent teeth must be maintained either permanently or, as is sometimes the case with first permanent molars, temporarily, while awaiting the eruption of other permanent teeth prior to active orthodontic therapy. A complicating factor in treatment is the state of apical development. As a rule, root closure in permanent teeth occurs three years after eruption. These teeth often present with large carious lesions involving the pulp prior to normal root closure. This makes conventional endodontic treatment impractical. It will be assumed here that such teeth require maintaining, if only over the short term, after orthodontic evaluation.

The treatment régimes applicable to young permanent teeth are: (1) Indirect pulp treatment; (2) Direct pulp capping; (3) Pulpotomy; (4) Pulpectomy—to induce root end repair of the open apex; and (5) Pulpectomy—when the apices are closed.

PULPOTOMY—VITAL PERMANENT TEETH WITH OPEN APICES
Technique

Large vital exposures in permanent teeth with incompletely formed apices warrant treatment by calcium hydroxide pulpotomy (*Figs. 142–145*). The aim is to remove the infected coronal pulp and place

241

calcium hydroxide over the healthy amputated radicular stumps. A calcific barrier should form in response to the calcium hydroxide and the radicular pulp should retain its vitality so that root closure can occur (*Fig. 144*). The coronal pulp chamber of the permanent molar is considerably deeper than in primary teeth. In fact, using normal length burs, there is little chance of perforating the pulpal

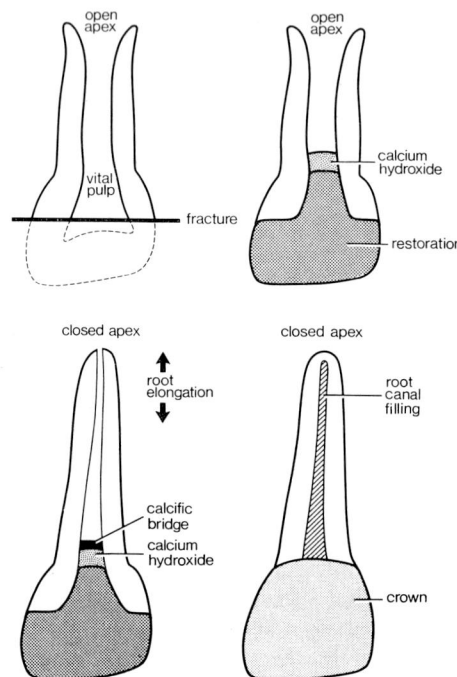

Fig. 142.—*Top left*, Class 3 fracture, vital pulp; open apex. *Top right*, Calcium hydroxide pulpotomy. *Bottom left*, Apical closure after calcium hydroxide pulpotomy. *Bottom right*, Completed root-canal treatment.

floor of a permanent molar. Long-shanked burs may be required to remove all coronal pulp. The level of amputation in permanent incisor pulpotomy is at the estimated cemento-enamel junction. Haemorrhage should be arrested with cotton pellets prior to placement of calcium hydroxide/methyl cellulose mixed with water or saline. Final restoration can be placed at this same visit if time permits.

Follow-up

Clinical and radiographical follow-up is identical to the follow-up for pulpally treated primary teeth. Apical development is monitored

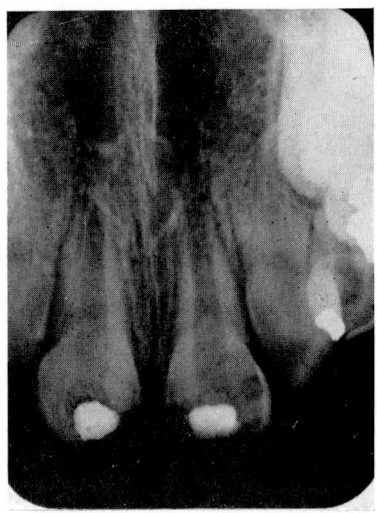

Figs. 143–145.—Treatment of young permanent teeth by calcium hydroxide pulpotomy, then root-canal filling.

Fig. 143.—Calcium hydroxide pulpotomies have been performed to treat exposed pulps when the apices are incompletely formed. The child was 7 years old.

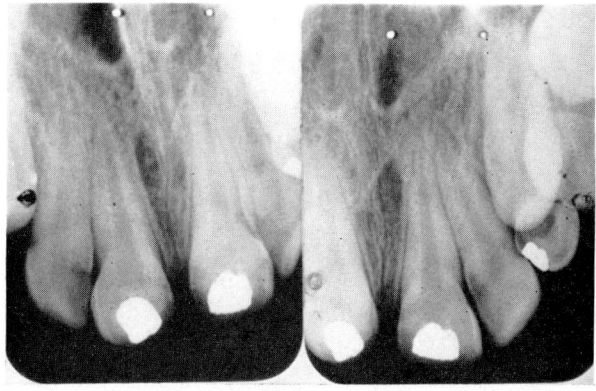

Fig. 144.—Radiographs 2½ years later show calcific bridges, continuation of growth in root length and apical closure. Root-canal filling is indicated to prevent further linear calcification along the canal.

by comparison with the preoperative periapical radiograph and where possible to a normal untreated antimere. Formation of a calcific bridge, continued apical development, absence of internal resorption and periapical radiolucency are radiographic evidence of

243

success (*Figs. 142, 144*). Often there is a linear calcification along the length of the root canal after formation of a calcific bridge. This has been labelled calcific metamorphosis and is considered to be a pathological rather than physiological process (Patterson and

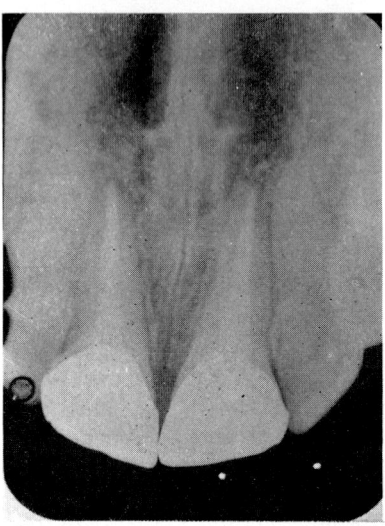

Fig. 145.—Radiograph taken 1 year after completion of root-canal therapy and crowning. Note well condensed root fillings and healthy periapical tissue. The child is now nearly 12 years old.

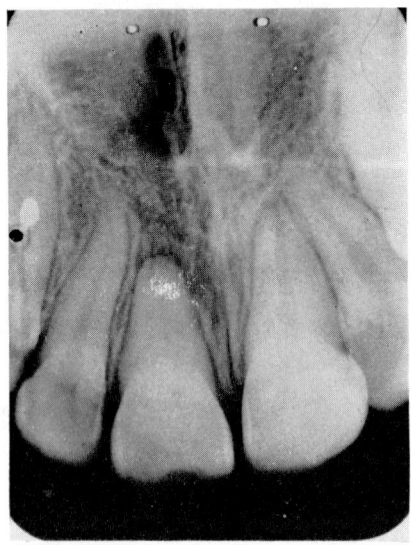

Fig. 146.—Calcified canal and periapical radiolucency: whenever linear calcification occurs, root-canal therapy must be considered.

Mitchell, 1965). It will progress until the canal will appear to be completely calcified radiographically. Many clinicians are content to call this nature's efforts at root filling. However, microscopical evaluation of such teeth reveals pulp remnants which slowly become non-vital through self-strangulation. Bacteria migrate within these root-canal spaces, which may be undetectable on the radiograph, and periapical pathology may result (*Fig. 146*). Of course, once the canal has calcified to this extent, it may be impossible to negotiate with instruments, even with the use of chelating agents such as EDTA (ethylene diaminetetra-acetic acid). This commits the tooth either to extraction or to apical surgery and retrograde root filling.

Calcium hydroxide pulpotomy should thus be considered as the first stage of treatment for vital cariously or traumatically exposed permanent teeth with incompletely formed apices, and the aim is to permit normal apical closure (*Figs. 142, 145*). The second phase of treatment is conventional root canal filling, once the apices have been closed; in addition to apical closure, the root continues its normal growth to assume normal length. The state of apical development and the speed of calcific metamorphosis will decide the exact timing of pulpectomy and root-canal therapy. It should be re-emphasized that watchful waiting can result in subsequent inability to instrument a calcified canal.

INDUCTION OF ROOT-END REPAIR—NON-VITAL PERMANENT TEETH WITH OPEN APICES

General Considerations

The permanent tooth with a vital degenerating or non-vital pulp and with incompletely formed apices presents a severe problem. The open apex and so-called 'blunderbuss canal' defy attempts at conventional root-canal therapy because the apical dimensions of the canal exceed those at the coronal access area. The treatment alternatives are root-canal therapy followed by apical surgery or induction of root-end repair followed at a later stage by conservative root-canal therapy.

The techniques of root-canal filling and apical surgery are described in texts on Endodontics. However, this approach is not recommended as the first choice of treatment for several reasons: First, surgical techniques are to be avoided whenever possible in young children. Second, the thin apical walls of the young permanent tooth make apical surgery even more difficult. If a retrograde filling procedure is necessary to obtain an adequate apical seal, these thin walls do not lend themselves to undercutting to obtain retention or to condensation pressure if amalgam is used. Finally, the root, which is already short because of its incomplete

245

formation, is further reduced by apical surgery. This has potentially far-reaching effects in terms of adequacy of periodontal support.

For these reasons, the non-surgical approach of induction of root-end repair is indicated for non-vital permanent teeth with incompletely formed apices. The principles of treatment are to débride and sterilize the canal before filling it with a calcium hydroxide paste; saturating the periapical tissues with calcium ions, together with the elimination of bacteria, stimulates physiological calcific

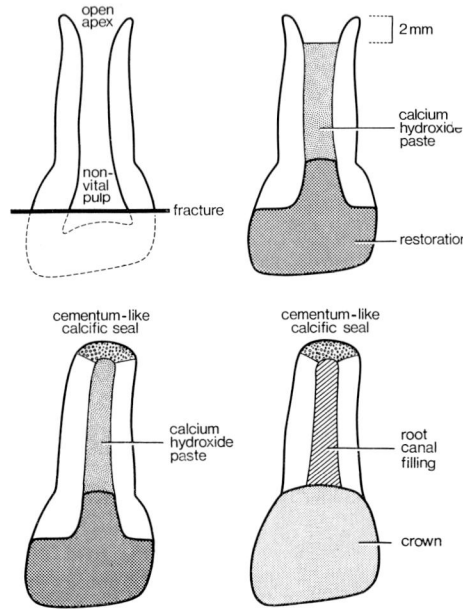

Fig. 147.—Apexification. Induction of root-end repair.

repair at the apex. When repair is complete, conventional root-canal therapy can be performed using lateral and apical condensation against the repaired calcified apical tissue (*Figs. 147–148*).

This treatment is often required in incisors rather than in molars because of the prevalence of untreated Ellis Class II fractures (involving dentine) in 7 and 8-year-olds, whose incisor apices would be incompletely formed. Subsequent pulp death may occur prior to apical closure.

Technique
Preoperative assessment includes clinical evaluation of colour, mobility, tenderness to percussion, and swelling. Periapical radiographs may demonstrate the preoperative root length, the extent of

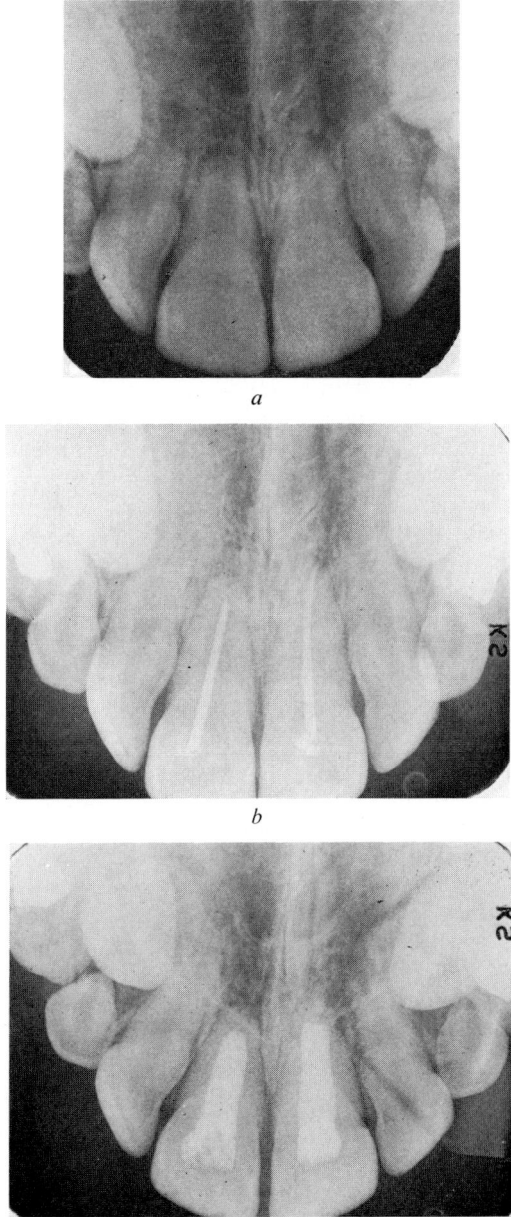

a

b

c

Fig. 148.—Apexification. *a*, Preoperative, age 8. *b*, Calcium hydroxide paste in canal on loosely fitting G.P. point. Apices closing. *c*, Final root-canal fillings.

247

apical development, the possibility of root fractures, the integrity of periodontal membrane and lamina dura, and the existence of periapical radiolucency.

Preoperative swelling warrants drainage through the canal; neither local anaesthesia nor rubber dam application is indicated when opening such a tooth. Drainage, as with primary molar pulpectomy, is supplemented when indicated by antibiotic therapy and local measures, such as warm saline mouthrinses, and should occur for no longer than 24 hours. The presence of haemorrhagic exudate should not alarm the student who may interpret this as vital tissue— rather, it is blood-tinged inflammatory exudate draining from the periapical lesion. When acute signs and symptoms are absent, instrumentation is recommended at the first visit, using local anaesthesia and rubber dam isolation. Even though the tooth may be non-vital, there may be tags of vital tissue in the apical parts of the canal. This vital tissue may in fact be ingrowing granulation tissue, which is as sensitive as vital pulp.

Barbed broaches are used to remove debris and necrotic tissue from the canal. A diagnostic radiograph must be taken with an instrument in the canal to assess the correct root length. Care should be exercised to avoid penetration of the apex, since the induction of periapical haemorrhage and the formation of a blood clot do not expedite periapical repair (Ham, 1969). The maxillary central incisor's normal root length is between 22 and 24 mm from incisal edge to apex. Since the root is incompletely formed, the clinician should place his diagnostic instrument appropriately short. After the diagnostic radiograph has been obtained the canal should be débrided to within 2 mm of the radiographic apex. The wide and diverging canal encourages the use of large instruments from the outset. Because of the divergent shape of the root canal, the file should be worked around the canal at the coronal access to ensure proper mechanical cleansing at the apex. Hedstrom files are used intermittently with copious irrigation by saline to remove infected dentine from the canal walls. The appearance of clean dentine filings should encourage the operator to terminate instrumentation. The canal is irrigated with saline and dried with paper points.

The canal should not be filled with calcium hydroxide until signs and symptoms are absent. The chances of success are greatly improved when the canal is filled in the absence of periapical inflammation (Ham, 1969; Steiner and Van Hassel, 1971). Therefore, avoiding overinstrumentation and using intracanal medication is advised. The canal is filled temporarily for 1–2 weeks with any antibacterial medicament. The following are commonly used: beechwood creosote, formocresol, camphorated monochlorophenol (CMCP), KRI liquid, or polyantibiotic paste (Friend et al., 1973).

It is unnecessary to obtain a negative culture prior to filling the canal with calcium hydroxide, provided that signs and symptoms are absent.

Pure calcium hydroxide is recommended for filling the canal(s) to within 2 mm of the radiographic apex, since its success has been well documented (Frank, 1966; Rule and Winter, 1966); the commercially available products (e.g. Dycal) cannot be recommended because of their short working time. The powder should be mixed with saline or camphorated monochlorophenol to the consistency of a creamy paste. The antibacterial properties of camphorated monochlorophenol may be of additional benefit, provided it does not irritate the periapical tissues. The paste can be introduced into the canal to the correct length with a rotary root-canal filler or with a large gutta-percha point. The latter technique lends itself to sealing the point in place at a predetermined distance, which assures that the calcium hydroxide paste is carried by the tip of the point. Since calcium hydroxide itself is not radio-opaque, it should be mixed with barium sulphate powder in equal quantities, to facilitate postoperative evaluation. Another material recommended for placing in the divergent canal is a polyvinyl resin* (Friend, 1967), although the periapical tissue reaction to it has been reported as severe in animals (Friend and Browne, 1968). Animal experimentation with a collagen calcium phosphate gel produces apical calcific repair faster than with calcium hydroxide (Nevins et al., 1976). At present there are no human studies with this product and so its use must be considered experimental. The canal opening should be obliterated.

Follow-up

Postoperative follow-up at 6-month intervals should include an evaluation of signs and symptoms as well as periapical radiographs. Comparison is made with the preoperative baseline radiograph to see if any change has occurred; the root appearance can also be compared with an untreated antimere. Frank (1966) described four types of repair:

1. The apex is closed with definite though minimum recession of the canal.

2. The apex is closed with no change in root space.

3. A radiographically apparent calcific bridge forms just coronal to the apex.

4. There is no radiographic evidence of apical closure but upon clinical instrumentation there is a definite stop at the apex, indicating some calcific repair.

---

* Diaket.

Since this apical calcification most frequently occurs in a horizontal, rather than vertical fashion, the term 'apical repair' is preferred to 'apical closure'. This latter term encourages the misinterpretation that the repair increases the root length. This seldom occurs, in contrast to the continued root growth after calcium hydroxide pulpotomy in vital young permanent teeth.

Calcific repair may be complete in 6 months postoperatively, although it may take as long as 2 or 3 years. Failure to see any radiographic change 1 year after initial placement of calcium hydroxide warrants re-entry into the tooth. The paste should be removed by further instrumentation and irrigation, the canal dried, and new paste inserted. A further diagnostic wire radiograph to assess root length is redundant because accurate records should identify the correct working length of the canal. Once calcific repair has occurred, the calcium hydroxide paste is removed, the canal is irrigated, and the final root filling placed. This can be done at one visit. Because of the wide canal, emphasis must be placed upon lateral condensation to adequately seal the canal. Fortunately the danger of overfilling is eliminated by the apical calcific barrier.

Histology

As identified from radiographic evaluation, root development is not normal. Rather, calcific material repairs the wide open apex in a horizontal fashion. Hertwig's root sheath has not been observed in animal histological sections (Ham, 1969; Steiner and Van Hassel, 1971); this may account for the lack of continued apical development in a vertical dimension. The calcified material is similar to cementum and continues with the cementum on the lateral root surfaces. Despite radiographic evidence of complete bridging, the calcific material has communicating channels between root canal and periapical tissues. This makes permanent root filling mandatory after apexification is complete to ensure a hermetic seal. While it is logical that the success of the completed root-canal treatment following apexification should be as high as conventional root-canal treatment, this assumption has yet to be clinically documented.

Success

There is abundant clinical evidence of the technique's success over the short term (Frank, 1966; Rule and Winter, 1966). However, the literature lacks evidence of continued success after completion of root-canal therapy against the repaired apical tissue. It is hoped that the success will be similar to that of root-canal therapy for teeth with normally closed apices; this awaits long-term documentation. It may therefore be wise to warn the parent that apical surgery may be required at some time. This forewarning is useful should surgery be required later. Also, the parent should understand the long-term follow-up that is required when induction of root-end repair is initiated.

MODIFIED FORMOCRESOL PULPOTOMY

Occasionally, a partially vital or non-vital permanent molar with open or closed apices must be maintained over the short term awaiting active orthodontic treatment. Conventional endodontics may be contra-indicated if investment of time is to be minimal.

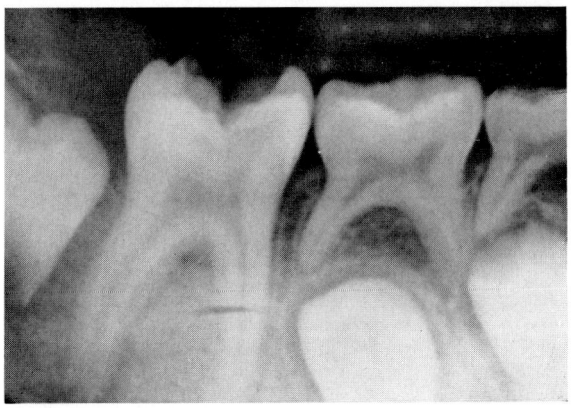

Fig. 149.—Preoperative radiograph of non-vital first permanent molar. The poor quality film just shows a radiolucency around the incompletely formed distal apex. For economic reasons a two-visit formocresol pulpotomy was performed in this uncrowded mouth, *see Figs. 150, 151.*

Success has been reported using a modification of the formocresol pulpotomy in these teeth (Trask, 1972). The technique is identical to that described for primary teeth, except that the formocresol pellet is sealed permanently in the tooth. Postoperative sensitivity, for 24 hours and controlled by aspirin, has been observed in vital treated teeth. According to Trask (1972), no deleterious effect has been reported from leaving the formocresol pellet in place for an extended time. On the other hand, a two-visit formocresol pulp-otomy can be performed (*Figs. 149–151*). The procedure is suggested as an alternative to extraction, and though it is no substitute for conventional root-canal therapy, it is an economic alternative. Its use can be encouraged in selected cases, prior to active orthodontic care, in the knowledge that the tooth can always be extracted if the treatment fails.

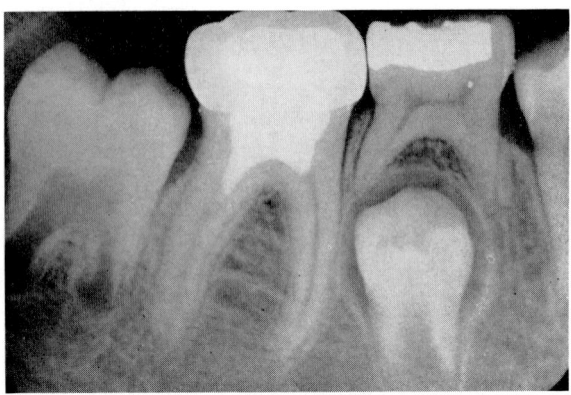

Fig. 150.—One year after a two-visit formocresol pulpotomy the radiolucency has disappeared and the distal apex has closed.

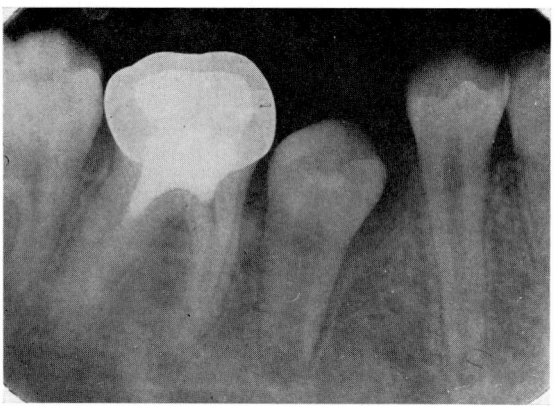

Fig. 151.—The case illustrated in *Figs. 149, 150,* three years later. Periapical tissues are normal. Linear calcification has occurred in the root canals.

PULPECTOMY—CLOSED APICES— PERMANENT TEETH

Once the apices have been closed and the pulp is non-vital, root-canal therapy should be instituted (see texts on Endodontics). It is also indicated in vital permanent teeth with exposures too large for pulp capping. Non-vital permanent teeth with periapical bone loss should always be treated conservatively before resorting to apical surgery. Such lesions will often repair in response to elimination of infection and effective sealing of the canal (*Figs. 152, 153*).

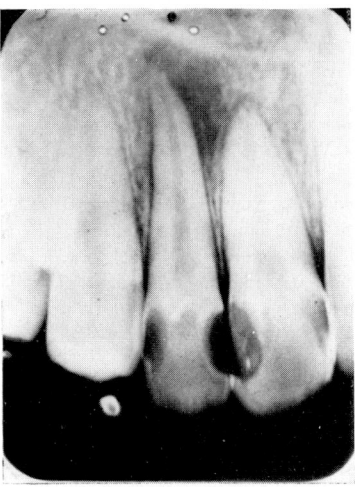

Fig. 152.—Twelve-year-old with non-vital permanent central and lateral incisors. Note size of preoperative radiolucency.

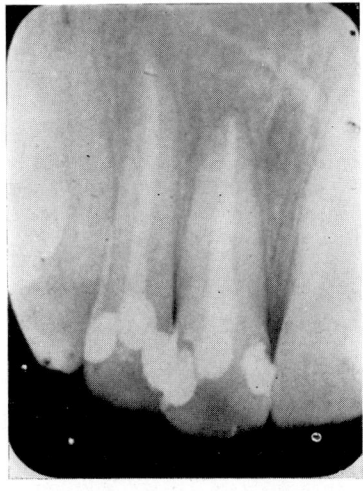

Fig. 153.—Both teeth were treated by pulpectomy and root canal filling. Six month postoperative radiograph demonstrates periapical bone repair.

REFERENCES

ANDREW P. (1955) The treatment of infected pulps in deciduous teeth. *Br. Dent. J.* **98,** 122.

BEAVER H. A., KOPEL H. M. and SABER W. R. (1966) The effect of zinc oxide-eugenol cement on a formocresolized pulp. *J. Dent. Child.* **33,** 381.

BERGER J. E. (1965) Pulp tissue reaction to formocresol and zinc oxide-eugenol. *J. Dent. Child.* **32**, 13.

CARTWRIGHT H. V. and BEVANS G. L. (1970) Management of two abscessed primary molars in a four-year-old child: Report of interesting case. *J. Dent. Child.* **37**, 230.

CRABB J. J. and ROCK W. P. (1971) Treatment planning in relation to the first permanent molar. *Br. Dent. J.* **131**, 396.

DIMAGGIO J. J. and HAWES R. R. (1963) Continued evaluation of direct and indirect pulp capping. *I.A.D.R. Abst.* **41**, 38.

DOYLE W. A. (1961) *A Comparison of the Formocresol Pulpotomy Technique with the Calcium Hydroxide Pulpotomy Technique.* Typed Thesis, Indiana University.

EASLICK K. A. (1943) Management of pulp exposure in the mixed dentition. *J. Am. Dent. Assoc.* **30**, 179.

EIDELMAN E., FINN S. B. and KOULOURIDES T. (1965) Remineralization of carious dentine treated by calcium hydroxide. *J. Dent. Child.* **32**, 218.

EMMERSON C. C., MIYAMOTO O., SWEET C. A. sen. and BHATIA H. L. (1959) Pulpal changes following formocresol applications on rat molars and human primary teeth. *J. S. Calif. Dent. Assoc.* **27**, 309.

FISHER F. J. (1972) The effect of a calcium hydroxide/water paste on micro-organisms in carious dentine. *Br. Dent. J.* **133**, 19.

FRANK A. L. (1966) Therapy for the divergent pulpless tooth by continued apical formation. *J. Am. Dent. Assoc.* **72**, 87.

FRIEND L. A. (1967) The treatment of immature teeth with non-vital pulps. *J. Br. Endodont. Soc.* **1**, 28.

FRIEND L. A. and BROWNE R. M. (1968) Tissue reactions to some root filling materials. *Br. Dent. J.* **125**, 291.

FRIEND L. A., GRIEVE A. R. and PLANT C. G. (1973) Tissue reactions to three root canal medicaments. *Br. Dent. J.* **134**, 11.

GELLER J. S., KLEIN A. I. and MCDONALD R. E. (1971) Association between dentinal sclerosis and pulpal floor thickness: television radiographic evaluation. *J. Am. Dent. Assoc.* **83**, 118.

GLASS R. L. and ZANDER H. A. (1949) Pulp healing. *J. Dent. Res.* **28**, 97.

GOULD J. M. (1972) Root canal therapy for infected primary molar teeth—preliminary report. *J. Dent. Child.* **39**, 269.

HAM J. W. (1969) *A Study of Induced Apical Closure in Pulpless Teeth with Open Apices.* Typed Thesis, Indiana University.

HANNAH D. R. and ROWE A. H. R. (1971) Vital pulpotomy of deciduous molars using N2 and other materials. *Br. Dent. J.* **130**, 99.

HARGREAVES J. A. (1959) A histopathological study following mortal amputation in seven deciduous teeth. *Odont. Rev.* **10**, 351.

HARGREAVES J. A. (1969) *Second Int. Symp. of Dent. for Child.* Proceedings, Sienna, p. 279.

HESS W. (1929) Pulp amputation as a method of treating root canals. *Dental Items of Interest* **51**, 596.

HOBSON P. (1970) Pulp treatment of deciduous teeth. *Br. Dent. J.* **128**, 232 and 275.

JEPPERSON, KRISTEN (1971) Direct pulp capping on primary teeth—a long term investigation. *J. Int. Assoc. Dent. Child.* **2**, 10.

JORDAN R. E. and SUZUKI M. (1971) Conservative treatment of deep carious lesions. *J. Can. Dent. Assoc.* **37**, 337.

KAKEHASHI S., STANLEY H. R. and FITZGERALD R. J. (1965) The effects of surgical exposures of dental pulps in germ-free and conventional laboratory rats. *Oral Surg.* **20**, 340.

KENNEDY D. B. (1971) *Formocresol Pulpotomy in Teeth of Dogs with Induced Pulpal and Periapical Pathoses.* Typed Thesis, Indiana University.

KERKHOVE B. C., HERMAN S. C., KLEIN A. I. and McDONALD R. E. (1967) A clinical and television densitometric evaluation of the indirect pulp capping technique. *J. Dent. Child.* **34**, 192.

KING J. B., CRAWFORD J. J. and LINDAHL R. L. (1965) Indirect pulp capping: A bacteriologic study of deep carious dentine in human teeth. *Oral Surg.* **20**, 663.

LAW D. B. (1956) An evaluation of vital pulpotomy technique. *J. Dent. Child.* **23**, 40.

LAW D. B. and LEWIS T. M. (1961) The effect of calcium hydroxide on deep carious lesion. *Oral Surg.* **14**, 1130.

LAWRENCE R. P. (1966) *A Method of Root Canal Therapy for Primary Teeth.* Typed Thesis, Enory University School of Dentistry.

LOOS P. J. and HAN S. S. (1971) An enzyme histochemical study of the effect of various concentrations of formocresol on connective tissues. *Oral Surg.* **31**, 571.

MASSLER M. (1978) Treatment of profound caries to prevent pulpal damage. *J. Pedodont.* **2**, 99.

MORAWA A. P., STRAFFEN L. M., MAN S. S. and CORPRON R. E. (1975) Clinical evaluation of pulpotomies using dilute formocresol. *J. Dent. Child.* **42**, 360.

MJOR I. A. (1967) Histologic studies of human coronal dentine following the insertion of various materials in experimentally prepared cavities. *Arch. Oral Biol.* **12**, 441.

NEVINS A. J. et al. (1976) Revitalization of pulpless open apex teeth in rhesus monkeys using collagen-calcium phosphate gel. *J. Endodont. Dent.* **2**, 159.

NICHOLLS E. (1963) *Trans. Third Int. Conf. Endodont.* **3**, 52.

NORDSTROM D. O., WEI S. H. Y. and JOHNSON R. (1974) Use of stannous fluoride for indirect pulp capping. *J. Am. Dent. Assoc.* **88**, 997.

PARKIN S. F., HARGREAVES J. A. and WEYMAN J. (1970) Children's dentistry in general practice. *Br. Dent. J.* **129**, 285.

PATTERSON S. S. and MITCHELL D. F. (1965) Calcific metamorphosis of the dental pulp. *Oral Surg.* **20**, 94.

PRUHS R. J., OLEN G. A. and SHARMA P. S. (1977) Relationship between formocresol pulpotomy on primary teeth and enamel defects on permanent successors. *J. Am. Dent. Assoc.* **99**, 698.

REDIG D. F. (1968) A comparison and evaluation of two formocresol pulpotomy technics utilizing 'Buckley's' formocresol. *J. Dent. Child.* **35**, 22.

RULE D. C. and WINTER G. B. (1966) Root growth and apical repair subsequent to pulpal necrosis in children. *Br. Dent. J.* **120,** 586.

SCHILDER H. and AMSTERDAM M. (1959) The inflammatory potential of root canal medicaments. *Oral Surg.* **12,** 211.

SPEDDING R. H. (1963) *The Effect of Formocresol and Hydroxide on the Dental Pulps of Rhesus Monkeys.* Typed Thesis, Indiana University.

SPEDDING R. H. (1973) Root canal treatment for primary teeth. *Dent. Clin. North Am.* **17:1.** Philadelphia, W. B. Saunders Co.

STARKEY P. E. (1973) Pulpectomy and root canal filling in a primary molar: Report of a case. *J. Dent. Child.* **40,** 213.

STARKEY P. E. (1974) Personal communication.

STEINER J. C. and VAN HASSEL M. J. (1971) Experimental root apexification in primates. *Oral Surg.* **31,** 409.

SWEET C. A. (1936) Treatment for deciduous teeth with exposed pulps. *Washington Univ. Dent. J.* **3,** 78.

SWEET C. A. (1963) *Trans. Third Int. Conf. Endodont.* **32,** 1963.

TRASK P. A. (1972) Formocresol pulpotomy on (young) permanent teeth. *J. Am. Dent. Assoc.* **85,** 1316.

TRAUBMAN L. (1967) *A Critical Clinical and Television Radiographic Evaluation of Indirect Pulp Capping.* Typed Thesis, Indiana University.

VENHAM L. L. (1967) *Pulpal Responses to Variation in the Formocresol Pulpotomy Technic: a Histological Study.* Typed Thesis, Ohio State University.

VIA W. J. jun. (1955) Evaluation of deciduous molars treated by pulpotomy and calcium hydroxide. *J. Am. Dent. Assoc.* **50,** 34.

WEISZ A. (1976) A comparative study of two techniques to fill the root canals of primary teeth. Typed thesis, Boston University.

WILLARD R. M. (1976) Radiographic changes following formocresol pulpotomy in primary molars. *J. Dent. Child.* **43,** 414.

WITTICH H. C. (1956) Treatment of pulps of deciduous and young permanent teeth. *J. Can. Dent. Assoc.* **22,** 142.

WRIGHT G. Z. and ALPERN G. D. (1971) Variables influencing children's cooperative behaviour at the first dental visit. *J. Dent. Child.* **38,** 126.

RECOMMENDED READING

BERGER J. E. (1965) Pulp tissue reaction to formocresol and zinc-oxide–eugenol. *J. Dent. Child.* **32,** 13.

FRANK A. L. (1966) Therapy for the divergent pulpless tooth by continued apical formation. *J. Am. Dent. Assoc.* **72,** 87.

HANNAH D. R. and ROWE A. H. R. (1971) Vital pulpotomy of deciduous molars using N2 and other materials. *Br. Dent. J.* **130,** 99.

JAFFE E. C. (1973) The endodontic treatment of primary molars. *Dental Update* **1,** 83 (July/August 1973).

KERKHOVE B. C., HERMAN S. C., KLEIN A. I. and McDONALD R. E. (1967) A clinical and television densitometric evaluation of the indirect pulp capping technique. *J. Dent. Child.* **34,** 192.

SPEDDING R. H. (1977) Endodontic treatment of primary molars. In: *Current Therapy in Dentistry,* Vol. 6. St. Louis, C. V. Mosby., p. 558.

GLOSSARY*

Amelodentinal Junction (Dentino-enamel Junction)—The line representing the junction of the enamel and the dentine.

Arch Length—The distance between the mesial surfaces of the first permanent molars measured around the arch of the erupted teeth.

Axial Wall—The wall of a prepared cavity in an axial surface of the tooth in a plane parallel with the surface in which the cavity is prepared.

Cavity Margins—The external surface of enamel wall of the finished cavity immediately adjacent to the restorative material.

Cavity Nomenclature—Includes the names of cavities, and of groups of cavities, including the several walls and their lines and points of junction. Cavities in the teeth take the names of the surfaces of the teeth in which they occur.

Cavity Preparation—All those operations required in the removal of carious material from cavities formed in the teeth by decay, and forming the cavities for restorations, with such extensions and preparations as seem most likely to prevent recurrence of decay.

Cavo-surface Angle—The angle formed by the junction of the wall of the cavity with the surface of the tooth.

Cervical Seat—The gingival floor of the step portion of a Class 2 preparation.

Coronal Pulp—The bulk of primary pulp extending up to the cemento-enamel junction in anterior teeth and root canal orifice in posterior teeth.

Dentine Wall—That part of a cavity wall consisting of dentine.

Dovetail or Lock—The occlusal extension of a Class 2 preparation; alternatively the labial or lingual extension of a Class 3 or Class 4 preparation.

Enamel Wall—That part of a cavity wall composed of enamel.

Fistula—An abnormal (pathological) passage joining one body cavity to another or one body cavity to the exterior.

High Speed—When the bur is used in an air turbine.

Isthmus—That area connecting the proximal and occlusal parts of the cavity.

Leeway Space—The difference in mediodistal widths of the primary canine, first and second primary molars compared to their underlying permanent successors.

Line Angle—Formed by the junction of two walls along a line and named by combining the names of those two walls.

Low Speed—When the bur is driven by a conventional motor, or belt driven.

Nomenclature of Cavities:
    Class 1—occlusal location.
    Class 2—approximal in posterior teeth.

---

* Some of these definitions are modified from Indiana University *Dental Student Handout* material: by courtesy of Dr. Paul Starkey, Indianapolis, Indiana, U.S.A.

Class 3—approximal in anterior teeth.

Class 4—approximal in anterior teeth involving also the incisal edge.

Class 5—cervical (gingival) location.

Outline Form—The finished shape of the cavity.

Point Angles—Formed by the junction of three walls at a point and named by joining the names of the three walls.

Primate Space—That space between primary canine and first primary molar in the mandibular arch—or between primary canine and primary lateral incisor in the maxillary arch.

Proximal Box—The mesial or distal proximal part of the cavity.

Pulpal Wall—That wall of a prepared cavity which is to the occlusal of the pulp and in a plane at right angles to the long axis of the tooth.

Pulp Horn—The extension of coronal pulp, located beneath the cusps.

Radicular Pulp—That pulp which fills the root canal.

Resistance Form—The shape of the cavity which protects the remaining tooth and the filling from the forces of mastication.

Retention Form—The shape of the cavity which prevents dislodgement of the restorative material.

Sign—A clinical observation of an abnormality made by the dentist, e.g. pulp polyp.

Symptom—A specific complaint made by a patient, e.g. pain when eating sweets.

Wall—One of the internal boundaries of a cavity.

INDEX

266